Cognitive-Behavioral Therapy for Bipolar Disorder

Cognitive–Behavioral Therapy for Bipolar Disorder

SECOND EDITION

Monica Ramirez Basco
A. John Rush

THE GUILFORD PRESS
New York   London

© 2005 The Guilford Press
A Division of Guilford Publications, Inc.
72 Spring Street, New York, NY 10012
www.guilford.com

Printed in the United States of America

This book is printed on acid-free paper.

Last digit is print number: 9   8   7   6   5   4   3   2   1

Library of Congress Cataloging-in-Publication Data

Basco, Monica Ramirez.
   Cognitive-behavioral therapy for bipolar disorder / Monica
Ramirez Basco, A. John Rush.— 2nd ed.
      p.   cm.
   Includes bibiographical references and index.
   ISBN 1-59385-168-5 (hardcover)
      1. Manic–depressive illness—Treatment.   2. Cognitive
therapy.   I. Rush, A. John.   II. Title.
RC516.B36   2005
616.89′506—dc22

                                                    2005008775

In memory of
David Walter Savage
1957–2003

About the Authors

Monica Ramirez Basco, PhD, is a clinical psychologist, author, lecturer, and Clinical Associate Professor of Psychology at the University of Texas Southwestern Medical Center at Dallas. She is an internationally recognized expert in cognitive-behavioral therapy (CBT) and a founding fellow of the Academy of Cognitive Therapy. Dr. Basco is the author of *Never Good Enough: How to Use Perfectionism to Your Advantage without Letting It Ruin Your Life* and coauthor of *Getting Your Life Back: The Complete Guide to Recovery from Depression.* She is also the author of *The Bipolar Workbook: Tools for Controlling Your Mood Swings,* a CBT guide for patients, to be released in 2006.

A. John Rush, MD, is Professor and Vice Chair for Research in the Department of Psychiatry at the University of Texas Southwestern Medical Center at Dallas. His work has focused on the diagnosis and psychotherapeutic, psychopharmacological, and somatic treatment of major depressive, bipolar, and other mood disorders. He has authored 10 books and over 400 journal articles. Dr. Rush's internationally recognized work has received numerous awards. Most recently, his research has focused on longer-term disease management programs, including multistep treatment algorithms for bipolar and major depressive disorders.

the development of clinical methods for preventing relapse and for helping patients to live with this illness. Its organization is different from that of the first edition, to allow more flexibility for clinicians. Rather than providing specific session-by-session instructions, it guides clinicians toward selecting methods that address the stage of illness and treatment and tailoring the intervention to the specific problems and needs of patients.

Our experience has shown us that people with bipolar disorder and their family members are often very active in seeking ways to improve their health, to stay abreast of recent developments in treatment, and to experiment with ways to control their symptoms. The members of the Depression and Bipolar Support Alliance groups across the United States as well as other self-help groups continue to make it their mission to support and educate themselves and one another, to convey hope, and to challenge the fields of psychiatry and psychology to assist them in finding new ways to improve the quality of their lives. Because people with this illness are able to play an active role in their care, they read about and make use of treatment methods available through therapy, in journal and magazine articles, through the visual media, and through books. As educated consumers, they often enter treatment already having implemented many of the methods we suggest in this book. The flexibility of the methods described herein will allow clinicians to bypass components of treatment about which the patient has knowledge and skills and move ahead to the more advanced methods offered for controlling depression and mania.

Before the cognitive-behavioral methods provided in this text can be of help, the patient must be ready to deal with the fact that he or she has a chronic and severe mental illness. This concept is very difficult for people to accept. Our natural inclination as human beings is to push away bad news. Thus, providing therapy and making it a successful experience is as much about the timing being right as it is about the methods being useful. If the patient is intellectually ready to learn to manage his or her symptoms but is not emotionally ready to fully grasp the meaning of having this life-long disorder, there will be many roadblocks on the path to recovery. Steps toward managing the symptoms may be followed by periods of frustration and anger with the enterprise, perhaps even the desire to give up on treatment altogether. It may be necessary to postpone psychotherapy or put it on hold while the person allows him- or herself time to grieve the loss of full mental health and of a life uncomplicated by depression and mania, medications and therapy, and doctors and hospitals. Patience is needed by both clinicians and patients to allow the normal process of acceptance to occur and adjustment to solidify. When the patient is ready, the cognitive-behavioral methods presented in this volume can help him or her to regain control, to prevent succumbing to the peaks and valleys of the illness, and to improve the quality of his or her life.

There is still much to be learned about the management of bipolar disorder, and our patients have much to teach us. If only we can maintain the sense of purpose as clinicians and researchers that brought us to the mental health field, we can persevere to find answers to the significant problems posed by this chronic and debilitating illness.

Contents

CHAPTER 1

Introduction
to the Second Edition

Much has happened since the writing of the first edition of *Cognitive-Behavioral Therapy for Bipolar Disorder*. The scientific world has grasped what patients and therapists have known for some time—namely, that psychotherapy can be a helpful adjunct to pharmacotherapy in the treatment of bipolar disorder. Studies have demonstrated the efficacy of cognitive-behavioral interventions in the treatment of bipolar disorder for improving outcomes and reducing the risk of recurrence (e.g., Cochran, 1984; Lam et al., 2000; Scott, Garland, & Moorhead, 2001). And, time and practice have allowed for refinement of the methods presented in the first edition.

In this second edition we offer an elaboration of the methods presented previously along with new strategies for preventing relapse, adaptations to the treatment of children and adolescents, ways to tailor the intervention to the specific needs of patients, and interventions for coping with common comorbid psychiatric and psychological problems.

The Therapeutic Alliance

It has become clear that the efficacy of cognitive-behavioral therapy (CBT) rests on the strength of the therapeutic alliance. For the clinician's part, respect for patients' preferences and needs, even when counter to clinical judgment, is a cornerstone of a strong collaborative relationship. For patients, trust in therapists, even when the feedback is not what the patient wants to hear, is critical to the task. Patients must feel comfortable telling therapists when symptoms are beginning to reemerge, and therapists must be able to give honest feedback to their patients when the warning signs are overlooked or when their actions place them at risk for relapse. Because of its pivotal role in the delivery of CBT, we begin this chapter with suggestions for building and maintaining a therapeutic alliance.

Commitment to Treatment

Unlike acute treatments for unipolar depression or anxiety disorders using CBT, the effective treatment of those who suffer from bipolar disorder requires a longer-term commitment. With its waxing and waning course, symptoms of bipolar disorder will remit spontaneously or with the aid of treatment and will recur with either precipitating events or on their own. The clinician's task is to not only help a person overcome the symptoms of the illness and recover from its psychosocial consequences but also to prepare for its inevitable return. This means that the course of therapy may follow an untraditional pattern. Visits usually occur weekly during the first phase of treatment when skills are taught and symptoms are reduced. As progress is made and patient distress decreases, the interval between visits is lengthened to biweekly and then again to monthly depending on the need of the patient. Once the patient is stable, therapy may take a pause for several months or perhaps years until the services of the therapist are once again needed. Cues to resuming therapy include a return of symptoms, stressful events, or life transitions. If therapy is discontinued for 6 months or more, it is helpful for continuity of care if the patient makes contact with the therapist to provide a progress update, either in writing or with a brief phone call. This helps the therapist to track the progress of the patient and stay aware of major life transitions. When and if therapy resumes, the therapist can help the patient pick up where he or she left off in the story. Rather than following the "no news is good news" rule, therapists should encourage their patients to call in when things are going well or when they have good news. This positive feedback provides positive reinforcement to the therapist for previous therapeutic efforts and communicates to the patient that he or she is of interest as a person not just as a disorder or problem. While in large practices this may seem impossible, a short note or brief phone mail message that takes only a small amount of clinician time will be returned with a better therapeutic bond that can be important when the patient is having difficulties with adherence to treatment or control of symptoms.

Stability and Structure

Psychotherapy is often a stabilizing force in the lives of patients. Therapy visits can provide a structure for marking the passage of time, for monitoring progress, and for achieving goals. Feedback from therapists on changes seen since the last visit or since beginning treatment can help patients gauge their progress and feel good about their accomplishments. Regularly scheduled visits where patients report on their progress between sessions provide opportunities for patients to be accountable, thereby increasing the chance that they will implement the plans made in therapy. Regardless of the time interval, anticipation of therapy visits cues patients to be self-observant and to identify difficulties they hope to address with the therapist. Most people who are not involved in psychotherapy do not regularly take the time to monitor their feelings and actions, nor do they make time to identify personal problems and set goals for improvement. Psychotherapy that focuses on symptom monitoring, goal setting, and relapse prevention provides a structure for self-improvement.

Symptoms and Therapy

There is interplay between a patient's symptoms and his or her experience in the therapy session. Cognitive and affective symptoms have the greatest impact on the therapy process. When concentration is poor or the person is easily distracted, it is hard to accomplish much in session. Sometimes it is necessary to shorten sessions, limit the agenda, or give the patient a mental break between topics of discussion. If the individual's outlook is colored by depression, efforts at reviving hope must be intertwined with other agenda items. Hypomania can begin with subtle cognitive changes. Increased optimism or desire to accomplish more may appear to be within normal limits, especially if it comes on the heels of a depressive episode. This enthusiasm can be very seductive for the therapist who wants the patient to feel better and achieve his or her goals. You might find yourself agreeing with the patient's numerous plans before realizing that the improvements in energy and optimism may be symptomatic.

If the patient has racing thoughts, it is possible that he or she will forget any plans made before the next session occurs. Note taking can help to cue the patient's memory between visits and can help the therapist to keep track of the number of plans made or homework assignments given within a session.

When a patient with bipolar disorder is hypomanic, therapy sessions can be quite enjoyable. There is often an injection of humor that may have been missing when the patient was depressed. The rate of speech is usually faster, perhaps an improvement over psychomotor retardation that may have made prior sessions seem to drag on. The quicker thinking of the patient and fluidity of new ideas can give the impression that time is being used more efficiently. These sessions often leave the therapist feeling more optimistic and perhaps energized.

In contrast, when patients are depressed and demonstrate some psychomotor retardation, therapy sessions can be slow and difficult for both parties. The therapist may feel compelled to help the patient more, fill in the blanks when word-finding difficulties occur, or show more enthusiasm in hopes that it might brighten the mood of the patient. A clinic day with several patients in a depressed state can leave the therapist feeling drained, discouraged, and useless. It takes some self-monitoring on the therapist's part not to communicate the impotence they may feel in the face of the patient's severe depression. Students of CBT who are instructed to set an agenda and accomplish tasks within session often feel particularly compelled to push their depressed patients to accept interventions, may resort to giving advice when the collaboration is slow, or may feel the urge to give up on CBT altogether.

CBT methods work just as well for therapists as they do for their patients. Therefore, when feeling internal distress during therapy sessions, therapists should be mindful of their automatic thoughts, search for thinking errors, and correct their distortions in logic before they have a negative effect on the therapeutic process. A recent doctoral student was treating a middle-age woman with chronic depression. The student's internal monologue was something like, "This woman is so sick. I can't begin to help her. She probably needs to be in the hospital. I have no idea what I'm doing here. She is bringing me down with her negativity. How much longer do we have until I can get out of here?" While the therapist was able to maintain composure and not show the distress, this train of negative thinking kept the student from selecting a CBT strategy that might have been useful. Instead, there was an overreliance on reflective listening.

Seeing the Person Separate from the Illness

The phenomenon of bipolar disorder can be so overwhelming to the patient and to care providers that it dominates the focus of therapy. It is easy to depersonalize the conceptualization of the problem or to organize treatment around remediation of individual symptoms and lose sight, to some extent, of the impact on the person. People who

suffer from bipolar disorder have difficulty knowing where their symptoms end and their personality begins. As one patient put it, "Am I an
impatient person and judgmental toward others or do I have an illness
that makes me act that way?" Another asked, "I think I am a natural
pessimist given all the tough times I went through as a kid. But on the
other hand, could it be that I have been depressed for so long, that I'm
just accustomed to thinking negatively?"

People try to understand themselves and their experiences. They
want to know what is stable and permanent in their lives and what is
likely to be transient or a product of their mental illness. They also
want others to see them as people, not as patients, or a case of bipolar
disorder, or an oddity. Attention to non-illness-related topics during
therapy sessions is one way of communicating to patients that we are
interested in them as people. During the first few minutes of most
therapy sessions there is time for chitchat or storytelling—disclosures
unrelated to illness that give clues to the happenings of patients' lives.
Some patients are too verbose and allowing too much time for storytelling can detract from the work of therapy. However, eliminating
such discourse altogether in the interest of time may send a message of
disinterest in the nonpathological elements of the patient's life.

To keep the focus on the individual and not just the illness,
inquire about patients' lives before the illness began, what they are
like between episodes, and what stays the same in them regardless of
how they feel. Characteristics such as intelligence, sense of humor,
social comfort, interests, sources of pleasure, and preferences for activity are elements of the person that are independent of the illness.
Other clues about the person behind the illness can be gleaned from
knowing about the family of origin, how other members of the
patient's family function, and what would have been expected from
life had the illness not intervened. When a therapist takes the time to
inquire about these things, he or she is showing interest in the person
and communicates a value for the patient's personal life.

Preexisting Coping Skills

CBT is a skills-oriented form of psychotherapy. Therapists are
equipped with a number of tools for helping patients to manage their
moods, restructure their thinking, and cope with their problems. It is
easy to assume that the patient is a blank slate and that the skills to be
introduced are not part of the individual's behavioral repertoire. As
clinicians, we sometimes forget that the people we treat have managed
to get along in life long before therapy came along. They may not have
managed in an optimal manner, but chances are they possess some

skills and have learned from their experiences along the way. When we assume that people have preexisting coping skills and we communicate that either verbally or through our actions, they get the message that we think they are competent, able to solve problems, and smart enough to know when to ask for help. Validation of this type enhances the collaborative nature of the therapeutic bond—an essential in CBT.

People who are distressed probably coped better with life at times when they were not distressed. Skills do not disappear when the symptoms of bipolar disorder emerge. However, the emotional upheavals, confusion, and loss of motivation and energy can make it difficult for people to access their skills. Many, in fact, forget they even possess coping skills. Their distress coupled with an eagerness to help can lead the therapist to introduce CBT methods before assessing the patient's existing coping skills. Some suggested questions for tapping into patients' skills include the following:

- "If you were not so distressed, how might you handle this problem?"

- "Have you run into this problem/symptom before? What has been helpful to you in coping with it in the past?"

- "What do you think would be a good way to deal with this?"

- "How do you imagine other people cope with things like this? Would that work for you?"

- "What advice would you normally give to a friend if they had a similar problem?"

As will be discussed in Chapter 7, one of the first steps in CBT for bipolar disorder is to get patients to avoid doing things that will make them feel worse. Interestingly, most patients quickly respond with a list of actions, thoughts, and situations that would likely made them more depressed or more manic. They have figured these things out from their experiences with the illness. Likewise, if the clinician inquires about things that might make their situation better, they will very likely come up with at least a few ideas. If reasonable, the clinician should go with their ideas first (e.g., visit with a friend instead of being alone), and then work on adding to their existing coping skills. If their coping ideas sound unreasonable (e.g., take sleeping pills in the early evening and sleep rather than face the loneliness of the evening), get patients to elaborate on their reasons for choosing such an intervention and then ask them to consider the disadvantages. Often there are short-term advantages for coping choices, such as allowing avoidance of stressful situations, but longer-term disadvantages (i.e., the problem never really gets solved).

If time in psychotherapy is limited, never sacrifice attention to the therapeutic alliance in order to teach another CBT skill. In the long run, if the patient does not feel respected or doubts the compassion of the therapist, he or she will not use the skills outside the therapy session.

A Reformulation of CBT
for Bipolar Disorder

The first edition of *Cognitive-Behavioral Therapy for Bipolar Disorder* provided a 20-session protocol including session procedures and homework assignments. That structure was omitted in this second edition to make the intervention applicable to a broader range of individuals with bipolar disorder. Instead, we present and discuss cognitive and behavioral skills for management of the symptoms and problems associated with bipolar as well as some guidelines for selecting the interventions that best meet the patient's needs. When we originally developed the CBT protocol for bipolar disorder we wanted to define the procedures of the protocol in such a way that they could be tested empirically. In the world of clinical research, procedures must be specified with enough detail to be easily replicated across clinicians with varying levels of training and skill. Therefore, it seemed necessary to provide session-by-session instructions. The first edition accomplished this goal. These session-by-session instructions are provided in the Appendix for anyone interested in using the standardized treatment protocol. With that goal accomplished, we now turn our sights toward providing an intervention that is flexible enough and complete enough to be useful with a broader range of patients, including those who have been recently diagnosed, those who have mastered the management of the illness, and those who struggle day to day to achieve symptom remission.

Patients' therapeutic needs will vary depending on their level of acceptance of the illness, experience with symptom management, and degree of symptom control. For example, basic education will be necessary for the patient who is unfamiliar with the illness but may be unnecessary for those who have dealt with it for many years. CBT techniques may be helpful to someone who realizes that his or her thoughts and feelings vary with the course of the illness but may be too complex for a person who is still questioning the accuracy of the diagnosis. In the sections that follow, suggestions for treatment are provided for three patient groups, those who are newly diagnosed, those who are experienced with the illness but have not yet reached stability, and those who are in sustained remission. Table 1.1 provides an overview of suggested interventions for these three groups of patients.

The Newly Diagnosed Patient

It is not unusual for a patient to have suffered through several episodes of depression or mania before the illness is diagnosed (Suppes 2001). Unless they are severe enough to include psychosis, a dramatic decline in functioning, or behaviors that draw the attention of law enforcement or health care providers, the first few episodes of depression and mania often go undetected or are misdiagnosed as stress reactions or medical conditions, such as the flu. This underestimate of the severity of the situation may be reinforced by the presence of stressful life

TABLE 1.1. Suggested Interventions by Patient Group

Newly diagnosed

    Education

    Instructions on lifestyle management

    Symptom Summary Worksheet

Experienced, but not yet stable

    Mood Graphs

    Symptom Summary Worksheet

    Controlling triggers

    Management of cognitive symptoms

    Management of behavioral symptoms

    Compliance training

Symptomatically stable

    Relapse prevention

    Maintenance of adherence

    Achievement of life goals

events, which is often associated with the first few episodes of depression or mania (Brown & Harris, 1978). In children, the symptoms of mania can be easily mistaken for conduct or attention problems, while depressive symptoms may be attributed to the child's temperament.

Although it may not always coincide with the first episode of illness, a new diagnosis of bipolar disorder is still often received with alarm and disbelief. The patient and his or her significant others may know very little about the illness but often fear the worst. In addition to feeling badly and having difficulty with attention and concentration, the newly diagnosed patient experiences confusion about the treatment, can have misconceptions about the nature or cause of the illness, and is usually uncertain about what to do next. As the reality of the illness begins to settle in, there are usually questions about the impact of bipolar disorder on the patient's life, such as the ability to work or care for family and the prospect of regaining stability. A reasonable reaction to receiving a lifetime diagnosis of a chronic and severe psychiatric illness is denial of its severity, chronicity, or the need for intervention (Dell'Osso et al., 2002; Swanson et al., 1995).

The therapist can be most helpful to the newly diagnosed patient by addressing patient and family member concerns and questions about the illness, the treatment, and the long-term consequences. As the patient and his or her loved ones begin to grasp what has happened, the therapist can help them to connect their observations and experience with the onset and symptoms of the disorder.

> John's wife, for example, knew that something was wrong with her husband, but could not get John or anyone else to listen to her. She knew that he was not acting like his normal self, not treating others with his usual kindness, and even physically changing from lack of sleep and appetite. When he was finally diagnosed with depression, she was relieved that he was getting the care he needed and furious that it had to reach the point of attempting suicide before she could get him the help he needed. John, though clearly depressed for several months, thought it was just work stress. Now that he had a diagnosis, he tried to rethink the past few months to connect what he had been through with what he was being told about depression.

The Experienced but Not Yet Stable Patient

Sandra, like many people who suffer from bipolar disorder, was compliant with her medication on an intermittent basis. People do not usually fluctuate between full adherence to their medication regimens and discontinuation altogether. Studies assessing compliance rates among people who suffer from bipolar disorder have shown that the majority of individuals periodically skip or alter doses, omit some but not all types of medications, or discontinue use for short periods (Keck et al, 1996; Scott & Pope, 2002a, 2002b; Weiss et al., 1998). Because non-compliance appears to be the rule rather than the exception (Basco & Rush, 1995; Svarstad, Shireman, & Sweeney, 2001), clinicians working with those who have not yet achieved consistent stability of remission should raise the issue for discussion.

> In Sandra's case, her extraordinarily busy home life did not follow a daily routine with regular work hours, meal breaks, or a set bed-time. She was a "soccer mom" with three young children whom she drove to school, piano lessons, sporting events, and tutoring in varying combinations each day. Because she was so intelligent, well organized, and compulsive with her kids and home life, it was easy to assume that she also was organized about taking medica-tions. But her evening schedule varied from day to day, and she often did household chores long into the night. By the time she went to bed she was exhausted and would forget to take her medi-cations. When Sandra reported continued problems with racing thoughts, distractibility, anxiety, and insomnia, her psychiatrist reevaluated her medication regimen and started her on a new mood stabilizer before assessing her degree of adherence with the old treatment plan. When she would not respond to treatment, more changes were made in the regimen. To improve her symp-tomatic control, Sandra would need to make modifications in her adherence to treatment.

CBT can help this type of patient in a variety of ways. Early goals might include improving adherence to treatment by helping Sandra apply her existing organizational skills to herself. Finding cues to remind her to take medications more consistently might be a start. Chapters 4 and 5 provide a number of interventions for managing treatment compliance.

Another way in which CBT can help the experienced yet still symptomatic patient is to help him or her become familiar with the factors that influence mood swings through "mood graphs," as described in Chapter 6. Once becoming sensitized to these changes, cognitive and behavioral interventions can be taught to help improve coping, regulate sleep, achieve goals, and eliminate distorted thinking patterns. Chapters 7 through 10 cover these interventions.

Work with the symptomatic patient most closely resembles cogni-tive therapy for acute depression in that skills are systematically taught to help control symptoms and homework is assigned to generalize skills outside the therapy session. Skills are presented in order of complexity beginning with simple mood, cognitive, and/or behavioral monitoring. Their effect on symptom reduction is closely monitored and success is reinforced. As skills are gained and symptoms remit, the frequency of visits can decrease perhaps from weekly to biweekly to monthly and so on. If symptoms begin to return, the frequency of visits can increase until the patient feels more confident in his or her newfound abilities in symptom management.

The Patient in Sustained Remission

Once the illness is under control, the focus of treatment is the maintenance of gains and improvement in quality of life. Continued psychotherapy can be useful to aid the patient in the surveillance of the illness and prevention of relapse. The content of therapy for the symptomatically stable patient, however, may shift away from symptom resolution to stress management, relationship problems, life decisions, and existential issues as well as relapse prevention.

Patients in sustained remission will usually come to treatment following a psychosocial stressor or present with some life management problem such as marital or job difficulties. In those situations, the illness may not be the initial focus of treatment. However, such a presenting problem does pose an opportunity to inquire about the person's management of his or her illness. Should information or training in relapse prevention be needed, it can be incorporated into the ongoing treatment.

Those who "graduate" from the skills training phase of treatment can be followed at less frequent intervals to help sustain remission and to facilitate their adaptation to the illness, once remission has been achieved. It is not unusual for patients to visit their therapist a few times each year to review progress, set goals for the future, assess symptoms, or seek support for life decisions or changes. Sometimes they use therapy to help themselves stay well when they fear a return of symptoms.

Regardless of the phase of adjustment to the illness and control of symptomatology, the primary focus of CBT is relapse prevention. The hope is that in augmenting medication treatment with CBT, recurrences of mania and depression will occur less frequently, will be controlled earlier in their course, and will remit more rapidly. Adjustment to the illness should mean more time feeling well, less time feeling ill, fewer disruptions in normal routines, and improved quality of life. To achieve these goals, we present various strategies, exercises, and methods throughout the book for (1) helping patients to better understand the nature of the illness; (2) developing an early warning system that symptoms are returning; (3) control of the cognitive, behavioral, and affective symptoms of depression and mania; (4) enhancement of treatment adherence; and (5) management of stress and resolution of psychosocial problems.

While the sequence of presentation of each component of CBT may vary across patients depending on their needs and abilities, a new patient might find it most helpful to begin with education and symptom detection before moving on to the other areas. Skills for symptom management can be combined with interventions for solving psychosocial problems. It is best to inquire early in treatment about medication adherence problems, as inconsistencies in dosing could preclude control of symptoms with psychotherapeutic methods.

Clinical judgment is needed to help the patient set and prioritize treatment goals. In the interest of developing a collaborative therapeutic alliance, it is generally best to begin therapy by addressing the most pressing problem identified by the patient. In this way, the patient will get the clear message that he or she will play an active role in the therapeutic process and that the therapist is taking his or her concerns seriously.

Table 1.2 gives the reader a preview of interventions to be covered in this book. It can be used to select interventions to address specific patient concerns. Although we suggest a structure for sequencing interventions, it is acceptable to pick and choose interventions that meet the needs of patients at the time of intervention and/or are possible to teach within the time constraints of the therapy. Even if clinicians can spend only a short time with patients at each visit, such as a medication visit, introduction of a few interventions at a time still can add up to a relapse prevention program.

Key Points for the Therapist to Remember

♦ The efficacy of CBT rests on the strength of the therapeutic alliance.

♦ The clinician's task is not only to help a person overcome the symptoms of the illness and recover from its psychosocial consequences but also to prepare for its inevitable return.

♦ Psychotherapy is often a stabilizing force in the lives of patients. Therapy visits can provide a structure for marking the passage of time, for monitoring progress, and for achieving goals.

♦ Psychotherapy that focuses on symptom monitoring, goal setting, and relapse prevention provides a structure for self-improvement.

♦ CBT methods work just as well for therapists as they do for their patients. Therefore, when feeling internal distress during therapy sessions, therapists should be mindful of their automatic thoughts, search

TABLE 1.2. Summary of Common Problems and Interventions

Problem	Suggested intervention	Chapter(s)
Does the patient understand the nature of bipolar disorder and its treatment?	Provide education. Complete Life Chart	1, 2, and 6
Does the patient need more information about his or her medication?	Provide information	3
Is the patient in denial?	Provide information. Challenge inaccurate views with Socratic questioning.	4
Is the patient having difficulty accepting the illness and treatment?	Identify stage of adjustment to having the illness, address automatic thoughts, facilitate grieving the loss of mental health.	4
Is the patient angry about having the illness?	Validate feelings. Do not move too quickly to intervention.	4
Is the patient engaging in a bargaining process by self-adjusting medications?	Explain process of adjustment that includes bargaining. Normalize the process. Allow patient to have input in regimen planning.	4
Is the patient's adherence to treatment inconsistent?	Provide education about adherence. Complete compliance contract.	4 and 5
Does the patient know his or her symptoms of depression, mania, hypomania, and mixed states?	Complete Symptom Summary Worksheet	6
Is the patient aware of when his or her mood is climbing or dropping and the factors that influences mood swings?	Complete Mood Graphs	6
Is the patient unsure if symptoms are returning?	Review the Symptom Summary Worksheet.	6
Does the patient engage in activities that seem to worsen mood or other symptoms?	Identify mood triggers and make plan to avoid them.	7
Has the patient stopped engaging in healthy habits?	Increase one positive and decrease one negative.	7
Does the patient have poor sleep habits?	Teach sleep hygiene	7
Is the patient isolated from others?	Increase social contact.	7 and 12

cont.

TABLE 1.2. *cont.*

Problem	Suggested intervention	Chapter
Does the patient engage in any enjoyable activities?	Use activity scheduling to add positive activities.	7
Does the patient feel overwhelmed and unable to take effective action?	Increase activity with graded task assignment or A list/B list.	8
Does overstimulation affect the patient's behavior?	Reduce or control hyperactivity with goal setting or A list/B list.	8
Is the patient's attitude overly negative or is he or she overlself-critical or pessimistic?	Teach Catch, Control, Correct interventions.	9
Does the patient fail to see his or her strengths or fail to see risks of his or her actions?	Address Tunnel Vision by examining the evidence and generating alternative explanations	9
Does the patient seem to be jumping to conclusions or making assumptions?	Address Making Guesses by examining the evidence and generating alternative explanations	9
Is the patient blowing things out of proportion or minimizing?	Address Misperceptions by getting feedback from others and monitoring symptoms.	9
Is the patient overly rigid in his or her thinking?	Address Absolutes with the cognitive continuum, weighing advantages and disadvantages, or problem solving.	9
Is the patient depressed about having bipolar disorder?	Use the Catch, Control, and Correct methods to cope with negative thinking.	9
Does the patient have difficulty coping with psychosocial problems?	Teach problem-solving, decision-making, and coping skills.	10
Is the patient having difficulty concentrating, organizing thoughts, or making decisions?	Teach the Slow It, Focus It, Structure It interventions.	10
Is the patient stressed?	Teach stress management skills.	11
Is the patient having problems with his or her relationships?	Teach CBT skills for improving interpersonal communication.	12

for thinking errors, and correct their distortions in logic before they have a negative effect on the therapeutic process.

♦ When the clinician assumes that people have preexisting coping skills and communicates that either verbally or through actions, they get the message that the clinician thinks they are competent, able to solve problems, and smart enough to know when to ask for help. Validation of this type enhances the collaborative nature of the therapeutic bond—an essential in CBT.

Points to Discuss with Patients

♦ For patients, trust in therapists, even when the feedback is not what the patient wants to hear, is critical to the task. Patients must feel comfortable telling therapists when symptoms are beginning to reemerge and therapists must be able to give honest feedback to their patients when the warning signs are overlooked or when their actions place them at risk for relapse.

♦ People who are distressed probably coped better with life at times when they were not as distressed. Skills do not disappear when the symptoms of bipolar disorder emerge. However, the emotional upheavals, confusion, and loss of motivation and energy can make it difficult for people to access their skills.

CHAPTER 2

Cognitive–Behavioral Therapy for Bipolar Disorder

AN OVERVIEW

When one thinks of bipolar disorder an image of mania often comes to mind—the wild look of insanity, the nonsensical ramblings of a person whose mind is racing from one idea to another, seeing visions, and conversing with unknown visitors. And although this image can characterize a person at the peak of mania, it does not capture the whole of the illness. In fact, while there are standard descriptions of bipolar disorder in the fourth edition of the *Diagnostic and Statistical Manual of Mental Disorders* (DSM-IV; American Psychiatric Association, 1994a), the presentation of the illness and its course varies greatly across individuals, as does the corresponding level of impairment.

What is common among the 1% of people who suffer from bipolar disorder in this country is its recurrent nature (Goodwin & Jamison, 1990; Zis & Goodwin, 1979). Once diagnosed, the individual can count on future episodic bouts of depression and/or mania that may present in times of stress or change or may recur without provocation. Although some fortunate individuals will have very few episodes of mania and depression in the course of their lives, most will have an increased frequency of recurrences as they age, with periods of wellness shortening and episodes of illness lengthening (Angst, 1981; Roy-Byrne, Post, Uhde, Porcu, & Davis, 1985; Zis, Grof, Webster, & Goodwin, 1980). As pharmacotherapies improve and more methods are found to enhance compliance with treatment, this progressive pattern should improve. Certainly as people are diagnosed earlier in the development of their illness, opportunities are provided for altering the overall course of the illness. And although the suicide rate remains high, there is reason to be hopeful that the increasing availability of psychotherapeutic interventions to augment medication treatment may lead people to help before reaching the unbearable pain that makes the taking of their lives seem like a reasonable solution.

What varies greatly across patients is the quality of their moods, the actions they take in response to symptoms, and the sequence in which their symptoms emerge. Even within individuals the symptoms of mania and depression can change from one episode to the next. For example, a person can have difficulty sleeping in one episode of depression, and in another be hypersomnic.

Every year there are new developments in the treatment of bipolar disorder. Medications are safer, cause fewer side effects, and provide more positive effects (e.g., Calabrese et al., 1999; Zarate, 2000). Psychotherapies have been developed that enhance outcomes, reduce relapse, and aid adaptation to the illness (e.g., Lam et al., 2003). Despite our greater understanding of the psychobiology of bipolar disorder we are only beginning to learn how to encourage patients to consistently use their pharmacological, psychosocial, and psychotherapeutic resources.

Symptoms of Depression and Mania

When depression begins, mood can change from euthymic to sad, blah, blue, empty, anxious, hopeless, or irritable. People describe feeling impatient, edgy, nervous, lost, misunderstood, disinterested, sensitive, angry, "stuck," or empty. Very often they find that they don't care anymore about their activities, the people around them, accomplishing tasks on time, or their personal appearance. They feel neutral, unaffected, and indifferent rather than sad, hurt, or fearful. They carry on with life because they "have to," but if their fate should lead to a sudden and untimely death, it would be fine with them.

The attitude shifts in depression may also include excessive negativity. Everything seems difficult and overwhelming. Patients are convinced that there is no point in trying to accomplish anything because a negative outcome is inevitable. Setbacks can feel insurmountable. Other people are perceived as insincere, unconcerned, or clueless. Self-criticism increases, life failures are recounted, regrets are reviewed, and self-esteem plummets. The depressed person does not see these as overly negative thoughts but, rather, realistic and easily supported by their view of the facts. In reality, there may be some amount of truth to their observations, but contradictory evidence is generally ignored, the circumstances surrounding events forgotten, and achievements undervalued.

If symptoms are not yet severe, people can usually keep up their work routine and manage the minimally required home responsibilities even when depressed. But they stop having fun, lose interest in hobbies, quit exercising, and stop calling on their friends. When asked, they claim to be too tired or too behind in chores to play. Extra efforts at work or home are curbed and more time may be spent in front of the television or other solitary activity. Eventually, minimal effort is not enough. Poor work performance comes to the attention of supervisors. Neglected household maintenance creates tension in the family. Declined invitations to socialize leads to isolation from others. Jobs may be threatened, debt builds, and the person who is depressed can do nothing but let it happen.

There is sometimes a temporary relief in these situations. When a job is lost, the immediate stress is gone; no one is making demands; the individual can be left alone to suffer in silence. Unfortunately, any relief is short-lived. The realities of daily life creep back in, and the stress that comes with self-awareness and sleepless nights of worry worsen the depression. It is a self-perpetuating cycle. Symptoms create impairment. Impairment causes problems. And problems increase stress and exacerbate depressive symptoms.

In contrast, the mood changes in mania can be positive, hopeful, excited, euphoric, "on top of the world," or exhilarated. For few patients are manic episodes always pleasant. Most have had periods of feeling extremely irritable, agitated, anxious, tense, and fearful. For some, the pleasant or euphoric mood evolves into irritability as the mania progresses and worsens.

In mania, the cognitive changes also vary greatly across patients but generally consist of changes in cognitive processing, changes in quality of cognitions, and changes in thought content. At the extremes, we are familiar with delusions of grandeur and paranoia. But more common are the subtle changes that fall within the realm of normal at first, such as more interest in life, optimism, and better self-esteem. If hypomania or mania falls on the heels of a lengthy period of depression, the switch may not be noticeable until the changes in thought process begin to interfere with optimal functioning. As the person's mood begins to lift there is often an improvement in sense of humor. Amusing ideas occur more frequently and the person is able to laugh at him- or herself. As mania progresses, humor can take on a more hostile, dark, or sarcastic tone. This change is unusually not noticeable to the patient but can be quite apparent to others.

The speed and efficiency of cognitive processing can improve early in the evolution of mania but disintegrate as thoughts increase in number and speed. Some people with bipolar disorder say they have their best ideas when hypomanic. Feeling free from the inhibiting nature of depression, the mind is open to new ideas and possibilities. Creativity during hypomania can result in taking chances at success otherwise inhibited by pessimism and low self-confidence. There is often an urge or need for stimulation that comes from changes in routine or activity. If judgment becomes impaired, the changes can create new problems for the individual such as quitting a job before having a new one available. If the quality of cognitions declines, and the person becomes disorganized or unfocused, changes are initiated but often not completed. More often, however, the urge for change in the early phases of mania or hypomania manifest themselves in more benign forms such as changing hairstyle, clothing, or jewelry, or rearranging furniture at home or work. There can be a shift in interests so that more time is allocated to planning or research on the Internet or accumulating resources for a new project.

Content changes in thought can also include sexually related ideas, interests, and observations of others. Sexual preferences can even temporarily change. Shopping may seem more interesting and stimulating and purchases may be more easily justified although less practical. Stores avoided when too depressed to shop, too self-conscious to try on clothes, or too full of shoppers to be comfortable suddenly feel inviting, curious, or too good to pass up.

With the onset of mania or hypomania people experience a change in their social interests. Rather than avoiding others, social contact is desired and sought out. As humor increases, people find themselves the center of attention at parties or other gatherings. No longer inhibited by anxiety or depression, they can allow themselves to be the life of the party. With the advent of the Internet, chat rooms and online support groups provide new outlets for the urge to talk and be heard.

It is apparent that changes in thought content and process with mania lead to changes in behavior. These behaviors can initially be quite positive. Some people report that they are quicker, physically and mentally, when mania is beginning to emerge. If not impaired by distractibility or racing thoughts, they can be more efficient than usual, able to multitask, and have the stamina to put in the added time needed to take on new activities or persist at old ones. Unfortunately, the activities stimulated by mania are not without problems. If not placed in check, the socializing and increased sex drive can lead to dangerous liaisons, infidelity, or actions that will be greatly regretted when the mania remits and the self-deprecation of depression returns.

Activity can become disorganized as thoughts become difficult to organize. The numerous starts of new projects without completion overwhelm the individual when he or she returns to a euthymic or depressed state. Money spent on shopping sprees leads to accumulated debt. Changes of residence, jobs, or relationships may be greatly regretted.

As mentioned previously, each patient can have a unique presentation and sequence of affective, cognitive, and behavioral symptoms during periods of depression and mania. Chapter 6 covers methods for assessing each patient's unique symptoms. There are several standardized methods for assessing the symptoms of bipolar disorder, which we briefly review in the following section.

Establishing the Diagnosis of Bipolar Disorder

To establish the diagnosis of bipolar I or II disorder, clinicians should be trained and experienced in recognizing and diagnosing psychiatric conditions, as well as general medical conditions that may cause a mood disorder which looks like but are not, in fact, bipolar I or II disorder. In addition, an accurate history is essential to making the diagnosis. It is best to obtain this history from both the patient and a close friend or relative who has known the patient well for at least several years. The most common problem in obtaining an accurate history is that people do not recognize or report manic or hypomanic episodes. In fact, they often do not seek treatment when manic or hypomanic; they seek treatment when depressed. But the nature of the depressive episode itself does not distinguish between bipolar I and II and major depressive disorders. By carefully questioning their past history of symptoms, a far clearer and more accurate history can be obtained, which is essential.

Misdiagnosis has serious consequences. The wrong medicine may be given, the prognosis can be wrong, and the overall management of the patient will suffer. The three most common diagnostic errors are (1) mistaking recurrent major depressive episodes for normal reactions to life's difficulties, (2) failing to detect manic or hypomanic episodes, and (3) judging the patient to have schizophrenia instead of bipolar disorder with psychotic features during manic, mixed manic, or major depressive episodes.

Finally, it is very common for patients with bipolar disorder to abuse alcohol, stimulants (amphetamines, cocaine), or other substances episodically (or chronically, though this is less common). In some, this is an attempt to self-medicate. For others, these substances precipitate specific episodes. Thus, the presence or history of substance abuse should not discount the diagnosis of bipolar disorder. On the other hand, if all of the manic or hypomanic episodes are caused by substance abuse and largely end when the abuse stops, the diagnosis of bipolar disorder should not be made.

Self-Report: Mood Disorders Questionnaire

The Mood Disorders Questionniare (Hirschfeld, 2002) is a brief screening questionnaire that can be completed by patients. It was developed to aid in the detection of bipolar disorder in patients seen in primary care settings. A copy of the questionnaire is available on the Depression and Bipolar Support Alliance website (*www.dbsalliance. org*). It able to correctly detect about 70% of bipolar patients and rule out approximately 90% of those who do not have the disorder (Hirschfeld et al., 2000). It is not intended to be a diagnostic instrument per se but, rather, to cue patients and providers to more fully assess the symptoms of the disorder and confirm the diagnosis.

Clinician Evaluation:
Structured Clinical Interview for DSM-IV

The Structured Clinical Interview for DSM-IV (SCID; First, Spitzer, Gibbon, & Williams, 1996) is a structured interview organized to assess DSM-IV criteria for diagnoses in a systematic fashion. First et al. (1996) have developed a clinician-friendly version of the SCID (SCID-CV). It simplifies the interview by providing an administration book with the structured questions and corresponding DSM-IV criteria and a separate score sheet for recording answers. Decision rules for determining mood and psychotic disorders are included in the score sheet. This format reduces the amount of paper used for each administration, making the method more cost-effective. A numbering system that corresponds questions in the administration booklet with answers in the score sheet helps the interviewer keep his or her place. DSM-IV criteria are included alongside the questions intended to assess a given symptom. This allows the interviewer to immediately assess whether or not a patient's answer is sufficient to meet the criteria in question.

Numerous studies have attested to the reliability of the SCID in its various forms in patients with substance abuse problem, mood disorders, psychotic disorders, and anxiety disorders (e.g., Kranzler et al., 1995, Kranzler, Tennen, Babor, Kaden, & Rounsaville, Skre, Onstad, Torgersen, & Kringlen, 1991; Steiner, Tebes, Sledge, & Walker, 1995). It is intended for use in adults over the age of 18 and has demonstrated reliability in even older adult populations (Segal, Kabacoff, Hersen, Van Hasselt, & Ryan, 1995).

Basco et al. (2000) used the SCID to diagnose psychiatric outpatients with severe mental illnesses in a community mental health setting. Comparing the nurses' diagnoses using the SCID with the diagnoses generated by the doctoral level research clinicians, reliability estimates were fairly high, with a kappa ranging from .61 to .64 depending on the specificity of the diagnosis. If the SCID evaluator was allowed to incorporate the information in patients' medical charts along with the SCID, the kappa agreements with skilled diagnosticians rose to .76–.78. These findings suggest that structured interviews using the SCID supplemented by information in the medical record could greatly improve diagnostic accuracy over routine psychiatric practices even in severely ill patient populations.

Diagnostic Interview for Children and Adolescents

The Diagnostic Interview for Children and Adolescents (DICA) is a semistructured interview that was originally designed to match the Diagnostic Interview Schedule (Robins, Helzer, Ratcliff, & Seyfried, 1982) and assesses lifetime history of DSM-IV diagnostic criteria for child and adolescent disorders. It has been found to have good test–retest reliability (Welner, Reich, Herjanic, Jung, & Amado, 1987; De la Osa, Ezpeleta, Oomenech, Navarro, & Losilla, 1997) and shows evidence of construct validity, particularly for children with bipolar disorder (Reich, 2000).

Assessment of Symptom Severity

Inventory for Depressive Symptomatology

The Inventory for Depressive Symptomatology (IDS; Rush, et al., 1986) clinician report (IDS-C), was designed to measure specific signs and symptoms of depression; to include measures of endogenous symptoms, melancholia, and atypicality; and to assess vegetative symptoms, cognitive changes, mood disturbance, endogenous symptoms, and anxiety symptoms. The IDS has been revised to include atypical symptoms of leaden paralysis and rejection sensitivity. Each of the 30 items is rated on a 0–3 scale, with higher scores representing increased severity of symptoms. A self-report version of the IDS is also available. The mean score for the IDS self-report version in a sample of patients with major depression was 36, which are significantly different from normal controls (2.1) and support the construct validity of the measure (Rush et al., 1986). The internal consistency of the IDS-C is high, with Cronbach's alpha of .88. The IDS-C correlates highly with the Beck Depression Inventory (BDI) (r = .61–.78) and the Hamilton Rating Scale for Depression (HRSD) (r = .67–.92; Rush et al., 1986).

In a sample of patients participating in research on depression, interrater reliability for the IDS-C was .96 for the 30-item version (Rush, Gullion, Basco, Jarrett, & Trivedi, 1996). When adding remitted depressed and normal control subjects to create a larger sample (N = 552), Cronbach's alpha was .93 for the 28-item version of the IDS-C and .94 for the 30-item version. (Rush et al., 1996). The self-report version was highly correlated with the BDI (r = .78) and the HRSD (r = .67), as was the clinician rating (r = .61 with the BDI and r = .92 with the HRSD). A factor analysis on 353 patients completing the self-report version of the IDS and clinicians completing the IDS-C showed three dimensions: cognitive/mood symptoms, anxiety/arousal symptoms, and vegetative symptoms (Rush et al., 1996). The IDS-C improves on the weaknesses of the HRSD by assessing endogenous and melancholic symptoms and atypical and anxious symptoms. It also provides uniform scaling across items and reduces assessment of multiple symptoms on single items.

Bech–Rafaelsen Mania Scale

The Bech–Rafaelsen Mania Scale (BRMS; Bech, Bolwig, Kramp, & Rafaelsen, 1979) is a clinician-rated scale designed to quantitatively assess the severity of the manic state in diagnosed patients. It consists of 11 items rated on a 5-point scale, with the total score comprising a summation of all items. The BRMS has an interrater reliability correlation of .95 using the Kendall coefficient of concordance, and the interobserver reliability correlation ranges from r = .97 to r = .99 (Bech et al., 1979). Homogeneity of the BRMS ranges between r = .72 and r = .94 on 10 of the items; sleep has an r = .48 when correlated to total scale score (Bech et al., 1979).

Young Mania Rating Scale

The Young Mania Rating Scale (YMRS; Young, Biggs, Ziegler, & Meyer, 1978) is one of the most widely used clinician rating scales for measuring severity of manic symptoms. It is not a diagnostic measure, but it consists of 11 items that are criteria for mania including changes in mood, cognition, and behavior. It is based on clinician observations supplemented by an unstructured inquiry regarding symptoms that are not readily observable. Young et al. (1978) report an interrater reliability of .93 for the total measure and scores ranging from .66 to .92 for the individual items. Its validity has been demonstrated through correlations of other mania measures (e.g., r = .71–.89) and through its prediction of hospitalization length of stay (Young et al., 1978).

The Cycle of Symptoms

There is a cycle in hypomania and mania where the new ideas and interests coupled with a loosening of inhibitions and increased energy leads to actions that overstimulate the person. This can further escalate the mania, which, in turn, stimulates more ideas, interests, and activities. An excellent example is sleep loss from nighttime activities such as socializing, working on projects, or surfing the Internet. People with bipolar disorder often have a preference for nighttime activity. They stay up late and miss out on sleep, which has been found to exacerbate mania, and their symptoms escalate. Figure 2.1 illustrates the progression of cognitive, emotional, and behavioral symptoms, their

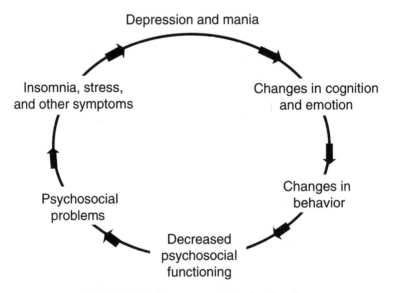

FIGURE 2.1. The course of bipolar disorder.

effect on psychosocial functioning, and, in turn, the effect of psychosocial problems on the perpetuation of episodes.

Keeping an early bedtime schedule is a significant sacrifice for a night person, particularly those who are tired and sluggish in the morning and only begin to find their pace in the late afternoon. If the evening dose of prescribed drugs causes sleepiness, it is often delayed and later forgotten or consciously omitted altogether to avoid the drowsiness that can interfere with activities. Without the protection of mood-stabilizing medications, a recurrence of full-blown mania is almost certain.

After years of observation and experimentation, many people with bipolar disorder learn to work with the ups and downs in their mood. They may allow a short flurry of hypomania but know when to put on the breaks, regulate their medication, get some sleep, and slow down their lifestyle. This is accomplished with varying levels of success. Some wait too long to intervene because they want to enjoy the high or because they do not recognize the mania until they have gotten into trouble or begin to decompensate. Most hate the lows but feel helpless to stop their progression. More mood-stabilizing medication may not help and can leave them more sluggish. Antidepressants run the risk of inducing mania. Getting medical attention as soon as symptoms of depression begin to emerge is complicated, if not impossible, for most who do not have the advantage of private care and for many who do.

Even people who consistently adhere to their medication regimens for bipolar disorder will likely suffer from symptom breakthroughs periodically (Gelenberg, Carroll, Baudhuin, Jefferson, & Greist, 1989). They may avoid full recurrences of depression and mania but will have enough symptoms to warrant attention from their health care providers. Unfortunately, despite having considerable experience with the illness, not all patients in this category are skilled at identifying the signs of relapse. Early intervention is generally considered the key to control. Waiting until symptoms cluster into a syndrome more likely predicts a difficult course back to normalcy.

How Can Therapy Help?

Psychotherapy for bipolar disorder is considered a luxury in a climate of managed care, where such treatment is unavailable or limited at best. Those with the most difficult-to-manage forms of the illness, who have few psychosocial resources and an abundance of problems, have the least access to psychotherapy. Affordable clinics that charge on sliding scales are often staffed by trainees or people with less therapeutic experience than is needed to provide an adequate intervention for an illness as challenging as bipolar disorder.

Psychotherapeutic interventions are delivered outside a traditional long-term weekly psychotherapy format as often as within one. Insurance companies often limit the length of treatment. Psychiatrists, who are likely to be the primary mental health provider for people with bipolar disorder, do not have the time to provide an hour of psychotherapy along with medication management. And community mental health centers rarely have the resources to provide psychotherapy for the people they serve. Therefore, the cognitive-behavioral interventions described throughout this book should be thought of as adjunctive to ongoing treatments. Given this framework, how can CBT help people who suffer from bipolar disorder?

When the first edition of this book was published, psychotherapy for bipolar disorder was a new concept. It had previously been believed that a psychosocial approach to the treatment of bipolar disorder was a waste of time. People diagnosed with bipolar disorder were considered to be unmanageable, self-destructive, and unable to participate in the therapeutic process. However, with better detection methods and improved efficacy of medical treatments, symptom control has become commonplace. People with bipolar disorder can and do actively participate in psychotherapy and learn to manage their illness. Psychotherapy is one vehicle for teaching patients the skills they need to cope with the symptoms that medication does not fully remedy. In addition, psychotherapy can bolster the effect of medication by providing strategies that help people to be more consistent in taking their medication. Given the episodic and recurring nature of bipolar disorder, psychotherapies, such as CBT, can aid in the anticipation and prevention of future episodes by teaching early detection methods, stress management, and problem solving.

Efficacy of CBT

Since we wrote the first edition a few controlled studies have been conducted to examine the efficacy of CBT for bipolar disorder. Although differing somewhat in methodology, all have shown evidence for its feasibility and usefulness. Cochran (1984) conducted the first CBT study of adherence. She evaluated the efficacy of CBT against standard outpatient clinic care by targeting thoughts and beliefs that interfered with lithium compliance. After a 6-week intervention the CBT group was significantly more compliant (as defined by appointment attendance and medication adherence) than patients receiving standard care. At 6 months posttreatment, the CBT group still demonstrated better adherence than the standard care group. Overall, the CBT group was less likely to terminate treatment against medical advice, had fewer hospitalizations, and had fewer noncompliance precipitated episodes of depression and mania.

In addition to improving treatment adherence, Lam et al. (2000) found that 12–20 sessions of CBT delivered over 6 months ($N = 13$) was superior to standard outpatient treatment ($N = 12$) in reducing the frequency of episodes and improved coping with prodromal symptoms. Results were maintained at 6-month follow-up, and fewer patients in the CBT group required neuroleptics than in the control group.

Testing CBT in a more challenging group of patients with bipolar disorder and comorbid personality disorders and strong histories of medication nonadherence, Scott et al. (2001) found that after 6 months, the CBT group ($N = 21$) showed significantly fewer symptoms and more improved social functioning than a wait-list control group. When wait-listed patients were subsequently provided with CBT, they showed similar improvement in symptoms and functioning from pre- to post-CBT and had significantly fewer hospitalizations at 12 months posttreatment relative to the 6-month wait-list period prior to receiving CBT.

With a focus on control of residual symptoms Fava, Bartolucci, Rafanelli, and Mangelli (2001) provided CBT for 15 patients who had relapsed while on lithium prophylaxis. Patients were initially treated with antidepressants or antipsychotics. These medications were tapered off as CBT began. The patient's participating in 10 30-minute CBT sessions resulted in significantly decreased residual symptoms and an increased number of months to the next relapse following CBT relative to baseline levels. All 15 patients had relapsed within 30 months of initial lithium therapy and prior to beginning any psychosocial interventions. Only five of these patients relapsed within 30 months after CBT was initiated.

Perry, Jarrier, Morriss, McCarthy, and Limb (1999) provided 6–12 months of CBT for patients with bipolar disorder in conjunction with standard medication treatment. These individuals were compared with patients receiving standard treatment only over an 18-month observation period. The patients in the CBT + Standard Treatment group had fewer manic episodes, spent fewer days in the hospital, had a longer time of wellness before relapse, and had significantly better psychosocial functioning.

Medication treatment of bipolar depression always runs the risk of inducing mania (Altshuler et al., 1995). Therefore an alternative, such as CBT, if efficacious, could provide an alternative to antidepressant therapy. Zaretsky, Segal, and Gomar (1999) compared response to CBT in bipolar depressed patients ($n = 11$) and a matched group of patients with unipolar depression ($n = 11$). All were moderately depressed and had a history of multiple depressive episodes. After 20 sessions of CBT, bipolar and unipolar depressed patients had a reduction in depressive symptoms. Although limited by a lack of a bipolar control group, the results suggest that CBT combined with mood stabilizers may be helpful in treating acute episodes of depression in bipolar patients without the risk of mania that comes with antidepressant medication.

These early studies suggest that CBT can be beneficial in increasing medication adherence, managing symptoms, and improving psychosocial functioning in people with bipolar disorder. Although demonstrating the feasibility of psychotherapy with this patient population, larger and more stringent studies will be needed to test the limits of CBT efficacy.

Key Points for the Therapist to Remember

◆ What varies greatly across patients is the quality of their moods, the actions they take in response to symptoms, and the sequence in which their symptoms emerge. Even within individuals the symptoms of mania and depression can change from one episode to the next.

◆ Symptoms create impairment. Impairment causes problems. And problems increase stress and exacerbate symptoms.

◆ Despite having considerable experience with the illness, not everyone is skilled at identifying the signs of relapse. Early intervention is generally considered the key to control. Waiting until symptoms cluster into a syndrome more likely predicts a difficult course back to normalcy.

◆ The expectation is that by reading this book either therapists will experiment with the psychotherapeutic methods described herein and learn to provide psychotherapy for their patients with bipolar disorder or clinicians of a variety of types, including psychiatrists, will implement selected interventions with their patients in the limited time available during a medication visit, crisis intervention session, inpatient or day treatment groups, or the course of another type of therapy.

Points to Discuss with Patients

◆ What is common among the 1% of people who suffer from bipolar disorder in this country is its recurrent nature. Once diagnosed, the

individual can count on a future of episodic bouts of depression and/
or mania that may present in times of stress or change or may recur
without provocation.

♦ Reasons for hope: Every year there are new developments in the
treatment of bipolar disorder. Medications are safer, cause fewer side
effects, and provide more positive effects. Psychotherapies have been
developed that enhance outcomes, reduce relapse, and aid adaptation
to the illness.

♦ Symptoms of depression and mania.

♦ Given the episodic and recurring nature of bipolar disorder, psychotherapies, such as CBT, can aid in the anticipation and prevention of
future episodes by teaching early detection methods, stress management, and problem solving.

CHAPTER 3

Medication Treatments for Bipolar Disorder

This chapter provides a brief overview of the use of medications, their side effects, and commonly encountered issues surrounding short- and longer-term management of bipolar disorder. This type of information is important for patients to know. It is the responsibility of the prescribing person to provide this information to the patient. However, nonphysician clinicians who are interacting with patients with bipolar disorder should also be generally informed about common medication issues. In particular, these clinicians can reinforce the need for careful medication adherence by patients, clarify issues of concern to the patient, help to identify early symptom breakthrough or side effects, and, importantly, encourage patients when appropriate, to seek medical counsel and possible medication revisions. Just as the management of diabetes requires lifestyle adjustments, careful symptom monitoring, and occasional changes in the doses or types of medication, so too does bipolar disorder. The nonphysician clinician can contribute in a major way to the longer-term medication management, lifestyle changes, and timely pursuit of help by the patients when medication adjustments may be called for.

On the other hand, nonphysicians are not responsible for providing in-depth pharmacological consultation to patients. Rather, by helping patients to identify questions and problems, symptoms, and possible side effects, nonphysician clinicians can ensure both the timely and efficient use of physician time in addressing these key patient concerns.

The information in this chapter is a snapshot (circa 2004) of how medications are used for bipolar disorder. In the last decade, a remarkable number of new medications have been developed and tested for bipolar disorder. One can expect that even within the next 2–3 years more information and more medications will become available. Thus, the following is only a synopsis of what we now know. At least some of the information herein will change sooner rather than later.

Overview of Medication Management

Medications are used in bipolar disorder to treat manic (antimanic or mood-stabilizing agents) or depressive (antidepressant agents) episodes or both. The proper, safe, and effective use of medication requires patient collaboration and, if possible, support by significant others (e.g., wife, husband, sibling, parent). With such collaboration, the chances are high that pharmacotherapy will control both manic and depressive symptoms, acutely and in the longer term. With sustained symptom control, most patients are able to return to their usual level of function, to avoid subsequent hospitalizations, and to avoid prolonged or significant disability. Improperly administered treatments, however, will fail to control symptoms, thereby leading to a poorer long-term course (prognosis), and may also lead to undesirable or even life-threatening side effects.

To enhance patient collaboration, it is essential that patients understand the reason a medication or combination is being used; what the expected outcome is; if successful, when success can be achieved; what side effects are likely; and, importantly, why and when specific laboratory tests are needed either to guide the proper dosing of the medications (e.g., when and how to obtain lithium or divalproex blood levels) or to monitor for adverse events (side effects) (e.g., obtaining white or red blood cell counts for patients taking clozapine [Clozaril]).

We recommend that the prescribing clinician, as well as the nonprescribing clinician, review with the patient (and significant other whenever possible) the signs and symptoms of mania, hypomania, and depression. Second, when a medication is prescribed, patients should be told the reason for its use and common side effects so that they can help determine whether the medication is working correctly or not, and so they can be on the lookout for and report salient side effects in a timely manner.

Third, patients (and significant others) should be taught how to monitor, measure, and record manic and depressive symptoms, so when it is time to see the prescriber, he or she will have a clear picture of what the effects of the medication were and will thereby be better able to make appropriate adjustments (see Chapter 6). Fourth, the prescribing person needs to be available by phone and should see the patient often enough to make timely adjustments in dose or medication type.

A range of effective antimanic and antidepressant medications is available. Typically, a single mood stabilizer (e.g., lithium, valproate, or carbamazepine) is the initial treatment. As with the treatment of other general medical conditions (e.g., arthritis, diabetes, heart disease, and hypertension), medication selection is, in part, a trial-and-error effort. Some patients respond well to and find few side effects with one medication while others do better on a different medicine or combination of medicines. The best way to determine whether a specific medicine is right for a particular patient is to try it out. Thus, one medication is prescribed and the tolerability and beneficial effects are evaluated. This medication, if tolerated but only partially successful, is augmented with a second medication, or if unsuccessful or very poorly tolerated, is switched to another medication. Again, the benefits and tolerability of this second step are evaluated. This stepwise sequence, over time, leads to medication or a combination of medications that provides optimal symptom control with minimal side effects.

This series of suggested steps requires substantial collaboration between the prescribing clinician and the patient. Because medications do not work fully for several weeks, the selection of an optimal treatment for a particular patient usually requires the evaluation of symptomatic outcomes over periods of weeks. Once the patient's condition is stabilized, treatment visits for medication become less frequent. However, continued symptom monitoring is essential to ensure that stabilization persists or that a timely revision in the medication type or dosage is undertaken to address symptom breakthrough should it occur.

For the medication management of bipolar disorder, we can divide treatment into two phases: acute and maintenance. Acute treatment is for patients who are in an episode of mania, hypomania, or major depression. In acute treatment, the first and most important objective is to control or eliminate the symptoms. If symptom elimination is achieved, the patient typically returns to a normal level of interpersonal, occupational, and social functioning. Acute phase treatment may be as brief as 6 weeks (if the first medication is effective and well tolerated) or it may last as long as 6–9 months. Longer-term acute phase treatment is often needed to sort through several different medications to find the medication or combination of medications that provides optimal benefit with minimal side effects.

Once the symptoms are under good control, the acute phase medications are continued, typically at the same dose to maintain the asymptomatic state by preventing the return of the most recent mood episode (i.e., mania, hypomania, or depression). Early in the maintenance phase, psychosocial, rehabilitative, or psychotherapeutic treatments are often added to enhance psychosocial functioning, or to teach patients to manage stresses and other day-to-day issues to help eliminate symptoms and/or improve function.

Later in the maintenance phase, one aim is to prevent the onset of a new mood episode (i.e., mania, hypomania, or depression) typically by continuing the same medications. As with other chronic medical conditions, such as diabetes or arthritis, patients with bipolar disorder are maintained on medication(s) to control the symptoms of their illness for prolonged periods of time. For nearly every patient with bipolar disorder, maintenance treatment lasts a lifetime. Prolonged symptom control results in continued optimal functioning on a day-to-day basis.

For both acute and maintenance phases of treatment, patients must take the prescribed medication(s) on a daily basis. Unlike aspirin, for example, which is taken for the treatment of headache only when a person actually has a headache, medications for bipolar disorder must be taken regularly—on both good days and bad days—at the same dosage. In addition, it is not uncommon during longer-term treatment for some symptoms to return even if the patient is taking the medications diligently. For example, winter in northern latitudes may be associated with the appearance of some depressive symptoms, or spring or fall may be associated with the development of some hypomanic symptoms. For other patients, life stresses, frequent travel through multiple time zones, the use of some over-the-counter medications, or the development of a viral illness may lead to a waxing and then subsequent waning of symptoms. Thus, maintenance treatment often requires some adjustments of medications, which if made early and in a timely fashion, can easily avert symptomatic worsening (see later section on long-term management issues).

What Patients Need to Know about Medication Management

To obtain optimal patient adherence, it is helpful for clinicians to explain to patients with bipolar disorder several general principles about the effective use of antimanic and antidepressant medications:

1. The objectives of medication treatment are, first, to control symptoms and, second, to maintain the asymptomatic state for prolonged periods of time. These objectives usually require some adjustment of medication type, dosage, or both.

2. To obtain optimal benefit, patients should diligently follow the prescribed treatment, carefully monitor their symptoms and side effects, and report both symptoms and side effects to the prescriber at each medication visit, as well as how they may have modified the recommendations as to dosing or types of medications to be taken.

3. If side effects develop, patients and their families, who are often the first to notice the problems, should report them to the physician as soon as possible to avoid prolonged discomfort. Most people will not take medications that cause significant side effects for very long. Therefore, if side effects are significant, even patients with a recurring severe illness, such as bipolar disorder, are likely to discontinue the medications or to change the dose. Therein lies a major danger—the manic or depressive episodes will return and hospitalization may be needed. Clearly, patients should be strongly encouraged to report side effects early so that physicians can deal with them aggressively and prevent poor patient adherence.

4. Other prescribed medicines, as well as drugs of abuse (e.g., alcohol, cocaine, amphetamines, hallucinogens, and narcotics), are known to directly and significantly affect the efficacy of the prescribed medications, and they may well increase side effects. For optimal control of bipolar disorder, patients should report all other medications they are taking for both general medical and psychiatric disorders to ensure that none are contraindicated or adversely interact with drugs prescribed for bipolar disorder. Importantly, medications may interact (both prescribed or illicit medications) such that effective medications may lose efficacy or normal doses can become toxic in the context of other medications.

5. Antimanic medications (lithium and anticonvulsants especially) may adversely affect the development of the fetus. Lithium may be the least teratogenic of these three medications. Whenever possible, women who wish to become pregnant must discuss these plans with their doctor so that the safest medications can be selected before she becomes pregnant.

6. Sometimes adjunctive medications (such as sleeping pills or antianxiety medicines) are used to augment the effect of antimanic or antidepressant medications.

7. In addition, adjunctive medications are often used for short periods to manage a breakthrough of symptoms of mania or

depression. While safe, these adjunctive medications are often not necessary over prolonged periods of time.

In sum, the key to effective and safe medication management of bipolar disorder involves early detection and careful monitoring of symptoms and side effects, diligent adjustment of the dosages or types of medications, and early detection and reporting of potential symptom breakthrough as well as side effects. Each step requires an active collaborative relationship between physicians and patients, as well as significant others, to work together for long-term successful management of this condition.

The next section of this chapter reviews the specific medications used to treat mania and depression. Commentary on medications in special patient groups (medically ill, children/adolescents) is provided. We then discuss drug–drug interactions and brain stimulation treatments. We briefly discuss medication algorithms (specific step-by-step sequences used to identify the best medication or combination for each patient). The final portion of this chapter discusses long-term disease management issues for bipolar disorder.

Medications Used to Treat Mania

As noted previously, the last decade has witnessed a rapid increase in the number of medications found to be of use in the treatment of mania and hypomania, as well as depression in bipolar disorder. Many antimanic agents are called mood stabilizers because they control *both* manic and depressive symptoms. Most mood stabilizers, however, are a bit *more* effective in the treatment of either the manic or the depressed phases of bipolar disorder. For example, lithium, a mood stabilizer, is an excellent antimanic drug, and it also has pretty good, but not quite as strong, antidepressant effects. Other mood stabilizers, like lamotrigine (Lamictal) are especially effective for depression, but it also has some antimanic activity, especially in the longer run. Lamotrigine is effective in preventing mania/hypomania, but it is not very useful as an acute antimanic treatment as the dose of the drug must be titrated (raised up) over several weeks, which typically takes too long to help the acutely manic patient in a reasonable time period.

In the treatment of both mania and depression, clinicians use agents—some of which have approval from the U.S. Food and Drug Administration (FDA), and some of which do not. Some of these nonapproved agents have been or are being studied with the aim of achieving FDA approval. For these medications, clinical research reports may suggest safety and efficacy, but the available data are not yet sufficient to achieve FDA approval. As a general principle, it is better to initially select agents that have FDA approval before moving to agents that are less well studied because the research evidence supporting FDA approved agents is typically better than the evidence for agents without FDA approval. That said, however, clinicians often must use drugs "off label" (i.e., without FDA approval) because the approved agents may prove to be ineffective, unsafe, or poorly tolerated by some patients. Even now some antimanic and antidepressant agents are under FDA review, so this synopsis is sure to be dated rather quickly. In addition to discussions with their presenting clinician, patients or families may want to contact the Depression and Bipolar Support Alliance (*www.dbsalliance.org*) or seek further information from reputable websites (e.g., WebMD—*www.WebMD.com*; or pharmaceutical company websites) in order to stay up to date.

Table 3.1 summarizes the most commonly used antimanic medications. They include lithium, certain anticonvulsants, and selected atypical antipsychotic medications. All these agents, save for lamotrigine, have efficacy in the acute phase treatment of mania (i.e., they resolve the manic episode). In some cases, as shown, some of these medications also have evidence suggesting or proving that they prevent recurrences of hypomanic or manic episodes. Sometimes, some of these agents will prevent or lessen the severity of relapses/recurrences of major depressive episodes (e.g., lamotrigine) (see Table 3.2). Lithium seems to have more antidepressant activity than does either carbamazepine or valproate. The atypical antipsychotic agents have less antidepressant activity than most antidepressants. Often, more than one antimanic medication are used together to treat acutely manic symptoms.

The antimanic or mood-stabilizing medications that are successful in acute treatment for a patient are typically continued in the maintenance phase. However, over time, effort is usually made to reduce the dose or even eliminate some antimanic medications to reduce side effect burden. However, all patients with bipolar disorder need to stay on at least one mood stabilizer (antimanic agent). This is crucial to control the long-term outcome of this illness.

Lithium

The best-studied antimanic medication is lithium. In 1949, an Australian physician, John Cade, discovered that lithium was effective when treating a severely disabled, manic patient in a state hospital who was

TABLE 3.1. Medications Used to Treat Mania

Drug[a,b]	Brand name	Usual dose for adults	Maximum dose/level	Common side effects	Initial labs	Monitoring	Warning	Efficacy in maintenance
Lithium[a,b]	Eskalith Lithane Lithotabs Lithium Citrate Syrup EskalithCR	0.7–1.2 mEq/liter	1.2 mEq/liter plasma level	Nausea, vomiting, diarrhea, tremor, weight gain, polyuria, polydypsia, acne, cognitive slowing	Kidney function Thyroid function EKG Blood count	Lithium levels Thyroid and kidney function	Lithium toxicity	++
				Anticonvulsants				
Carbamazepine Carbamazepine extended release	Tegretol Tegretol-XR	800–1,000 mg/day 4–12 µg/ml (target blood level)	1,600 mg/day level (up to 12 µg/ml)	Sedation, dizziness, GI distress, balance problems, poor liver function, cognitive slowing	Blood count Urinalysis Liver function	Blood count Liver function	Anemia Low white cell count	+
Divalproex[a,b] Valproic acid	Depakote Depakene	50–150 mEq/liter	Level of 150 mEq/liter	Nausea, vomiting, weight gain, hair loss	Blood count Liver function	Blood count Liver function	Liver toxicity Pancreatitis	++
Lamotrigine[b]	Lamictal	Not recommended for acute mania	Not recommended for acute mania	Headache	None	For serious rash	Serious rash (Stevens–Johnson syndrome)	++
Oxcarbazepine	Trileptal	600–2,400 mg/day in divided doses	2,500 mg/day	Fatigue, nausea, vomiting, dizziness, sedation, low sodium	Kidney function	Sodium levels	None	+/–

cont.

TABLE 3.1. *cont.*

Drug	Brand name	Usual dose for adults	Maximum dose/level	Common side effects	Initial labs	Monitoring	Warning	Efficacy in maintenance
				Atypical Antipsychotics				
Aripiprazole	Abilify	15–30 mg/day	30 mg/day	Gastrointestinal distress, somnolence, restlessness	None	None	None	+
Clozapine	Clozaril	100–900 mg/day in divided doses	900 mg/d	Sedation, salivation, sweating, rapid pulse, weight gain, diabetes, low blood pressure, constipation	Blood count	Blood count	Low blood pressure, low WBC count, seizure, myocarditis	−
Olanzapine[a,b]	Zyprexa	10–20 mg/day	40 mg/day	Somnolence, weight gain, dizziness, dry mouth, increased blood lipids, diabetes	None required Body weight Fasting blood sugar Lipid profile suggested	Weight Fasting blood sugar Lipid profile	None	++
Quetiapine[a]	Seroquel	100–800 mg/day	800 mg/day	Somnolence, dry mouth, weight gain, dizziness	None	None required	None	−
Risperidone[a]	Risperdal	3 mg/day	6 mg/day	Somnolence, gastrointestinal distress, motor activation	None	None required	None	−
Ziprasidone	Geodon	40–160 mg/day	160 mg/day	Somnolence, dizziness, motor restlessness	None	None required	None	−

[a]FDA approved for acute mania.
[b]FDA approved for maintenance treatment.

38

TABLE 3.2. Medications Used to Treat Depression in Bipolar Disorder

Drug	Brand name	Usual dose for adults	Maximum dose/level	Common side effects	Initial labs	Monitoring	Warning
Lithium	Lithobid Eskalith Lithane Lithium Citrate Syrup	600–1,800 mg/day (0.7–1.2 mEq/liter)	1.2 mEq/liter	Nausea, vomiting, diarrhea, sedation, weight gain, polyuria, polydypsia, acne, psoriasis	Kidney function Thyroid function EKG Blood count	Lithium levels Thyroid and kidney function	Neurotoxicity Low thyroid or kidney function Cardiac conduction problems
Tricyclic antidepressants							
Norepinephrine reuptake inhibitors							
Desipramine	Norpramin Pertofrane	100–250 mg/day	250 mg/day	Dry mouth, blurred vision	None	None	None
Maprotiline	Ludiomil	100–225 mg/day	225 mg/day	Dry mouth	None	None	None
Nortriptyline	Pamelor Aventyl	50–150 mg/day	150 mg/day	Dry mouth, blurred vision	None	None	None
Protriptyline	Vivactil	15–60 mg/day	60 mg/day	Anxiety	None	None	None
Mixed norepinephrine–serotonin reuptake inhibitors							
Amitriptyline	Elavil Endep	100–250 mg/day	250 mg/day	Dry mouth, blurred vision	None	None	None
Amoxapine	Asendin	150–400 mg/day	400 mg/day	Dry mouth	None	None	None
Clomipramine	Anafranil	150 mg/day	200 mg/day	Dry mouth	None	None	None
Doxepin	Adapine Sinequan	100–300 mg/day	300 mg/day	Sedation	None	None	None

cont.

TABLE 3.2. cont.

Drug	Brand name	Usual dose for adults	Maximum dose/level	Common side effects	Initial labs	Monitoring	Warning
Mixed norepinephrine–serotonin reuptake inhibitors (cont.)							
Imipramine	Tofranil	100–250 mg/day	250 mg/day	Dry mouth, blurred vision	None	None	None
Trimipramine	Surmontil	100–300 mg/day	300 mg/day	Sedation, dry mouth	None	None	None
Monoamine oxidase inhibitors							
Phenelzine	Nardil	60–90 mg/day	90 mg/day	Low blood pressure	None	Blood pressure	Dietary precautions
Tranylcypromine	Parnate	40–60 mg/day	60 mg/day	Low blood pressure	None	Blood pressure	Dietary precautions
Atypical antipsychotics							
Olanzapine	Zyprexa	5–15 mg/day	20 mg/day	Somnolence, weight gain, dizziness, dry mouth	None	Weight Blood sugar Lipids*	Observe for early weight gain; glucose dysregulation
Olanzapine–fluoxetine Combination	Symbyax	Olanzapine: 6–12 mg/day Fluoxetine: 25–50 mg/day	Olanzapine: 12 mg/day Fluoxetine: 50 mg/day	Drowsiness, weight gain, appetite increase, swelling, tremor, feeling weak, trouble concentrating	None required	Weight Blood sugar Lipids*	None
Anticonvulsants							
Divalproex (valproic acid)	Depakote Depakene	1,000–1,500 mg/day	1,500 mg/day	Nausea, vomiting, sedation, weight gain	Blood count Liver function	Blood count Liver function	Liver toxicity Pancreatitis

40

able to return to normal functioning with lithium. (In fact, the patient died only recently, in his 80s, having had a successful career while he continued to take lithium.) Lithium is a salt and is quite inexpensive. It appears in very minimal amounts in everyone's body; therefore, allergies to it are very rare. Table 3.1 shows the available lithium preparations.

Lithium is an effective antimanic and antidepressant medication, though it has been most widely evaluated as an antimanic agent in both acute and maintenance phase treatment studies. Lithium is approved by the FDA for both the acute and maintenance treatment of mania. Patients with typical manic episodes generally respond rapidly, within 1–3 weeks. The response rate in patients who take lithium alone for the acute phase treatment of mania is approximately 50–75% (Goodwin & Jamison, 1990). By contrast, patients with dysphoric manic episodes (i.e., manic episodes accompanied by substantial irritability or depressive symptoms) or those with a rapid cycling course (i.e., four or more manic, depressive, or hypomanic episodes per year) seem to have lower response rates to lithium alone—less than 50% of these patients improve significantly. If lithium alone is not fully effective in the acute phase treatment of mania, it is often combined with other antimanic medications (listed in Table 3.1) (e.g., atypical antipsychotic or anticonvulsant medications) to achieve fuller symptom remission. The depressed phase of bipolar illness may also respond to lithium alone, although the response may not occur until the third or fourth week of treatment.

Lithium must be taken at a dosage that results in a blood level within a specific therapeutic range (i.e., 0.7–1.2 mEq/liter), as determined by measurements on blood samples that must be drawn 10–12 hours after the last oral dose. The oral dosage needed to obtain this level varies among different individuals. When beginning lithium, levels are usually checked often (e.g., every 1–2 weeks), and the dose is adjusted to achieve the therapeutic blood level. Once a therapeutic level is attained, periodic blood level determinations are still essential to ensure that each patient is taking a therapeutic but not a toxic amount of lithium over the longer term.

Specific clinical situations that also call for lithium level checks include the following: after a change in the dose of lithium (5–10 days later); during major weight changes (e.g., diet); during treatment with diuretics (water pills often used to treat hypertension or other cardiac conditions); during a change in mood (both to check compliance and because lithium levels decrease in mania and increase in depression); during general medical illnesses, including the flu (which may disturb fluid and electrolyte balances); or if lithium toxicity is suspected (Preston, O'Neal, & Talaga, 1994).

In maintenance phase treatment, the therapeutic blood levels of lithium are the same as those found to be effective in acute phase treatment. Alone, lithium is an effective maintenance phase treatment for 30–60% of patients with bipolar disorder. Other patients, however, may experience some breakthrough of manic or depressive symptoms on lithium alone in the maintenance phase, even if the lithium level is appropriate. In such cases, another antimanic agent is often added, or sometimes substituted for lithium.

The difficulty with lithium is that patients may take too little or too much. Too little lithium provides little or no therapeutic benefit. On the other hand, too much lithium causes significant side effects (Table 3.1), the most common of which are thirst, excessive urination, weight gain, fatigue, and dry mouth. The most distressing side effects are weight gain, cognitive slowing, excessive urination, nausea, and fatigue. In some cases, lithium may affect the function of the thyroid gland or the kidneys. Lithium decreases the production and release of thyroid hormone by the thyroid gland. Some 1–3% of patients taking lithium will develop hypothyroidism (i.e., low thyroid function). Women are at higher risk than men for lithium-induced hypothyroidism. Lithium may also affect the tubular system in the kidney, interfering with the kidneys' ability to concentrate urine and, thus, increasing both the amount and frequency of urination in some patients. This increased urination is not life threatening, because it is not due to progressive destruction of the kidney.

Lithium has a low therapeutic to toxic ratio. That is, the therapeutic dose is only a bit lower than the toxic dose. Toxic effects of lithium are usually seen at blood levels of 1.5 mEq/liter. Thus, when more than therapeutic amounts of lithium are used, they will produce toxic reactions. The earliest signs of toxicity often include a tremor (often progressing from a fine to a coarse tremor), diarrhea, nausea, and poor balance (ataxia). If the clinician recognizes the toxic reaction at this stage and reduces the dosage, damage is rare. At higher levels (i.e., above 1.8 mEq/liter), mental confusion, impaired alertness, cardiac arrhythmias, unconsciousness, and even death can occur. Immediate recognition and treatment of these more severe signs and symptoms is essential.

There are no absolute contraindications to the use of lithium, but several general medical conditions and concurrent uses of certain medications require caution. Impaired kidney function is a relative contraindication, because the kidney clears lithium from the body. It is best to avoid lithium in cases of dementia, because these patients seem particularly sensitive to the effects of lithium on the central nervous system. Lithium may worsen the muscular weakness seen with myasthenia gravis. Certain diuretics and some other medications taken in conjunction with lithium increase (or decrease) lithium levels, thus requiring even more careful monitoring for safe therapy.

Anticonvulsants

Carbamazepine

In the 1970s and early 1980s, Japanese and American investigators found that carbamazepine, an anticonvulsant, was an effective treatment for mania. In addition to carbamazepine (Tegretol), other anticonvulsants such as valproate (Depakote, Depakene) are also effective antimanic agents (Bowden et al., 1994) (see below). Once again, patients can take too little or too much carbamazepine, but clinicians often monitor the level of carbamazepine in the blood. The target blood level is well established. Carbamazepine, however, can lower white or red blood cell counts, which should be monitored. The side effects of carbamazepine differ from those of lithium. Side effects include dizziness, poor coordination, double vision, gastrointestinal distress, or slowed thinking, all of which are dose related. Dose adjustments are needed to minimize side effects, while preserving the antimanic effect. If properly regulated, however, carbamazepine usually has few side effects for most patients.

A rare, but very important, possible side effect is a decrease in the ability of bone marrow to produce white blood cells to fight infection and platelets to help blood to clot. The incidence of this bone marrow suppression (agranulocytosis) is estimated to be between 1 in 40,000 and 1 in 125,000 patients (Post et al., 1983).

Carbamazepine is an effective acute phase treatment in 30–60% of patients with mania. It also appears to be effective (though less well studied) in maintenance phase treatment. That is, carbamazepine appears effective in the prevention of relapses or recurrences into mania or hypomania, but it may be less effective in preventing relapses or recurrences into depression. Carbamazepine may be more effective than lithium in the acute treatment of dysphoric mania and rapid cycling forms of bipolar disorder. Thus, carbamazepine represents a useful alternative to lithium for patients with dysphoric mania or a rapid cycling course. Carbamazepine also appears to work very well when it is added to lithium, if lithium alone is not fully effective, or vice versa.

The average oral dosage for carbamazepine is 800–1,000 mg/day, although therapeutic effects can be seen at dosages from 400 to 1,200 mg/day. Most laboratories report the therapeutic blood level to be 4–12 mEq/liter for carbamazepine, even though the relationship between blood level and therapeutic response is not well established (Post et al., 1983). Because of its short half-life, patients usually take carbamazepine two to three times per day. By dividing the dose over the day, a more constant blood level and lower side effects are achieved. Although carbamazepine is free of many of the side effects of lithium, it can cause a variety of side effects of potential concern. As always, the risks and benefits must be weighed.

Carbamazepine also induces liver enzymes such that the metabolism of carbamazepine itself and some other medications is actually increased. Therefore, over time (3–8 weeks), a fixed oral dosage of carbamazepine may result in subtherapeutic medication levels. In most cases, carbamazepine doses need to be raised to maintain a therapeutic blood level. In addition, carbamazepine often lowers the blood levels of other oxidatively metabolized drugs (such as tricyclic or other antidepressants or birth control pills), so that the doses of these agents need to be increased when patients are taking carbamazepine. Note that carbamazepine may make birth control pills ineffective by increasing their metabolism.

Carbamazepine—Extended Release

This preparation allows for less frequent dosing (usually twice a day) than carbamazepine (usually three to four times a day), thereby enhancing adherence.

Oxcarbazepine

This agent is an anticonvulsant that is taken twice a day. It does not have FDA approval for use in bipolar disorder. Its structure is very similar to carbamazepine. Evidence suggests somewhat better tolerability than carbamazepine.

Divalproex

There is now strong evidence that divalproex (valproic acid; Depakote, Depakene) is effective in the acute treatment of mania, even in cases in which lithium is ineffective or only partially effective (e.g., when dysphoric mania or a rapid cycling course is present; Rosenbaum, Fava, Nierenberg, & Sachs, 2001; McElroy, Keck, Pope, & Hudson, 1988). A mildly abnormal electroencephalogram (McElroy, Keck, & Pope, 1987) is another potential predictor of a positive response to valproate in bipolar disorder.

The oral dose of divalproex should be sufficient to achieve blood levels of 50–150 ug/ml, although within the therapeutic range the blood levels of divalproex may not correlate with therapeutic efficacy. This agent potentiates the effects of gamma-aminobutyric acid (GABA), an important inhibitory neurotransmitter in the central nervous system. Enhancing the effects of GABA potentially decreases electrical activity and, therefore, it has an antiseizure effect. GABA, along with lithium, may also affect the messenger systems inside cells (McElroy et al., 1988).

Divalproex is well tolerated and usually has fewer and milder side effects than carbamazepine. The most common side effects are nausea, diarrhea, mild tremor, and sedation. Weight gain and hair loss are less common but troublesome. The enteric-coated form (Depakote) reduces or eliminates nausea as compared to valproic acid. Although bone marrow suppression, which is associated with carbamazepine, does not occur with valproate, a rare but severe liver condition has been reported in children treated for seizures with valproate. In adolescents and adults, however, valproate has not caused these severe liver problems.

Lamotrigine

Lamotrigine (Lamictal) is the newest anticonvulsant to receive FDA approval as a preventive treatment for both the depressive and manic phases of bipolar disorder. It appears to be effective in some patients with treatment-resistant major depressive episodes, possibly for both major depressive and bipolar disorders (Barbee & Jamhour 2002; Frye et al., 2000). It is thought to work through a different neurotransmitter system (glutamate) than other mood stabilizers or antidepressants.

Lamotrigine is not clinically useful in the acute treatment of mania because the dose of this drug must be gradually built up over several weeks in order to reduce the chance of a skin rash, which can be very serious in a small number of people. Some of these drug-induced skin rashes are associated with a systemic toxic reaction known as Stevens–Johnson syndrome—which can be fatal (seen in 1 in 1,000 patients). The therapeutic dose of lamotrigine is 100–400 mg/day, but the drug must be initiated at 25 mg/day for 2 weeks. The rash, if it is to develop, typically occurs in the first 8–10 weeks of treatment as the dose is raised. Once in the therapeutic range, lamotrigine is typically very well tolerated with minimal side effects.

Lamotrigine is more effective in preventing depressive relapses/recurrences, but it also seems to be effective in preventing manic/

hypomanic relapses. Lamotrigine may also used in the acute treatment of the depressed phase of bipolar disorder. It requires no initial laboratory testing or ongoing laboratory monitoring.

Antipsychotic Medications

Typical Antipsychotic Medications

Sometimes older antipsychotic (neuroleptic) agents, but more often newer antipsychotic agents (so-called atypical antipsychotics), are useful in the acute phase treatment of mania. Chlorpromazine has FDA approval for the acute treatment of mania. Older agents, such as haloperidol (Haldol), thioridazine (Mellaril), and chlorpromazine (Thorazine), are often combined with lithium or an anticonvulsant to help control hallucinations (voices or visions) or delusions (fixed irrational beliefs), to induce sleep, to reduce inappropriate grandiose thinking, or to decrease irritability or impulsive behaviors that are frequently part of manic episodes. Antipsychotic medications are usually not needed to treat hypomanic episodes, however. Antipsychotic medications are not always necessary in maintenance phase treatments even in patients with psychotic symptoms if they are on another mood stabilizer. On the other hand, quite a few patients who are psychotic when acutely manic may require small dosages of antipsychotic medications over prolonged periods to ensure that their delusions, hallucinations, or other symptoms of mania do not return.

The older antipsychotic medications (neuroleptics) reduce psychomotor agitation, but they may be less effective for some other core features of manic episodes. Acute akathisia (motor and subjective restlessness), cognitive impairment (e.g., trouble concentrating), anticholinergic side effects (e.g., blurred vision, dry mouth, and difficulty urinating, especially for men), and, after chronic use, tardive dyskinesia (an involuntary movement disorder) are common problems in the use of older antipsychotic medications. These problems can be reduced or avoided by using the lowest necessary doses of the neuroleptics whenever clinically feasible, or they can be reduced by using newer atypical antipsychotic medications.

Atypical Antipsychotic Medications

In the last decade, a number of atypical (also called second-generation) antipsychotic medications have received FDA approval for the treatment schizophrenia. Recent research has evaluated these agents in the acute and longer-term treatment of mania (with or without psychotic symptoms). At the moment, olanzapine (Zyprexa), risperidone (Risperdal), and quetiapine (Seroquel) have FDA approval for the acute treatment of mania. Of these, only olanzapine has FDA approval for maintenance phase treatment of mania/hypomania in bipolar disorder. It is easy to use clinically, but it is associated with substantial weight gain in 25–30% of patients, which typically occurs within 6–10 weeks. The two newer atypical agents (aripiprazole [Abilify] and ziprasidone [Geodon]) are under study as acute or potentially maintenance treatments for bipolar disorder.

The FDA has recently issued a warning about the increased risk of high blood sugar and diabetes with all atypical antipsychotic agents. Whether some of these medications are more or less likely to cause such problems is still under study, but they do seem to differ in the probability of weight gain, which is thought by some to contribute to these problems. Aripiprazole and ziprasidone have the lowest likelihood of weight gain, while clozapine and olanzapine have the greatest likelihood (American Diabetes Association, 2004).

Clozapine (Clozaril). This agent was the first atypical antipsychotic. It has FDA approval for schizophrenia, should other first-line treatments fail. It is a highly effective agent, and it has been found to be effective in a controlled trial of treatment-resistant bipolar disorder (manic or mixed manic phase) (Suppes et al., 1999). While the efficacy of clozapine for difficult-to-treat bipolar disorders, especially for manic or mixed-state patients, is well accepted, it does not have FDA approval for bipolar disorder. On the other hand, clozapine has a significant side effect profile, including the possibility of reducing white cell counts into the dangerous zone. Clozapine also lowers blood pressure. It requires regular monitoring of blood cell counts (weekly for the first 6 months, then every other week), and it can be sedating and cause weight gain (see Table 3.1). Thus, clozapine is not a first choice among the atypical antipsychotic medications, but it may well help when other atypical antipsychotic agents have failed (Suppes, Phillips, & Judd, 1994).

Combination Treatments

As noted earlier, using a combination of two or more medications is common in the management of bipolar disorder, particularly to control mania (e.g., lithium and atypical antipsychotic medications are frequently used together). However, very few randomized, controlled, prospective studies have evaluated the safety and efficacy of different medication combinations. Because toxic as well as nontoxic but troubling side effects are likely to increase when medication combinations are used, careful monitoring of both clinical responses and side effect burden is especially important when combinations are used. Whether one combination is better than another is not known.

Medications Used to Treat Depression

As with antimanic medications, antidepressant medications have an important role in both acute and longer-term phases of treatment of bipolar disorder. Table 3.2 summarizes the antidepressant medications based on the major neurochemical effects thought to account for their therapeutic action. The first antidepressants were the tricyclic (three-ring) antidepressant compounds (TCAs; including imipramine, amitriptyline, desipramine, doxepin, and nortriptyline) and the monoamine oxidase inhibitors (MAOIs; phenelzine and tranylcypromine). Both classes were discovered in the 1950s. The newest tricyclic is clomipramine (Anafranil). Newer antidepressant medications, introduced in the early 1970s, sometimes called the heterocyclic (multiring) or unicyclic (one-ring) agents, include amoxapine, maprotiline, trazodone, and bupropion. The newest group, the selective serotonin reuptake inhibitors (SSRIs), includes citalopram, fluoxetine, fluvoxamine (FDA approved in the United States as a drug for obsessive–compulsive disorder), paroxetine, S-citalopram, and sertraline. In addition to these specific antidepressant medications, recall that some antimanic medications (especially lithium and selected anticonvulsants) also have some antidepressant activity. All antidepressant medications can induce manic or hypomanic episodes in patients with bipolar disorder, particularly if the patient is not taking a mood-stabilizing agent along with the antidepressant medication.

No one antidepressant medication is known to be preferentially effective in bipolar disorder. Furthermore, in prescribing any antidepressant medication, it is possible to (1) start with too high a dose, (2) increase the dosage too quickly, (3) not increase the dosage rapidly enough, or (4) not give the antidepressant medication enough time to achieve efficacy. Because all antidepressant medications appear to be equally effective, and all take several weeks to work fully, side effects play a key role in selecting among these various treatments. As is the case with the treatment of mania, a trial-and-error approach is often used to select the most effective, best-tolerated antidepressant for a particular patient. In general, if a patient fails to respond to one class of drugs, he or she will often tolerate and respond to a different class. Interestingly, intolerance (i.e., development of intolerable side effects) to one agent in a class does *not* necessarily mean that the patient will not tolerate another drug in the same class.

Side Effects

The side effects of an antidepressant medication are due to pharmacological effects that may not be related to its presumed therapeutic mechanism. For example, for the TCAs, anticholinergic side effects include dry mouth, blurred vision, constipation, sedation, and difficulty urinating), which is not needed for the therapeutic effect. Older patients are especially likely to suffer these anticholinergic side effects. Newer drugs (e.g., bupropion, the SSRIs, mirtazapine, and venlafaxine) have fewer anticholinergic side effects.

It is important to help patients who are taking antidepressants to distinguish depressive symptoms from the side effects of the antidepressant medication. It is always useful for physicians to discuss side effects with patients before prescribing any antidepressant medication. Patients should know (1) which side effects are more or less likely, (2) which side effects are dangerous, (3) which side effects will gradually disappear over time, and (4) what methods can be used to counter side effects should they occur. For example, depression often comes with a dry mouth, trouble sleeping, and sexual dysfunction. On the other hand, some antidepressant medications can actually cause or worsen these symptoms based on the medication side effects. Therefore, it is important for patients to note the specific symptoms they have *before* beginning an antidepressant; thus, if after taking the medication for a while they begin to report the same symptoms as side effects, a record of the type and severity of symptoms prior to the medication is available. A careful tracking of symptoms and side effects over time helps to distinguish medication side effects from lack of therapeutic effect.

Side effects are typically seen early (i.e., within a few days following drug initiation) or when the dose is raised. Some TCAs are sedating (although not all to the same extent), as are trazodone, nefazodone, and mirtazapine. Most physicians recommend that the sedating medications be taken at bedtime so whatever sedation occurs is maximized during sleep. Once-daily dosing with TCAs is as effective as divided dosages, and it is preferred to optimize adherence. Lower doses are associated with fewer side effects. Lowering the dose or more gradually raising the dose is often an excellent first step if side effects occur. Sometimes another medication can be used to treat the side effects. Switching to another drug is sometimes required, if dose adjustments do not result in better tolerance and good efficacy. Longer-term side effects are especially important in selecting among the available antidepressants. In general, the newer drugs (e.g., bupropion-XL, venlafaxine-XR, and the SSRIs) have fewer side effects in the short- and longer-run than older medications (e.g., TCAs).

Blood Pressure Effects

Dizziness on standing (postural hypotension) is a relatively common side effect with TCAs and MAOIs that is manifested by a drop in blood pressure when the person changes position, especially when standing up. Venlafaxine may cause increased blood pressure in higher doses.

Sexual Side Effects

Sexual side effects are common (decreased ability to maintain an erection and/or an orgasm) with the TCAs and MAOIs, and quite a few of the newer drugs (e.g., S-citalopram, venlafaxine, paroxetine, and sertraline). Some newer drugs (nefazodone, bupropion, mirtazapine) have few sexual side effects. Trazodone can cause priapism—a prolonged painful erection that occurs without sexual stimulation in 1 in 6,000 men.

Anxiety, Insomnia, and Restlessness

Some patients feel increased anxiety, restlessness, or insomnia with some of the more activating agents, such as bupropion, desipramine, or protriptyline.

Appetite and Weight Effects

Some TCAs (e.g., amitriptyline and imipramine), as well as olanzapine, fluoxetine, and mirtazapine, for example, may increase appetite and weight. Drugs least likely to cause weight gain include bupropion and the SSRIs (especially if used for brief periods).

Risk in Overdose

The TCAs and MAOIs can be lethal if as little as a 2-week supply is taken. The newer agents are far safer in overdose.

Risk of Rapid Cycling

Rapid cycling refers to a bipolar disorder that has at least four mood episodes in a year. A mood episode includes depressive, manic, mixed, or hypomanic episodes. These patients (more likely women, by the way) suffer greater impairment in function and require more aggressive antimanic/mood-stabilizer medications. One cause of rapid cycling can be antidepressant medications (apparently any antidepressant can do this). The treatment is to reduce the dose or to eliminate the antidepressant altogether.

Selecting the Best Dose

Generally, TCAs (and MAOIs) must be titrated up in dose over several weeks to minimize side effects. Thus, the clinician gradually increases the dosage over 7–14 days to the lower end of the therapeutic range. If there is no response at all after several weeks and side effects are minimal, the medication dosage is gradually raised up to the maximum shown in Table 3.2. If there is no response after 6 weeks of increasing dosages, the clinician may switch medications or obtain a blood level (for some TCAs) to determine if the dosage is adequate. Most newer agents (e.g., S-citalopram, bupropion, mirtazapine, and paroxetine) require fewer dose adjustments.

Monoamine Oxidase Inhibitors

Because of necessary dietary precautions, MAOIs are not commonly used to treat bipolar disorder. However, some evidence suggests that these drugs may be particularly useful in bipolar disorder when other groups of drugs fail (Himmelhoch, Thase, Mallinger, & Houck, 1991). The most common side effects of the MAOIs include postural hypotension, weight gain, sexual dysfunction, insomnia, energy slumps, nervousness, irritability, tremor, sweating, tachycardia, palpitations), edema (swelling), and muscle twitching.

Patients taking an MAOI should not use certain medications or eat certain foods. The proscribed medications include certain prescription medications, most drugs of abuse, and quite a few over-the-counter (nonprescription) medications.

If these proscriptions are not followed, blood pressure may increase suddenly, causing headache, nausea, vomiting, and the risk of stroke. Even if a food does not cause a reaction the first several times a patient eats it, there may be a reaction the next time. Moreover, the amount of proscribed food or medication taken determines the risk of this sudden increase in blood pressure (a hypertensive episode). For instance, four glasses of red wine are more likely to provoke a hypertensive reaction than are two. A headache often signals the onset of a hypertensive episode. It is typically severe and pounding, unlike a tension headache. Patients with such symptoms who are taking MAOIs should go to an emergency room to have their blood pressure checked and, if needed, treatment given.

Newer Antidepressants

These newer agents, due to their better side effect profile, as well as their safety in overdose and easier dose adjustment, have become popular agents. They largely lack anticholinergic side effects found with TCAs, but the SSRIs do cause gastrointestinal symptoms and interfere with sexual desire or function (e.g., delayed ejaculation and anorgasmia). The SSRIs (fluoxetine, sertraline, paroxetine, citalopram, S-citalopram) appear to be effective for the depressed phase of bipolar disorder. Some weight gain does occur in the longer run (6–12 months) in 6–20% of patients with these agents. Paroxetine is most likely of the group to cause weight gain. As with other antidepressant medications, the SSRIs can precipitate manic or hypomanic episodes in bipolar disorder.

Bupropion has no effect on serotonin, but it does affect both norepinephrine and dopamine. Some evidence suggests that bupropion is effective when the SSRIs are not. The longer-acting forms (Wellbutrin SR or Wellbutrin XR) can be taken twice or once a day, respectively, which helps with adherence. The long-term side effects of this drug are minimal and do not include sexual dysfunction or weight gain. If taken in overdose, the main risk is seizures.

Venlafaxine and mirtazapine are the newest among drugs that affect both norepinephrine and serotonin systems. The longer-acting venlafaxine XR is easier to take and is better tolerated than the shorter half-life venlafaxine. The doses often need to be titrated up. Hypertension can occur in 2–4% of individuals taking the drug, especially at higher dosages. There is evidence, on the other hand, that increasing the dose of this medication increases the likelihood of a response and/or the thoroughness of the symptom reduction caused by this agent.

Mirtazapine is easier to dose, but it does cause weight gain and sedation in a significant proportion of patients. It has minimal effects on sexual function.

Special Patient Groups

Three special groups deserve comment: those with psychotic symptoms when manic or depressed, children and adolescents, and the elderly or medically more fragile patients.

Patients with hallucinations or delusions when manic or depressed often require more intensive care, often inpatient treatment, until these psychotic symptoms are controlled. Often, antipsychotic medications (either the older neuroleptics or the newer atypical antipsychotic agents) are needed in the acute treatment phase. Once the psychotic symptoms are dispatched, the dose of the antipsychotic agent is reduced and in many patients, if subsequent good control of their mood episodes can be achieved with mood stabilizers, the antipsychotic agent may be discontinued, though the patient should still be closely monitored.

For children and adolescents, we have fewer studies to guide treatment. Lithium, divalproex, and carbamazepine all seem to be effective (Kowatch et al., 2000). Dosages are less well established for these pediatric patients. The TCAs are not indicated for these patients as they are not effective for unipolar depression in this age group. The MAOIs are particularly risky given the need for careful adherence and the risk of drug–drug interactions with drugs of abuse (e.g., cocaine plus MAOIs can cause a hypertensive crisis). Some SSRIs (e.g., fluoxetine) have been studied in depressed pediatric patients, but a number of newer agents (e.g., venlafaxine) have not been fully tested in this age group. Careful monitoring, frequent visits, and careful dose adjustments are all essential for these younger patients.

The older or medically fragile patient requires slower dose escalations and likely lower overall doses because many of the medications used for bipolar disorder, whether for mania or depression, are metabolized more slowly by older patients. Recent evidence also suggests that certain racial groups (e.g., Asians) may also metabolize some of these drugs more slowly. However, there is no evidence that older patients or those with medical illnesses will not respond to these medicines. Careful medical monitoring is needed for some agents (see Tables 3.1 and 3.2) for all age groups. This monitoring may be especially important for patients with compromised immune or cardiac systems. In addition, it is essential to monitor other medications that older patients may be taking for other problems (hypertension, gastrointestinal problems, etc.), as these medications can result in drug–drug interactions.

Drug–Drug Interactions

Most patients with bipolar disorder are taking multiple medications, either for their bipolar disorder or for other general medical conditions. Consequently, the psychopharmacologist must be aware of potential drug–drug interactions.

There are different types of potential drug–drug interactions. One involves protein binding and drug displacement by other drugs. One drug may displace another drug from circulating proteins. Protein-bound drugs are not able to enter cells and are, therefore, not active until they are made free or become unbound from the proteins in the bloodstream. One drug may displace another drug from binding to these proteins. The result is an increased level in the bloodstream of the displaced drug. More drug is now available to enter cells. For example, nefazodone displaces haloperidol from proteins in the blood, which in turn increases haloperidol bioavailability. This increased availability can cause more side effects or interfere with the therapeutic effect if the dose is not adjusted.

A second type of drug–drug interaction is the competition for the same enzyme systems that are involved in the metabolism and breakdown of the drugs. For example, fluoxetine and the TCAs compete for the same isoenzyme system in the liver. When fluoxetine is used with a TCA in the same patient, the circulating blood level of the TCA can be markedly increased (two- to fourfold) as compared to when the TCA is used alone. Thus, this combination increases the side effects of the TCA. The solution is to reduce the oral dose of the TCA, often with the assistance of blood-level measurements.

A third kind of drug interaction involves autoinduction. That is, some drugs can induce their own metabolism (e.g., carbamazepine can induce its own metabolism, and that of other drugs metabolized by the enzyme system that is involved in carbamazepine's metabolism). Therefore, over time, the dose of carbamazepine may have to be raised or the dosages of other medications may need to be increased when they are given with carbamazepine.

A fourth kind of drug interaction includes the combined effect of two drugs in the central nervous system at the level of the neuron. For example, TCAs and alcohol are more than additive in their ability to cause cognitive impairment, because both drugs are active at the level of the neuron in the same regions of the brain, which leads to impaired mental processing if both drugs are used in significant doses.

Our knowledge about the liver enzymes (proteins) that help us metabolize drugs has grown dramatically over the last decade, and this knowledge continues to rapidly expand. In helping patients with bipolar disorder to manage their illness, it is essential that they always tell every doctor, dentist, or pharmacist whom they see all the medications they are taking. When a medication change (in dose or type) is made, the prescribing clinician must evaluate what they are recommending given the other medications that patients are taking. This knowledge allows practitioners to properly gauge the safety of adding or subtracting an agent, as well as to knowledgeably modify the dose of the drug should it be found to be safe to be prescribed.

For example, the dentist may recommend codeine for tooth pain. But if the patient is taking a medication like fluoxetine or paroxetine, the codeine will not work because these two drugs each block a specific liver enzyme called P4502D6. For codeine to work, this enzyme must convert codeine to its active metabolite. With the enzyme blocked by either of these two drugs, no analgesia will occur when the patient takes codeine. Even some over-the-counter non-prescription as well as some natural or herbal medicines can affect the absorption, metabolism, or effect of prescribed medications. Any time a patient with bipolar disorder decides to take another medicine, he or she should check with the doctor before such a decision is made.

Brain Stimulation Treatments

Electroconvulsive therapy (ECT) is not usually a first-line treatment. It can, however, be extremely important for some patients with bipolar disorder, especially when the manic or depressive episodes do not respond to medication. Thus, candidates for ECT usually have had only a partial or no response to various earlier treatments during the manic or depressive episode. ECT is also effective for patients in a mixed (or dysphoric) manic episode.

There is substantial evidence that ECT works. In fact, it is approximately 70–90% effective in manic and severe depressive episodes that have failed to respond to medication treatments. So, although often not a first-line treatment, ECT can be life saving. ECT is typically used as an acute rather than longer-term treatment. Patients are placed on medication following acute treatment with ECT. Medication doses are adjusted as previously described.

New, better, and safer ways to stimulate the brain are under study. For example, giving a very brief electrical stimulus in ECT seems to reduce cognitive (memory) side effects. Other modifications, including using a magnetic field either to induce seizures (magnetic seizure therapy, or MST) or to simulate certain specific brain regions (repetitive transcranial magnetic stimulation, or rTMS), seem to both have much less to no effect on memory while still providing antidepressant and possibly antimanic effects.

Another stimulation method is called vagus nerve stimulation (VNS) therapy. Already FDA approved for use in epilepsy, VNS consists of very brief and mild intermittent stimulation of the left vagus nerve (which is in the neck and which provides signals to the limbic system or emotional brain). The stimulation is provided by a small stopwatch-size device, which is implanted under the chest muscles (like a heart pacemaker). VNS is under FDA review for treatment-resistant depression in both bipolar and major depressive disorders (Sackeim et al., 2001).

Medication Algorithms

The last 10 years have been a period of rapid explosion in the range of the types of treatments available for bipolar disorder. We are now faced with a new challenge—namely, to define the most efficient and effective way to select from among and, when needed, to appropriately combine, medications to achieve maximal control of the symptoms and maximal improvement in day-to-day function, while also minimizing side effect burden. Recently, using both scientific evidence and expert clinical consensus, a number of specific guidelines or more specific treatment step recommendations (called algorithms) have been put forth (American Psychiatric Association, 1994b; Kahn et al., 2001; Sachs, Printz, Kahn, Carpenter, & Docherty, 2000; Suppes, Rush, Kramers, & Webb, 1998; Suppes, Swann, et al., 2001). The best algorithm or guideline has yet to be identified. However, we already have evidence (Suppes et al., 2003) indicating that algorithm-based care may be more efficient or effective than current practice. Much research is ongoing to better define what the next best treatment steps are for persons with bipolar disorder who have not achieved a satisfactory response to one or more prior treatment attempts.

Most important for today's patient is the need for patients to carefully monitor, record, and discuss with their doctor the signs and symptoms of both mania and depression. By carefully tracking the effects of each step in the treatment plan, the patient can help the doctor make well-informed adjustments in the dose or types of medication being used. In addition, patients play a critical role in optimizing outcome by maintaining healthy appropriate lifestyle choices (see below) and by anticipating and preparing for potential issues that could affect how their bipolar disorder is to be managed (having surgery, becoming pregnant, etc.).

Just as is the case with diabetes, hypertension, and many other chronic general medical problems, it is the combination of both the medications *and* a well-regulated, day-to-day life that produces the best outcome. For example, how much, what type, and when to take insulin or other drugs for diabetes must be combined with appropriate management of the types and amounts of excessive, food intake, and other medicines being taken to achieve optimal control of diabetes. So too with bipolar disorder (see below).

Long-Term Management of Bipolar Disorder

The patient and his or her "significant other" (family member or friend) are essential to the optimal short- and long-term care of bipolar disorder. This section discusses what they can do to monitor the disorder, control biostressors, anticipate problems, and optimally manage the medicines. The first step requires patients to recognize that bipolar disorder requires long-term care, which, if properly implemented, can more often than not lead to a healthy, happy, and productive life. It simply takes focus, commitment, and initially a substantial effort. Over time, less effort is needed, but careful attention will always be needed to keep the conditions in check.

Defining the Disorder

The optimal management of bipolar disorder requires the diligent tracking, at least weekly and in some cases daily, of manic/hypomanic and depressive symptoms. It is these symptoms (the types of symptoms, their severity, and their impact on function) that guide the doctor in selecting, adjusting, and changing medications. In addition, a careful record of the types and severity of side effects is critical to the decision to modify medications.

Some patients have symptoms that change almost every day. In such cases, this mood lability or instability calls for changes in mood-stabilizing agents, or even reduction or removal of antidepressant medicines. In other cases, the patient may be taking another prescribed or over-the-counter drug that should be changed because it is causing mood instability. Thus in addition to tracking and recording manic and depressive symptoms and medication side effects, a record of all medicines being taken every day is essential to help the prescribing doctor.

It is also very useful to develop a clear picture of what symptoms occur and in what order for each individual patient who has entered a manic, hypomanic, or depressive episode. Some patients, as they become depressed, will first note fatigue, then insomnia, guilt, and finally loss of appetite. Other patients will report a different progression of symptoms. They may first note that they oversleep, then concentration problems arise, perhaps followed by loss of appetite and, finally, the development of sadness. The progression of symptoms is often the same for one patient as he or she enters one and then another depressive (or manic or hypomanic) episode. But the progression is often quite different across different individuals. It is almost like a "signature" for each patient. By recognizing and recording this signature based on prior history, the doctor and patient can often distinguish whether the patient is just having a few good or bad days from whether he or she is likely to be entering a manic or depressive episode in the future. In this way, premature medication changes can be avoided, while necessary medication changes can be made in a timely fashion.

In addition, significant others play a critical role in (1) helping to define the signature and (2) assisting the doctor in evaluating especially when hypomania may be occurring. One patient illustrates the point. He, when he was becoming manic, would go to bed earlier (10:00 P.M. instead of 11:30 P.M.), would arise earlier (4:00 A.M. vs. 6:00 A.M.), and would go to the Seven-Eleven convenience store to discuss world affairs with the clerk. The latter was noted by his wife. This signature allowed the doctor and patient to recognize very early when mania was becoming a risk.

Regular tracking of symptoms and a careful discussion with patient and significant other often identify other danger periods. For example, does the depression get worse or come on in the premenstrual phase of the patient's cycle? Is spring or fall likely to be associated with more mania or depression? For persons having to fly long distances, does crossing a number of time zones raise or lower the mood? Does it precipitate depression or mania? By recognizing what sort of events lead to dysregulation, lifestyle changes can be made, medications can be changed, or more frequent doctor visits can be scheduled when the risk of symptoms worsening is higher.

Biostressors

A variety of expectable events in addition to seasons and menstrual cycle phases is known to dysregulate or exacerbate bipolar disorder. This includes substance abuse, intercurrent viral or bacterial infections, and pregnancy and delivery, as well as psychological stresses such as moving residences, responding to deadlines, or becoming overextended or overcommitted to too many projects or people. Both alcohol and nearly all substances of abuse dysregulate bipolar disorder in two ways. First, they often change blood levels of therapeutic antimanic, antidepressant, or mood-stabilizing agents. Second, they can have a direct effect on the very brain systems already not functioning well in bipolar disorder. For example, appetite suppressants, or stimulants like amphetamine or cocaine, directly dysregulate norepinephrine and dopamine systems in the brain. As a result, even if the patient is on a proper medication regimen, it will fail to work if these additional chemicals are added. Thus, abstinence from illicit substances is essential. Alcohol intake should be *very modest* or eliminated. Very modest means one glass of wine or a beer a day.

Viral infections such as hepatitis or mononucleosis, as well as flu viruses, and even cold viruses, may in some (not all) precipitate a depression or worsen a depressed mood. The mechanism is not clear. But often the patient's history will reveal such a pattern. These are often brief depressions, but for some, they can be longer. Getting the flu vaccine yearly or getting vaccinated against hepatitis may be very useful for these patients. Further, if the episodes are not too severe or too long, then it may be wise to <u>not</u> add an antidepressant should such an event occur in the future.

Life stresses (deadlines, long and unpredictable work hours, dealing with large numbers of potential customers at trade shows, running for political office, etc.) can precipitate manic or depressive episodes, again in some but not other patients. History will often identify such patterns, especially if the significant other is invited to provide his/her observations. Which stresses cause mood dysregulation? Can they be avoided or managed in a constructive way? For example, can deadlines be planned for so the pressure to do everything in a very short period can be reduced? Can some duties be assigned to others in these high-pressure situations? After a multicity business trip, should the patient take a vacation day to wind down?

Pregnancy presents two issues: (1) how to manage the medications used for bipolar disorder and other chronic medications during pregnancy and delivery, and (2) how to anticipate and control the mood dysregulation that is likely in many during pregnancy and that is even more likely following delivery. The best rule of thumb here is to plan the pregnancy so that medications that are likely to cause birth defects can be stopped before conception. More frequent visits during pregnancy, provision of psychotherapy during pregnancy, and coordination with the obstetrician in terms of medication management are essential. Anticipating and treating prophylactically the expected and often severe postpartum depression is also very helpful, especially if there is a prior history of postpartum depression.

Medication Management

The most important rule for optimizing medication management, as noted earlier, is full disclosure to all prescribers of all medicines (prescribed, over the counter, natural or herbal products, alcohol, and illicit drug use). This policy minimizes the risk of drug–drug interactions. It also prevents inappropriate changes in the medicines used for bipolar disorder, because other medications can cause mood shifts by themselves. For example, appetite suppressants or decongestants may for some cause hypomania by themselves. The treatment in such cases is simply to stop the offending medicine rather than to add another antimanic agent. Clearly, a careful record of all drugs taken is essential.

In addition, such a record often helps the doctor to simplify the medication regimen over time in patients with stable and well-controlled bipolar disorder. This not only saves money but reduces unwanted side effects.

When to Call for Help

As each patient develops expertise in managing his or her bipolar disorder, when to call for help will become clear. The most important rule here is if the patient is not sure whether to call, he or she should call. It is far easier to have a brief phone call early in the course of mood dysregulation than to have to respond to a crisis. Sometimes the significant other will have a concern, but the patient will not recognize the issue. Or, it may be a false alarm. Either way, it is best to check it out rather than to worry and doubt. Is this just a bad day, which we all have, or is it the beginning of a clinical depression? Is this normal joy at getting promoted or is it excessive exuberance portending a manic episode? Here, judgments need to be made. But armed with the signature and a careful record of mood changes and medications, the doctor, patient and significant other can work together to decide what, if anything, needs to be done. This team approach is most effective and most likely to lead to maximal control of bipolar disorder. Medications are the mainstay of treatment for bipolar disorder. However, selection of the best medicine or combinations of medicines for a particular patient depends on individual responses. Clinicians, patients, and, whenever possible, significant others must work together to try out, carefully and diligently, one and sometimes several medications to get the best results. Because of symptom breakthrough, intercurrent illnesses, pregnancy, the use of medicines for general medical conditions, and a variety of other situations, medications need to be carefully adjusted over the months and years of treatment for bipolar disorder. Well-informed patients, knowledgeable about symptoms, side effects, and the general objectives of medication treatment, are essential members of the treatment team. While finding the right medication regimen can be time-consuming, the effort almost always pays off in a return to good functioning with minimal side effects. Patients are to be encouraged to ask, learn, and discuss all medication questions they have with the appropriate clinician in a timely manner.

Key Points for the Therapist to Remember

♦ Patients should be told the reason for the use of each specific medication and common side effects so that they can help determine whether the medication is working correctly, and so they can be on the lookout for and report salient side effects in a timely manner.

♦ The prescribing person needs to be available by phone and should see the patient often enough to make timely adjustments in dose or medication type.

♦ Most patients with bipolar disorder are taking multiple medications, either for their bipolar disorder or for other general medical conditions. Consequently, the psychopharmacologist must be aware of potential drug–drug interactions.

Points to Discuss with Patients

♦ It is essential that patients understand the reason why a medication or combination is being used, what is expected to be the outcome (if successful), when success can be achieved, what side effects are likely, and, importantly, why and when specific laboratory tests are needed either to guide the proper dosing of the medications or to monitor for adverse events.

♦ Patients and their significant others should be taught how to monitor, measure, and record manic and depressive symptoms, so when it is time to see the prescriber, he or she will have a clear picture of what the effects of the medication were and will, thereby, be better able to make appropriate adjustments

♦ For both acute and maintenance phases of treatment, patients must take the prescribed medication(s) on a daily basis—on both good days and bad days—at the same dosage.

♦ Patients should know (1) which medication side effects are more or less likely, (2) which side effects are dangerous, (3) which side effects will gradually disappear over time, and (4) what methods can be used to counter side effects should they occur.

♦ Patients need to carefully monitor, record, and discuss with their doctor the signs and symptoms of both mania and depression. By carefully tracking the effects of each step in the treatment plan, the patient can help the doctor make well-informed adjustments in the dose or types of medication being used.

♦ Patients play a critical role in optimizing outcome by maintaining healthy appropriate lifestyle choices and by anticipating and preparing for potential issues that could affect how their bipolar disorder is to be managed (having surgery, becoming pregnant, etc.).

CHAPTER 4

Enhancing Adherence

Placing Adherence in Perspective

Adherence is a multidimensional concept. Many factors influence a patient's degree of adherence; it changes form over time; and the decisions that affect a patient's choice to comply are sometimes emotional and at others times quite rational. Clinicians often have misconceptions about the complexity of the treatment process for people who suffer from chronic mental illnesses. There is a tendency to oversimplify by classifying people as compliant or not. To be helpful to their patients clinicians must place adherence in its proper perspective. Understanding how common nonadherence is, the challenges that patients face, and the patterns of nonadherence will prepare clinicians for intervening with adherence problems.

Noncompliance Is as Much the Norm as the Exception

Surveys of literature on medication compliance in psychiatric (Basco & Rush, 1995) and general medical populations (Meichenbaum & Turk, 1987) have found that most patients are either fully or partially noncompliant with treatment. Compliance is most likely to occur when treatment is short and health problems produce discomfort and is least likely to occur for prophylactic treatment, when symptoms are in remission, or before significant complications have occurred (Meichenbaum & Turk, 1988). Among patients with bipolar disorder, estimates of noncompliance vary depending on the data collection method. For example, taking a global look at compliance, Svarstad et al. (2001) examined Medicaid drug claims to assess the frequency with which medication prescriptions were filled by patients with severe mental illnesses over a 12-month period. They found that 33% of the 67 patients diagnosed with bipolar disorder irregularly filled their medications prescriptions. Keck et al. (1996) found that of 101 patients hospitalized for mania, 64% had been noncompliant with pharmacotherapy in the month prior to admission. Basco and Rush (1995) found that across studies of patients with mood disorders, the probability of compliance varied from .53 to .63 for pharmacotherapy.

Compliance Is Not an All-or-Nothing Phenomenon

Patients are often described clinically as compliant or noncompliant, as if it were a trait and not a behavior. Studies on compliance rates with pharmacotherapy show that most patients tend to miss some but not all doses of medication, while a smaller minority discontinue treatment altogether (Keck et al., 1996; Scott & Pope, 2002a). For example, Weiss et al. (1998) examined the compliance rates of 44 patients with bipolar disorder. Depending on the medication types, compliance rates for individual patients ranged from 66% to 100%. However, only 21% of patients taking lithium were completely adherent to treatment and 13% of patients taking lithium and 8% of those taking valproate reported taking medication less than one-third of the time. The varying rates of compliance across patients, as well as its limited association with any predictors of compliance, suggests that it may be more accurately viewed as a continuum of behavior rather than a trait.

Compliance Is More Difficult Than It Looks

The mental confusion and disorganization caused by depression, mania, and mixed states, as well as external distractions in the patients' environment, make compliance harder to accomplish than it might appear. Furthermore, patients are often requested to abide by complicated and expensive treatment recommendations that produce uncomfortable side effects and involve complicated dosing schedules.

While physicians prescribe medications and therapists assign homework with the assumption that their directions will be followed, it is naïve to assume that patients will adhere to a treatment plan just because clinicians say it will work. Acceptance of this fact will help clinicians lower their expectations to more realistic levels and plan ahead for noncompliance rather than assume it will occur or to hope for the best. Approaching patients with a matter-of-fact discussion of the complexities of compliance (e.g., "It is hard to stick with treatment for long periods of time.") opens the door to frank discussion and proactive planning (e.g., "What do you think could interfere with you following this treatment plan?" "What can we do about it?").

You Cannot Always Predict Who Will Comply

Clinical studies have shown that degree of adherence with treatment is an important predictor of outcomes for patients with bipolar disorder (Craig, Fennig, Tanenberg-Karant, & Bromet, 2000; Ghaemi, Boiman, & Goodman, 2000; Kulhara, Basu, Mattoo, Sharan, & Chopra, 1999; Scott & Pope, 2002b; Tsai et al., 2001), with full compliance leading to the best overall outcomes, as would be expected. However, there does not appear to be a consistent association between compliance and illness characteristics such as length of episode, age of onset, or polarity of episodes (Aagaard & Vestergaard, 1990; Colom et al., 2000 et al., 1982; Danion et al., 1987; Frank et al., 1985; Jacob et al., 1984).

The most consistent finding across studies is that greater psychiatric comorbidity has been associated with lower compliance rates. For example, patients treated for bipolar disorder who have substance abuse problems or personality disorders have more difficulty following treatment plans (Aagaard & Vestergaard, 1990; Colom et al., 2000; Danion et al., 1987; Jacob et al., 1984; Brown et al., 2001). Unfortunately, the majority of people who have been diagnosed with bipolar disorder suffer from one or more secondary psychiatric problems. More than 65% of these individuals have at least one comorbid Axis I diagnosis, and about 43% have two or more comorbid Axis I disorders (McElroy et al., 2001).

The Best Predictor of the Future Is the Past

Scott and Pope (2002a), in their examination of plasma blood levels of mood stabilizers in patients with bipolar disorder ($N = 78$) and major depressive disorder ($N = 20$), found that one of the best predictors of incomplete adherence to treatment was a prior history of noncompliance. Specifically, 84% of patients reporting a past history of noncompliance acknowledged that they had been only partially compliant with their medication in the month prior to evaluation and 47% had been noncompliant within the week prior to the evaluation.

There Is More to It Than Simply Denial

A common clinical assumption is that patients who are not cooperative with treatment are in denial about their problems. There is some limited empirical evidence that, in fact, noncompliance with treatment may be related to denial of illness in patients with bipolar disorder (Greenhouse, Meyer, & Johnson, 2000; Keck et al., 1996; Peralta & Cuesta, 1998; Scott & Pope, 2002a). Dell'Osso et al. (2002) found that inpatients with bipolar depression, mixed states, or manic episodes had less insight into their illness than those with unipolar depression. Manic patients more often reported that medications were unlikely to help their symptoms subside and had less insight regarding the social consequences of bipolar disorder compared with bipolar depressed and mixed patients (Dell'Osso et al., 2000), and more often deny that their symptoms are a sign of mental illness (Swanson et al., 1995).

While this research confirms clinical common sense, the magnitude of the relationship between clinical features or denial/acceptance and adherence to treatment is minimal, accounting for only about 16% of the variance (e.g., Greenhouse et al., 2000). This is insufficient to explain why adherence waxes and wanes or what to do about it. To fully understand the nature of adherence with treatment, one must look more closely at the decision points between treatment prescription and daily implementation. At a minimum, there are two requirements for daily compliance with treatment: (1) patients must recall that a treatment-related behavior is to occur, such as taking a pill, and (2) they must make a decision to engage in that treatment related behavior.

The Illness Interferes with Adherence

Recollection of treatment recommendations can be affected by the impaired concentration and memory associated with depression and mania, and there is recent evidence from empirical studies that decision making is impaired when patients are in manic or depressive states (Murphy et al., 2001; Rubinsztein et al., 2001). However, even when relatively asymptomatic, people who are prescribed medication for bipolar disorder often decide to discontinue its use. A better understanding of patients' decisionmaking processes is critical to solving the puzzle of noncompliance.

Rethinking Adherence

A more accurate depiction of adherence is that it is a behavior that waxes and wanes over the course of time. According to the health belief model (Becker, 1974), the decision to comply with treatment is initially dependent on whether or not patients find the prescribed treatment understandable, acceptable, and manageable. Even if these prerequisites are satisfied, however, numerous factors can influence adherence. Such obstacles include intrapersonal factors such as symptoms, denial, or forgetfulness (Keck et al., 1996). Interpersonal difficulties with providers, staff, or health care facilities can also keep people from adhering to treatment (Gitlin, Cochran, & Jamison, 1989.) Social system influences in the form of competing advice from other health care providers, discouragement from family, or negative publicity in the media all can influence a person's decision to take medication or participate in psychotherapy (Meichenbaum & Turk, 1988). Side effects or inconveniences caused by the treatment itself, including costs, regimen complexities, and lack of transportation to clinics or pharmacies, also represent potential obstacles to adherence (Gitlin et al., 1989; Keck et al., 1996; Nilson & Axelsson, 1989).

The connection between treatment obstacles and adherence is not usually direct. Family members do not generally restrict patients' access to medications, most symptoms do not preclude treatment, clinicians do not force patients to discontinue treatment, and inconveniences are not always impossible to overcome. Instead, the intrapersonal, interpersonal, social system, and treatment-related obstacles seem to affect patients' perceptions of treatment, which, in turn, influences their decisions to engage or not engage in the recommended intervention. According to decision theory, these perceptions help shape heuristics, or general rules of thumb, for treatment decisions made by the patient (Tversky & Kahneman, 1974) and are impressionistic rather than formal evaluations of the costs and benefits of treatment.

Ideally, to facilitate adherence, treatment should be convenient, comfortable, and affordable. Family, friends, and providers should be supportive and encouraging. The reasons to comply should be compelling and the decision should be obvious and easily made. Unfortunately, as often as not the circumstances surrounding treatment are far from perfect and the nature of the illness itself and its sequelae create conflict and complexities at all levels. With multidose regimens and perceived constriction in lifestyle required to manage the illness, patients with bipolar disorder are in the position multiple times daily of deciding whether to comply with the instruction of their doctor and take their medication or take their chances that skipping a dose will be OK.

The Decision to Comply or Not to Comply with Treatment

Decision research, a branch of social–cognitive psychology, explores theories of decision making that may help us to better understand the problem of nonadherence in bipolar disorder. For example, it is believed that people use unsystematic and personally biased heuristics to make decisions (Plous, 1993). These heuristics are formed by one's conceptualization or mental model of a problem or situation and may not be based completely on facts or logic. For example, if a person negatively stereotypes the mentally ill as criminals or the homeless, he or she may reject a diagnosis of bipolar disorder as not fitting with his or her self-view. If attitudes toward psychiatrists are shaped by media portrayals of them as incompetent or unethical, then any advice or recommendations for treatment will be viewed as suspect. If a person trusts only homeopathic remedies, then prescribed medications may be viewed as harmful.

In psychiatry and other areas of medicine, the views or heuristics used by doctors to make treatment decisions are likely to be quite different from the views or heuristics used by laypersons (Byram, Fischhoff, Embrey, de Bruin, & Thorne, 2001; Morgan, Fischhoff, Bostrom, & Atman, 2002; Silverman et al., 2001).

Nonadherence with treatment can therefore be defined as a discrepancy between treatment recommendations derived from clinicians' conceptualization of illness and patients' acceptance of those recommendations, which is based on their unique mental model of illness.

Some preliminary research with clinical populations has shown a relationship between the discrepancy in clinicians' and patients' mental models and compliance levels. Cohen, Tripp-Reimer, Smith, Sorofman, and Lively (1994), using hemoglobin A1c (HbA1c) values as indicators of patient compliance with treatment, attempted to correlate the degree of discrepancy between patient and provider views and compliance. Correlations did not reach statistical significance in this small sample of 14 patients for whom HbA1c levels were available but showed a trend toward greater discrepancy associated with higher HgA1c levels, an indicator of degree of adherence to treatment and control of the illness. Specifically, 68% of those patients whose mental model was congruent with practitioners mental models had normal HbA1c levels, compared to only 52% of those with minor discrepancies, and only 50% of those with major discrepancies between patient and practitioner mental model. In a sample of depressed patients in a primary care setting, Brown et al. (2001) found that patients' mental models of their disorder were associated with help-seeking, symptom-coping strategies and medication adherence. To better address compliance issues with patients, it may be helpful to know the types of thought processes that lead a patient to or away from treatment. Decision theory provides some clues to explain this process.

For example, according to "satisfice" theory (Simon, 1956), patients will choose a path that satisfies what they believe to be their most important need even if the choice is not a good idea. For some people the choice to avoid or discontinue treatment may not be ideal but may satisfy the need to feel normal and not be labeled mentally ill. For others the decision to comply with pharmacotherapy may satisfy the need for emotional stability, even though medications may cause uncomfortable side effects.

According to "prospect theory" (Kahneman & Tversky, 1979), once people actively engage in treatment, the decision to continue may be dictated by the aversiveness of potentially losing the stability previously gained, as the threat of losses is generally more influential than the prospect of positive gains. On the flip side, before symptom stability is achieved, the threat of financial losses due to the cost of medications may be more compelling than the promise of gains in mental health.

As noted previously, adherence to treatment is more likely to be partial than to be complete or absent (Greenhouse et al., 2000; Keck et al., 1996; Scott & Pope, 2002a). Patients often make choices to modify dosages or timing of some, but not all, medications in their regimen. They may substitute "natural" substances for prescribed drugs or may try to alter their lifestyles as a substitute for biological treatments. Which decisions are made may depend on the cognitive strategy employed by the patient. For example, if employing an "ideal point model" (Plous, 1993), people will choose the option closest to their ideal choice. Thus if not needing medications at all would be an ideal choice, they will vary their medication intake to get as close to that as possible.

Plous (1993) describes several decision-making strategies that can be used when multiple choices are available, such as multiple medication alternatives or the options to partially or fully adhere to treatment recommendations. If using a "conjunctive rule," patients will eliminate all treatment choices that fall outside a predefined boundary (e.g., refusing to take any medications that cause weight gain or considering only those medications that are reimbursed by their insurance company). Using the "disjunctive rule," each treatment alternative is evaluated in terms of its best attribute such as providing greatest symptom control, costing the least, or having the fewest associated side effects. With a "lexicographic" strategy the patient selects the most important attribute (e.g., potential for weight gain) and chooses the most desirable alternative on that attribute. Tversky (1972) described an "elimination by aspect" decision-making strategy in which one attribute at a time is reviewed and any treatment options not meeting that criteria are eliminated. For example, first drugs are rejected that cause weight gain, then those whose costs are prohibitive, then those that are not on their insurance formulary.

The framing of the necessity of treatment by clinicians may also influence patients' decisions to adhere or not adhere with treatment. If the likelihood of relapse without consistent treatment is described as inevitable, according to the "certainty effect" (Tversky & Kahneman, 1981), people are more likely to agree to treatment than if the risk were framed merely as likely or probable, particularly when the risks are described in detail (Tversky & Kahneman, 1982). And when risks are presented as catastrophic and are dreaded by patients and/or would be regrettable, preventive measures are more likely to be taken (Dunning & Parpal, 1989; Slovic, 1987; Stone & Yates, 1991). This may be particularly true when the patients can easily recall prior experiences when discontinuing medication led to a severe relapse of depression or mania (Tversky & Kahneman, 1974). Of course, denial can also color people's recollections of non-adherence-related relapses, and when such reference points are unavailable and the risks are difficult to image, the probability of adherence would decrease.

It is human nature to try to make sense out of our experiences. However, conclusions drawn can sometimes be erroneous, patterns can be falsely seen in random events, or unusual occurrences can be perceived as commonplace and likely to recur. In the case of medication treatment for bipolar disorder, an illness that naturally waxes and wanes in severity, missing a few doses with little consequence can lead to the assumption that skipping pills is always safe. What has been forgotten are the times when decreasing medication dosages led to a worsening of symptoms and prompted resumption of treatment.

Human beings are prone to errors in judgment even when thinking is not impaired by symptoms. We believe in winning streaks, think that all things will average out in the end, ignore the base rates of events, and disregard information that is contrary to our beliefs (Plous, 1993). Probability estimates are more influenced by positive outcomes than by negative outcomes (Plous, 1993). So for patients with bipolar disorder the notion that they will "be fine" given nonadherence with treatment is more believable than the idea that they will "get sick" if nonadherent. These types of erroneous conclusions can lead to risky choices of action, nonadherence to treatment in this case, and bad outcomes.

Given the many potential influences on patients' decisions to follow their prescribed treatment plans, it is important that clinicians explore each patient's reasons for adhering or not adhering with treatment. If their decision-making algorithms are better understood, then interventions can be focused on correcting faulty views of illness and its treatment and education can be provided so that decisions are based on a balanced view of the facts.

There is no formal exercise for learning more about patients' decisions to adhere to pharmacotherapy that can replace listening for clues and inquiring about both the positive and negative aspects of treatment. If an environment has been created for an honest and open discussion of compliance, clinicians will learn over time how patients make those daily decisions about treatment.

Measurement of Compliance

The simplest way to assess compliance is to ask patients if they have taken all their medication, if they have missed any doses, and if they have taken their doses at the correct times of day. Questionnaires can also be helpful because they provide a standard format for measuring self-perceived, self-reported compliance and make it possible for clinicians to compare the compliance scores of a given patient over time or the scores of several patients. Although they are simple, self-reports can be inaccurate because of memory deficits, recall bias, or deliberate distortion.

In scientific investigations and in some clinic settings, health care providers use "pill counts" to measure patient compliance. After dispensing a number of pills that may match or exceed the amount needed until the next visit, a clinician instructs the patient to return any unused pills at the following visit. The clinician then counts the remaining pills and compares the total to the number previously dispensed. Discrepancies are considered evidence of poor compliance. Pill counts are considerably more complex, but tend to be more accurate, than self-reports. When they compared self-reports of compliance and pill counts in the same patients, Park and Lipman (1964) found that 40% of the patients' self-reports did not match the results of the pill counts. They also found that minor discrepancies tended to occur more frequently than major deviations in compliance.

A more commonly used method for assessing treatment compliance is to measure the plasma concentrations or blood level of medications. A higher than expected ratio of prescribed dose to plasma drug level may suggest poor compliance. A comparison of dose to plasma level ratios in a given individual over time allows for individual variations in metabolism and avoids invalid accusations of poor compliance when the ratio in one patient is different from those observed in other patients. Changes in the ratio within an individual may be more likely to indicate poor compliance, provided that the timing of doses and blood sampling remains constant.

Although measuring medication blood levels appears to be a more accurate method than self-reports, the consistency with which blood levels reflect the dose ingested may vary with the type of medication (Hollister, 1982). Plasma concentrations of lithium, for example, may be fairly reliable indicators of patient compliance, assuming consistency in timing of doses and blood sampling. This method, however, is not foolproof as the following example illustrates.

> Mr. Fulton has been taking lithium for bipolar disorder over several years. Sometimes he is consistent with taking medication and sometimes he is not. He doesn't want his doctor to know that he is inconsistent with medications, so he either postpones his visits until he can get back into the habit of taking his lithium or if he is short on time, he just takes his medication very consistently for a few days just before his blood lithium level measurement. He figured out somewhat by accident that if takes his medications consistently for several days in a row, his blood test will show a lithium level in the therapeutic range. He sees this as harmless and it gets him out of receiving another lecture from his doctor on medication compliance.

Schwarcz and Silbergeld (1983) knew that patients such as Mr. Fulton could outsmart lithium level checks if they knew they were coming, so they conducted a study in which patients received unannounced blood tests to spot-check plasma lithium levels. Of the 26 lithium clinic patients who participated, 42% ($N = 11$) had lithium levels below the therapeutic range. These 11 patients received counseling about compliance with medication and more than half improved in their adherence to the treatment regimen.

The degree to which patients actively participate in treatment also indicates the level of their compliance. Appointment attendance, tardiness to sessions, level of involvement in the treatment sessions, and completion of homework assignments between sessions are all indicators of general compliance to treatment.

In clinical practice, assessment of compliance through conversations with patients is the most widely used method. In Chapter 5, we discuss methods for establishing a therapeutic environment where compliance can be discussed openly and the patient feels comfortable enough to reply honestly. This does not mean that assessment of medication blood levels is unnecessary. Although it may not be the best way to monitor compliance, it is often critical to pharmacological management of patients to determine if medication blood levels are within the expected therapeutic range and do not exceed medically safe levels.

The assessment of treatment adherence is not always practical beyond patient self-report. Clinically useful, accurate, reliable, and valid methods have not yet been perfected. In research studies in other areas of illness some simple self-report methods have been found to be useful. The measure illustrated in Figure 4.1 includes typical questions posed by clinical researchers to evaluate levels of compliance. A scoring key is provided. The points from each item are added up to derive a total score.

Couldn't It Just Be Denial?

Many clinicians assume that patients who are not cooperative with treatment are in denial about their problems, and there is some empirical evidence to support this idea (Greenhouse et al., 2000; Keck et al., 1996; Peralta & Cuesta, 1988; Scott & Pope, 2002a). Keck et al. (1996) found that denial and poor insight were common factors associated with poor medication compliance among patients admitted for mania, and Greenhouse et al. (2000) found a curvilinear relationship, where only high levels of denial were related to poor adherence with treatment.

Acceptance, however, is not the absence of denial. In fact, the two appear to be only moderately correlated (Greenhouse et al., 2000). To better understand the adjustment people make to having a chronic and life-altering illness such as bipolar disorder it is helpful to consider denial and acceptance as end points in a process such as the

Please (circle) the answer that best describes your recent experiences with taking medication.

1. Do you <u>always</u> take medication as prescribed?   Yes   No

2. Do you have <u>any</u> trouble taking your medications   Yes   No
   as prescribed?

3. Are you taking any prescriptions now for bipolar   Yes   No
   disorder?

4. Do you ever stop taking your medication when   Yes   No
   you feel better?

5. Do you ever stop taking your medication when   Yes   No
   you feel worse?

6. Do you sometimes forget to take your medication?   Yes   No

7. How many days in the past week were pills forgotten?

   0   1   2   3   4   5   6   7

8. How many days in the past week were pills not taken on purpose?

   0   1   2   3   4   5   6   7

9. What proportion of medications have you <u>missed</u> in the <u>last week</u>?

   None   Less than half   About half   More than half   All

10. What proportion of medications have you <u>missed</u> in the <u>last month</u>?

   None   Less than half   About half   More than half   All

   cont.

FIGURE 4.1. Basco Adherence Questionnaire. Derived from Choo et al. (1999); Keck et al. (1996); Kwon et al. (2003); Magura, Laudet, Mahmood, Rosenblum, and Knight (2002); Peveler, George, Kinmonth, Campbell, and Thompson (1999); Scott and Pope (2002b); and Sternhell and Corr (2002).

one proposed by Elisabeth Kübler-Ross (1970, 1974) to describe working through a significant sense of loss. In this way, acceptance of a diagnosis of bipolar illness and its treatment comes only after grieving the loss of the "normal" or mentally "healthy" self. Using Kübler-Ross's description of the phases of grief, denial is only the first phase that people go through when facing a loss.

Clinicians working with the newly diagnosed patient will note a

Scoring Key

Number in parentheses is the score to be given for each of the patient's answers.

1. Do you <u>always</u> take medication as prescribed?   Yes**(1)** No**(0)**

2. Do you have <u>any</u> trouble taking your medications as prescribed?   Yes**(0)** No**(1)**

3. Are you taking any prescriptions now for bipolar disorder?   Yes**(1)** No**(0)**

4. Do you ever stop taking your medication when you feel better?   Yes**(0)** No**(1)**

5. Do you ever stop taking your medication when you feel worse?   Yes**(0)** No**(1)**

6. Do you sometimes forget to take your medication?   Yes**(0)** No**(1)**

7. How many days in the past week were pills forgotten?

   0**(7)**   1**(6)**   2**(5)**   3**(4)**   4**(3)**   5**(2)**   6**(1)**   7**(0)**

8. How many days in the past week were pills not taken on purpose?

   0**(7)**   1**(6)**   2**(5)**   3**(4)**   4**(3)**   5**(2)**   6**(1)**   7**(0)**

9. What proportion of medications have you <u>missed</u> in the <u>last week</u>?

   None**(4)** Less than half**(3)** About half**(2)** More than half**(1)** All**(0)**

10. What proportion of medications have you <u>missed</u> in the <u>last month</u>?

   None**(4)** Less than half**(3)** About half**(2)** More than half**(1)** All**(0)**

Total Score: _____

0	5	10	15	20	25	30
Nonadherence			Moderate adherence			Full adherence

FIGURE 4.1. *cont.*

tone of disbelief in or disagreement with the diagnosis as evidence of denial. There is often a downplaying of the seriousness of impairment or behaviors that brought the patient to the attention of health care providers. Anger is Kübler-Ross's second phase. Our patients express fury with the unfairness of "getting" this illness. Their anger at having to take medication, modify their lifestyles, and be different from everyone else can come across as anger with the clinician or family members who either forced them into treatment or passed on the gene for the illness. Bargaining, the third step in the adjustment process usually takes place within the individual rather than between the individual and care providers, although the latter would be preferable. Self-adjustments in medication dosing and replacing antidepressants with vows to exercise and think more positively are examples of what people do during the bargaining phase. When no longer able to ignore the accuracy of a diagnosis of bipolar disorder or the need for medication or when faced directly with the life-altering consequences of the illness, depression, the fourth phase begins. Compliance with medication can begin to improve as the individual comes to grips with the necessity of treatment. Acceptance or adaptation to the illness and treatment is the end goal, but regression to previous stages is likely as the person encounters problems with treatment or unwelcome restrictions.

A patient's progress through the stages of grief may be evident in his or her comments about treatment or in affect shifts when the discussion moves to problems or treatment changes. Another indicator may be the thoughts verbalized by patients as they discuss their views of the disorder, symptoms, or health care providers. Table 4.1 provides some examples of the negative automatic thoughts and behaviors associated with each stage in the grieving process.

For those with newly diagnosed bipolar disorder, acceptance of the initial diagnosis is dependent on their view of the problem. Some find relief when what they have been living through is finally identified and treated. Those with a family history of bipolar disorder, particularly in first-degree relatives, may not be surprised by the diagnosis but are usually discouraged and disappointed. In these cases, denial that the illness exists may never be an issue, but ideas about control of the illness may be unrealistic. On the one hand, patients may intellectually comprehend the link between their genes, their biochemistry, and their mood symptoms. But on the other hand their behavioral noncompliance with treatment may indicate a lack of acceptance of the chronicity or severity of the disorder. Those who are not ready to accept a diagnosis of bipolar disorder will avoid the health care system. They may be court ordered to receive care but once released are likely to discontinue their medications.

TABLE 4.1. Automatic Thoughts and Behaviors Associated with Stages of Grief over the Illness

Thoughts	Behavior
Denial	
• "I don't have it. The doctor made a mistake. It must be because I've been drinking too much."	• Getting a second opinion.
	• Looking for other explanations for symptoms.
• "It will pass."	• Ignoring treatment recommendations.
Anger	
• "It's not fair that I have this illness"	• Refusing to listen to advice.
• "I can't deal with this right now."	• Refusing to discuss the illness.
• "Why me? What did I do to deserve this?"	• Losing temper with health care providers, pharmacies, or anyone else associated with treatment.
Bargaining	
• "I'll clean up my act."	• Adjusting doses. Changing the timing of doses.
• "I'll stop drinking, start waking up on time, start exercising, get a better job, and it will be OK."	• Trading active drugs for "natural remedies."
• "I'll make myself go on a diet, straighten out my sleep. It will get better."	• Staying up late to avoid taking sleeping medications.
• "I'll try natural remedies. I don't really need medicine."	• Drinking alcohol to avoid anxiolytics.
Depression	
• "I'll never have a normal life."	• Self-destructive behaviors.
• "No one will want me."	• Avoidance of stimuli related to the illness.
• "I hate myself."	• Withdrawal from others.
Acceptance	
• "I can work my way through this.	• Adherence with treatment.
• "It's not the end of the world."	• Open discussion of treatment options with clinicians before discontinuing medications.
• "I don't have to give up everything just because I have to take medication."	

Compliance among children and teenagers with bipolar disorder is largely dependent on the compliance of their caretakers in dispensing medication or supervising its usage. Parents can sometimes bargain with or coerce their children into taking medications, but they may not be able to force compliance with other self-management behaviors such as going to sleep at a reasonable hour or avoiding alcohol or street drugs. Young adults, who are no longer under parental control, may assert their independence by refusing medications and ignoring or "toughing out" symptoms. Others have not suffered enough consequences of their illness to accept the notion that continuous treatment is necessary, particularly if supportive family members protected and aided the individual until the episode remitted. Colom et al. (2000) found lowest compliance rates among people who suffered relatively few episodes of depression and greater rates for those who had suffered through more episodes of illness. In the first few years of the illness denial may be at its strongest. Acquiescence with family and doctor demands may only happen after life disruptions become too severe or too frequent to ignore.

Coping with Denial

Providing patients with a thorough explanation of bipolar disorder may be all that is needed for those ready and able to accept the diagnosis and its treatment. For those in denial, education about the illness is usually insufficient if they cannot accept the possibility that they have a chronic mental illness. Socratic questioning is one effective cognitive therapy method for aiding patients in addressing issues of denial. The goal is for patients to challenge their inaccurate views of bipolar disorder and replace them with a perspective that encourages self-care and compliance. Following is an example of the use of Socratic questioning to explore the issue of denial in a patient recently diagnosed with bipolar disorder.

Suzanne is a 24-year-old Hispanic female who was referred by her psychiatrist following hospitalization for major depression.

THERAPIST: What brings you to see me?

SUZANNE: Everyone thinks I need therapy.

THERAPIST: Everyone?

SUZANNE: Well, my mom, my doctor, and my sister.

THERAPIST: What do you think?

SUZANNE: I don't know. I guess everyone with bipolar disorder is supposed to need therapy.

THERAPIST: Do you agree with that?

SUZANNE: I guess. I'm not even sure I have it. I know I get depressed. I've been in the hospital twice for that.

THERAPIST: What makes your doctor think you have had mania also?

SUZANNE: I don't know. I guess I get a little weird sometimes.

THERAPIST: Weird?

SUZANNE: I have mood swings. I can get kind of hyper and silly. Like yesterday I started laughing at this stupid commercial on TV and then everything was funny. I started making jokes. My dad got irritated with me and told me I was getting high again.

THERAPIST: Being silly and laughing is not your normal self?

SUZANNE: Not really. I'm usually pretty quiet around my parents.

THERAPIST: Do you know what mania is?

SUZANNE: Yeah, but I don't get that wild.

THERAPIST: Do you know about hypomania?

SUZANNE: Yeah. But I'm not sure that's it either.

THERAPIST: How do you explain the mood swings?

SUZANNE: I can't. I thought maybe it was hormones, but that didn't turn out to be right. I got on birth control pills and stopped taking antidepressants for a month to see if that worked. I got really depressed, started coming up with ways to kill myself.

THERAPIST: So that convinced you that the depression was real. What would convince you that the hypomania was real?

SUZANNE: If I got really manic, like some people do when they spend a lot of money or do stupid things then I would have to believe I have bipolar disorder.

THERAPIST: So you'd have to be sick enough to get into trouble before you'd be convinced?

SUZANNE: I know that sounds pretty stupid. I don't want to lose complete control like that.

THERAPIST: Have you ever been close to that?

SUZANNE: Well, maybe. Last year my friends and I went on this trip to Cancun. We were having fun, drinking and dancing. Everyone else got tired and wanted to go back to the room, but I wasn't ready. I thought they were just acting like old ladies. They got me to leave around 3:00 in the morning, but I was too wound up to sleep. They thought I was on something but I wasn't. I didn't even drink that much. It kind of freaked me out because I wanted to sleep, my body was tired, but I couldn't fall asleep until about 9:00 in the morning. My mind would not shut off.

THERAPIST: Is that the only thing that happened on that trip that bothered you?

SUZANNE: The day before I stayed up all night we went to watch these cliff divers. I'm usually a big chicken, but one of my friends said, "I'll dare you to try that," and I was all for it. It is so unlike me to do anything unsafe, but I almost did it. What scared me is that part of my brain knew that it was a really bad idea and another part of my brain didn't care if I died trying. That sounds manic, doesn't it?

THERAPIST: Yes, it does.

As patients begin to digest the idea of having bipolar disorder, it is best to give them time to think about all that it means to them before beginning to intervene. A follow-up visit should provide an opportunity to inquire more about the patient's thoughts and feelings about the illness and begin educating her about its management.

Coping with Anger

Frustration and anger with may surface when patients have to confront the physical, financial, and psychosocial consequences of having bipolar disorder. It is not unusual for them to become frustrated with the trial-and-error approach to finding the right medication, the uncomfortable and unexpected side effects, and the imposition of symptoms and treatment on their lives. They lose faith in doctors when prescribed treatments fail. They remember what it was like to feel normal and associate this feeling with a time when they were not taking medications. The unfortunate conclusion drawn is that medication is the problem rather than the solution, and as a consequence, compliance wanes. As clinicians, we often underestimate the patience required to tolerate the lengthy, costly, and uncomfortable process of finding the best medication regimen for a given patient, particularly those with refractory illness. We want to be helpful and not hurtful but can also become frustrated with the process. Patients notice their doctors' facial expressions, body language, and subtle intonations that stem from this frustration but may misinterpret them as evidence of disapproval, discouragement with the process, or hopelessness that an appropriate medication can be found. Doctors' responses can reinforce patients' own frustration and sense of hopelessness about their illness.

Even after patients have worked through their anger about having the illness, it can flare up when they are reminded of the inconveniences it has caused, and how their quality of life has been compromised. Brenda provides an excellent example of this.

> Brenda is a 50-year-old advertising director who has struggled with bipolar disorder for over 25 years. She has mastered control over mood swings, is very consistent with taking medications, and has had a successful work life in spite of her illness. Her only regret is that she chose not to have children. She told herself that the stress of childrearing was more than she could handle since managing herself was a full-time job. But her real reason for not having children was that she would not be able to live with herself if she passed on the genes for bipolar disorder to a child. She believes the guilt would eat her up and the despair would plunge her into such a state of depression that she would be unable to function as a mother.
>
> Whenever Brenda thinks about how her life might have been different with children she feels enraged at her illness. Her mother had bipolar disorder, and of her six brothers and sisters she is the only one who inherited it. "I hate having this illness. Why me? I get around my beautiful nieces and nephews and later find myself cursing my mother and cursing myself."
>
> Brenda didn't need a pep talk or encouragement to count her blessings. She didn't need her negative thoughts analyzed. Instead, this type of patient needs validation of how hard it is to live with the ups and downs in mood, the medication side effects, and the embarrassment of having to disclose information about her illness to others. Although she knows she made the right life decisions, support for her choices and her sacrifices can be reassuring during these times of distress.

In response to anger, many clinicians would instinctively provide encouragement and support. This might include attempts at masking their own discouragement: "looking at the bright side" and offering hope in a less than convincing manner. An alternative strategy is to validate their feelings of frustration rather than move too quickly to dispel them. It is reasonable to confide one's own feelings of frustration about the slow process and the less than perfect effectiveness of treatment. Such an admonition can help to strengthen the alliance with the patient.

Bargaining for Treatment

As patients work through the adjustment process from denial to acceptance, they might imagine along the way that they can manage the illness through behavior change. If they can do this they can convince
themselves that perhaps the diagnosis is not entirely correct, a mild
version of the disorder is present, or mind can prevail over body. Each
makes the argument for reducing dependence on pharmacotherapy.
Although some people will attempt to negotiate with their psychiatrists, many will hold an internal debate in which promises of
improved self-care are made in exchange for reduction in need for formal treatments. Some might decide to reduce their alcohol consump-
tion and improve sleep and eating habits with the hopes that their
symptoms will improve. This type of bargaining can be interpreted as
acceptance of the illness without complete acceptance of the treatment.

Bargaining can also take the form of self-adjustments to medication regimens. For example, some patients may alter the timing or frequency of medication according to an unsystematic algorithm they
have created. This might include skipping medication doses, lengthening the interval between doses, or raising or lowering the dose to
achieve a more complete remission or fewer side effects. Other
patients replace some or all medications with "natural" remedies. The
bargain made is usually to resume the prescribed medication regimen if
the patient begins to feel worse. However, the desire to avoid medicine
as much as possible can lead to underestimation of symptoms until
they reach intolerable levels.

To help people recognize bargaining as a way of adjusting to bipolar disorder, the therapist can ask if changes the patient is making or
proposes to make result in his or her feeling any better about having
the illness. Allow patients time to consider the connection between
bargaining behavior and adjustment. This should be followed by normalizing the process of bargaining as a phase many people experience
until they are comfortable with treatment. Encourage patients to
express their feelings about the illness. Inquire about the impact it has
had on their lives and how it has changed their self view.

It is a judgment call whether to go along with patients' self-
adjustments or to insist on compliance with the prescribed plan.
Allowing patients to make the suggested changes is a way of express-
ing respect for their opinions. If the patient suggests an alternative
treatment that is contraindicated there may still be an opportunity
to negotiate for a plan that addresses his or her concerns but is still
clinically safe.

It is not unusual for patients to express their displeasure with medication treatment to a therapist but to fail to provide direct feedback to the psychiatrist. This may be due to the patient's lack of assertiveness, forgetfulness, or poor planning; perceived intimidation by the physician; or insufficient time during a medication visit.

The prescribing physician can encourage patients to describe the pluses and minuses of their treatment regimens. A therapist can teach the patient how to voice concerns through assertiveness training or role-play exercises. If necessary and with the permission of the patient, the therapist can call the treating psychiatrist directly to facilitate communication with the patient.

Depressed about Being Ill

As people progress through Kübler-Ross's stages of grief, working their way toward acceptance, they usually reach a point where they become fully aware of the meaning and depth of their mental illness and its potential for disrupting their lives. The costs of acknowledging the necessity of pharmacotherapy can leave them feeling overwhelmed, distraught, and hopeless about the future. Sadness after being given a diagnosis of a chronic and incurable psychiatric illness is not an emotion fueled by cognitive distortion but a reasonable response to what often feels like a life sentence. Depression is a necessary part of the grieving process and should not be dismissed or worked through too quickly.

Cognitive restructuring may be needed to help patients challenge their negative automatic thoughts and to set up experiments to test their assumptions about the future if the depression prolongs or if the patient's beliefs about their disorder become distorted. Attendance at support groups such as the Depression and Bipolar Support Alliance and numerous autobiographical books can provide models of successful living with the illness.

Receiving a diagnosis of bipolar disorder can have a damaging effect on a person's self-esteem. To regain confidence, individuals must revise their self-view to incorporate their premorbid personality with the changes caused by episodes of depression and mania. Some people view bipolar disorder as a character flaw or a permanent scar. They underestimate their abilities to cope, overlook successes, and underestimate the capacities of others to be accepting and supportive. A therapist can help people rebuild their self-esteem by challenging them to redefine themselves: "Who are you now? How are you different than before? In what ways are you just the same? Have you grown stronger than you were before?"

The Fantasy of Acceptance

Clinical lore would suggest that once people fully accept the conditions of their illness, they will eagerly cooperate with treatment. Unfortunately, just as acceptance is not always a prerequisite for compliance, achieving acceptance does not guarantee compliance. Practical problems such as forgetfulness, or lack of resources (Keck et al., 1996), intolerable medication side effects (Gitlin et al., 1989; Keck et al., 1996; Nilson & Axelsson, 1989), discomfort with health care providers (Gitlin et al., 1989), and family discouragement of pharmacotherapy, can interfere with even the best intentions to comply with treatment.

In the next chapter, we introduce strategies for coping with these and other obstacles to full compliance with treatment.

Key Points for the Therapist to Remember

♦ Adherence is a behavior that waxes and wanes over the course of time.

♦ Adherence to treatment is more likely to be partial than to be complete or absent.

♦ The best predictors of incomplete adherence to treatment are a prior history of noncompliance and psychiatric comorbidity.

♦ The magnitude of relationship between denial/acceptance and adherence to treatment is minimal, accounting for only about 16% of the variance.

♦ At minimum, there are two requirements for daily compliance with treatment. First, patients must recall that a treatment-related behavior is to occur, such as taking a pill, and second, they must make a decision to engage in that treatment-related behavior.

♦ If an environment has been created for an honest and open discussion of compliance, clinicians will learn over time how patients make those daily decisions about treatment.

♦ Acceptance of a diagnosis of bipolar illness and its treatment comes only after grieving the loss of the "normal" or mentally "healthy" self. Using Kübler-Ross's description of the phases of grief, denial is only the first phase that people go through when facing a loss.

♦ Achieving acceptance, however, does not guarantee compliance.

Points to Discuss with Patients

♦ Patients will choose a path that satisfies what they believe to be their most important need even if the choice is not a good idea. For some people the choice to avoid or discontinue treatment may not be ideal but may satisfy the need to feel normal and not labeled mentally ill. For others the decision to comply with pharmacotherapy may satisfy the need for emotional stability, even though medications may cause uncomfortable side effects.

♦ If the likelihood of relapse without consistent treatment is described as inevitable, according to the "certainty effect" (Tversky & Kahneman, 1981), people are more likely to agree to treatment than if the risk were framed merely as likely or probable, particularly when the risks are described in detail.

♦ Given the many potential influences on patients' decisions to follow their prescribed treatment plans, it is important that clinicians explore each patient's reasons for adhering or not adhering with treatment.

CHAPTER 5

Compliance Contracts

Establishing a Forum for a Discussion of Compliance Problems

Mrs. Munoz did not take her medication regularly. With all the things that she had on her mind, she often forgot. She had been relatively free of symptoms but knew that it was impossible to predict how much longer she would feel good before the pain of depression or the chaos of mania could come crashing down on her. Periodically, she vowed to become more diligent about taking her medication. Mrs. Munoz did not always tell her therapist, Dr. Mendez, the whole story. When he asked about it, she would answer, "Oh yes, Doctor, I'm still taking my lithium, and I'm feeling great. No problems with symptoms. I'm fine." Mrs. Munoz had come to like her doctor and to care what he thought of her. Dr. Mendez would be disappointed if he knew that Mrs. Munoz had not been adhering to her medication regimen. "He would just worry about me," she thought. "I'll be OK." Although Mrs. Munoz felt comfortable in talking with Dr. Mendez about most things, she believed that her failure to take her medication as prescribed would upset him. She feared his disapproval, rejection, and withdrawal of support. Thus, she withheld the information about her missed doses.

To avoid such problems, it is important to establish a precedent of discussing compliance issues at the outset of treatment. However, clinicians must first accept that patients are not always going to follow directions, even if the directions are clearly explained, are in the best interest of patients, and will greatly help their condition. Second, it is important to introduce the idea that full compliance can be difficult to achieve even when a person has the best intentions. For example, the clinician might say:

> "As you probably already know, this medication will be most helpful if you take it every day. A lot of people have trouble doing this. They forget or run out, or just decide they don't like it. I want us to be able to talk about any problems you might have in taking medication regularly or if you begin to have second thoughts about taking them altogether. This will give us a chance to develop a plan that helps you to be more consistent with medicines or to talk about making changes when either of us thinks a change is needed. Does this idea make sense to you? To accomplish this, you and I have to be comfortable talking about the times you miss your medicines."

Some clinicians are concerned that this type of discussion about compliance may inadvertently invite noncompliance from patients by implying that it is acceptable. It is much like the concern that inquiring about suicidal ideation may actually suggest suicide to patients. This theory has not been formally tested, but experience suggests that it has no basis in fact. To avoid such a suggestion, the message to patients must be that nonadherence to treatment is common but carries consequences for their well-being.

> After Mr. Silver complained about his medication's side effects, his internist suggested that he call his psychiatrist to ask about discontinuing the medication. Mr. Silver was feeling better, and he and his internist were concerned about the weight that he had gained since he had been taking lithium. Although patients typically discontinue medication without first seeking consultation, Mr. Silver called his psychiatrist for permission. The psychiatrist had made it a practice to discuss medication compliance with all patients, and this precedent, which was set during treatment, made Mr. Silver feel comfortable discussing the medication change before any action was taken.

If more than one clinician is treating a patient (e.g., a psychiatrist and a psychotherapist), it is best if each is aware of the other's treatment plan. In this way, they can work together to monitor a patient's progress and determine if noncompliance is a problem. It is not necessary to begin each visit with an interrogation: "Have you taken your medication this week? Are you sure you haven't missed a dose? Show me your medicine bottle and let me see for myself." A less accusatory approach is best. For example, "Have you had any problems in taking your medication lately?" If there is no indication that compliance has been a problem, there is no reason to continue the discussion. If the clinician has evidence that the patient has not been taking the medication (e.g., laboratory results that indicate a low plasma medication level), it is best to tell the patient directly that the laboratory findings were below the therapeutic level, which usually means the patient has missed some doses. The clinician can normalize the problem by reminding the patient that many people find it difficult to adhere to treatment over a long period of time.

The success of a treatment plan depends largely on its acceptability to the patient. The simplest way to determine the patient's response is to review the diagnosis and treatment with the patient and ask his or her opinion: "Does this diagnosis make sense?" "Do you think it describes what you have been experiencing?" "Do you think this treatment plan will work?" As the patient responds, the clinician listens for underlying beliefs or attitudes about treatment.

It is not unusual for patients to feel apprehensive about treatment. If they have lingering concerns, they might agree to follow treatment recommendations while in the office but fail to follow through at home. Inquiring about patients' feelings and concerns gives health care providers opportunities to address these issues before they interfere with treatment. Simple questions (e.g., "How long will I have to take the medication?") may suggest some concern about addiction, dependence, or expense of treatment. Nonverbal behaviors can also provide clues to underlying concerns. Looks of confusion, skepticism, or other facial expressions may suggest that they are troubled or are not paying attention. Verbalizing these observations (e.g., "You look confused") can open the door for discussion.

Although patients' fears or beliefs about treatment may seem illogical or absurd, it is better to validate their underlying concerns than to negate or dismiss them. If a patient says, "I feel like a drug addict when I have to take medication every day," inquire about his or her concerns and indicate that you understand this perspective. For example, clinicians may ask, "What do you think will happen if you keep taking this medication?" A less effective strategy is to invalidate the patient's concerns. "Don't be silly. These are prescribed mediations, not street drugs. They won't make you high and they won't cause addiction."

To be able to adhere to treatment, people must understand (1) the rationale for treatment, (2) the purpose of the intervention, (3) the outcome expected if the intervention is successful, and (4) their specific responsibilities. A person who does not understand the importance or purpose of the treatment has no reason to comply with it. Patients do not always realize that they need this type of information or that they have the right to ask questions. Clinicians can help their patients to be knowledgeable consumers by encouraging them to ask questions and to be as active in treatment planning as they are expected to be in the execution of the regimen.

The degree to which patients feel that they have the necessary resources to carry out an intervention also affects compliance. Resources can include money to buy medication or to pay for office visits, transportation to the clinic, the ability to remember to take multiple daily doses, and tolerance for side effects, as well as encouragement and assistance from others. Lack of resources is a common obstacle to adherence for people who are unable to work because of their illness. Assistance from financial caseworkers, social workers, and families can be particularly helpful in reducing this treatment obstacle.

Psychoeducation

People with psychiatric illnesses do not always receive sufficient information about their disorders or their treatment. Symptoms such as impaired concentration, racing thoughts, distractibility, and anxiety may not always be apparent to clinicians but can reduce a person's comprehension or retention of information. Likewise, clinicians may not effectively convey information or may not take sufficient time to educate patients. The jargon used in daily interactions among mental health professionals is often confusing to patients (e.g., "You are having a breakthrough of hypomania," or "You may be having a recurrence of major depression"). Patients can sometimes recall a diagnosis given in the past but may not understand what it means. They will not always ask for clarification because they are embarrassed to acknowledge that they did not understand a word or expression used to describe their illness or treatment. Sometimes health care workers fail to provide adequate information because they believe the patient is incapable of understanding, is uninterested, or has already been informed by a previous clinician. Despite good intentions, learning does not occur if information is not clearly sent and received.

In busy clinics or practices there is often little time for patient education. By necessity, clinicians must curtail their visits in order to see a large number of patients. While there may be many reasonable explanations for poor patient education, there are few legitimate excuses.

Why Patient Education Is Important

There is some evidence that patient education can improve adherence to treatment and ease adjustment to the illness. Peet and Harvey (1991) randomized 60 lithium clinic patients to either participate in an educational group that viewed a 12-minute videotaped lecture on lithium and received a written transcript or to receive standard pharmacotherapy. Measurements of patients' attitudes toward lithium and understanding of lithium treatment before and after the educational video showed a significant improvement after the educational lectures.

Van Gent and Zwart (1991) provided educational sessions to 14 patients with bipolar disorder and their partners. After five educational sessions and a 6-month follow-up, the patients' partners demonstrated more understanding of the illness, of lithium, and of social strategies for coping with their partners' symptoms. Patients' serum lithium levels did not change in the year following the education program from the levels achieved during the program. This suggests that the education program may have helped to prevent the deterioration in compliance over time often found in lithium-treated patients.

Altamura and Mauri (1985) and Youssel (1983) also tested the effectiveness of patient education in improving treatment compliance in depressed outpatients. Both studies indicated that patients who received information about their illness were more likely to follow the prescribed treatment regimen.

In a more elaborate patient education study, Seltzer, Roncari, and Garfinkel (1980) provided nine lectures for inpatients on their diagnosis, course of treatment, medication, side effects, relapse, and importance of social support. Based on diagnosis and current medication type, 44 patients with schizophrenia, 16 with bipolar disorder, and 7 with major depression were placed in either education groups or a no-education control group. Compliance was measured through pill counts or medication blood levels. Five months later, patients in the education groups demonstrated greater treatment adherence and were less fearful of side effects and drug dependency than were those in the control group. The noncompliance rate for educational group members was 9%, while the noncompliance rate for the control group was 66%.

These studies provide some examples of the value of patient education. It is difficult to say if the type of effect observed (e.g., decreased side effect and better compliance) is dependent on the type of information provided to patients. Psychiatric patients, like all other patients, can be better participants in the treatment process if they understand the nature of the disorder and their role in its treatment.

Why Family Education Is Important

Angela was diagnosed with bipolar disorder when she was in her first year of college but was able to control her illness fairly well and graduated with honors. After graduation she moved back home to live with her parents until she was well established in her new job in her dad's company and felt confident to live on her own. After several years had passed she was still living with her parents. She resented this arrangement but was fearful of being alone. Angela's parents viewed their daughter as "handicapped," unable to care for herself, and fragile. She was sheltered from stress and little was expected of her at home. She was not pushed to work full time or encouraged to set out on her own. When Angela took on a few challenges at work or by taking some graduate courses, she retreated at the first signs of discomfort.

When meeting for the first time with Angela, it became apparent that she had a number of misconceptions about the illness and her vulnerability to relapse. Her mother, a former nurse, fueled Angela's concerns that she would never lead a "normal" life. She felt the need to avoid exposing Angela to any stress or challenge.

Angela's situation is quite common and provides a good example of why it is important to educate both patients and their family members about the illness.

Most patients' families will have questions about the symptoms of mania and depression, the treatment, and the prognosis for the future. Educating family members about bipolar disorder serves two functions. First, it helps the family members cope with their own pain and suffering and prepares them for difficult times to come. Second, it enlists them as active participants in the treatment process.

Those who live with, have regular contact with, or who may be in a position to assist patients with treatment should be involved in the education process. Spouses, children, and parents are good candidates. Sometimes friends of the family are included as well. The real question is, who does the patient want involved in the treatment? It is necessary to tailor the involvement of significant others to the special needs of each individual. As always, it is important for the clinician to protect patients' confidentiality and to seek their permission before communicating clinical information to their family members.

When to Educate

Every contact with patients and their family members is an opportunity to educate them about living with bipolar disorder. The most obvious time is when the initial diagnosis is made. Often this occurs in an emergency room or inpatient unit when the patient is acutely ill. As patients' mental statuses clear, the education process begins.

After patients' discharge from the hospital, the education process continues. Because, as was mentioned earlier, the symptoms experienced during the acute phase of treatment may have interfered with patients' abilities to grasp all the provided information, clinicians responsible for outpatient follow-up care can probe for how much information was retained and fill in any gaps. Information will be better retained if everyday experiences are used to illustrate the concepts being taught. Each outpatient visit offers an opportunity for clinicians to inquire about the experiences their clients may have had with the symptoms of bipolar disorder and the treatment.

It is common for patients to change health care providers several times during the course of their lives. At each transition point, the education process begins again. Even if individuals previously received care from prominent clinicians with reputations for educating patients and their significant others, those who later care for patients should never assume that further education is unnecessary. Furthermore, as research continues to expand our understanding of the psychobiology and treatment of mood disorders, there will be new information to share.

Clinicians differ in their treatment philosophies. For example, some psychiatrists teach patients to make changes in their medication regimens when breakthroughs of depression or mania seem imminent. Others prefer to discuss any change in dosage with patients before any such adjustment. Patients may not know that there are different strategies for controlling symptoms of bipolar disorder, depending on their symptoms; their lifestyles; and the preferences, training, and comfort of the physicians. They may logically assume that a new psychiatrist will provide the same care as the former one. When treating new patients, clinicians can reduce misunderstandings by sharing their treatment philosophy. If that philosophy of care does not match the patients' needs, it is best to discuss this early in treatment and, if necessary, refer them elsewhere.

How to Educate

Informational materials on bipolar disorder are widely available in bookstores, through the Depression and Bipolar Support Alliance (DBSA)(*www.dbsalliance.org*), and through the National Institute of Mental Health. The Internet is an excellent source of information, from factual data on treatment options to anecdotal accounts of the illness. Online support groups have become popular as alternatives to group therapy. Local chapters of the DBSA conduct educational seminars and self-help groups for people who have bipolar disorder or depression and for their family members. Most organizations invite clinicians and researchers in the community to provide presentations to DBSA groups on a monthly basis.[1]

Methods for Enhancement of Treatment Compliance

The goal of CBT for bipolar disorder is to maximize adherence with pharmacotherapy and other forms of treatment over time. The emphasis on attenuation of compliance assumes that even under the best circumstances, most people will be unable to comply perfectly with treatment at all times, particularly if treatment is lifelong. If the goals and methods of treatment are acceptable to patients, the effort of CBT is to increase the likelihood that treatment will be followed as it is prescribed. This is accomplished by identification and removal of factors that can interfere with compliance.

Our approach uses a variation of behavioral contracting that is refined and augmented with the identification and resolution of obstacles to compliance. This critical element in the contract differs from standard behavioral contracting in that it helps people anticipate impediments to compliance before they appear. This "troubleshooting" process allows for open discussion of adherence with treatment as a mutually agreed on goal rather than as a mandate. Clinicians introduce the notion that full compliance with treatment would be preferable, providing a rationale for the need for consistent use of medication to maximize its effectiveness. If the patient does not agree with this logic, further discussion is necessary to clarify how psychotropic medications work and to determine whether patients have any misconceptions about pharmacotherapy. It is not unusual for people with bipolar disorder to have had bad experiences with medications, particularly if their symptoms had been severe enough to require emergency treatment or hospitalization or if medicines caused severe side effects. These types of experiences may leave patients suspicious about the intentions of their psychiatrists and about the usefulness of pharmacotherapy.

---

[1]Using newer technologies to deliver information on cognitive therapy for depression, Dr. Jesse Wright at the University of Louisville, Department of Psychiatry, has developed a DVD-ROM-based multimedia program that delivers 4–6 hours of cognitive therapy in an interactive format. The program is called "Good Days Ahead" and is available at *www.mindstreet.com*.

Another way in which the CBT approach to compliance differs from traditional behavioral contracting is that no external reward is provided. The focus of the intervention is on patients being consistent with treatment because it makes them feel better. Clinicians can help, but taking medications regularly is ultimately the responsibility of the patient. The consequences for noncompliance are internal and personal. The rewards for compliance must be as well.

The behavioral contracting intervention for improving compliance begins with a clear definition of treatment plans or goals. These include dose schedules for medications (e.g., take 300 mg of lithium in the morning, at noon, and at bedtime), appointment plans (e.g., attend appointment with doctor once each month, attend Alcoholics Anonymous meetings three times next week), and/or homework assignments (e.g., fill out a mood graph each day). To be successful, the patient and the health care provider must both understand and agree on the treatment plan. Once defined, they should be documented in a form that provides a record for both the patient and the clinician. Figure 5.1 provides an example of the first part of a behavioral contract where treatment plans are specified.

The second step in the compliance contract is to identify factors that could potentially keep the patient from taking medication daily. This would include things about the individual (e.g., mood, fears about medications, and forgetfulness) and external influences (e.g., family members discouraging use of medications and conflicting medical advice). Table 5.1 lists some of the common obstacles to adherence with treatment.

To help identify any potential roadblocks to compliance, therapists can inquire about past experiences in which the patient found it difficult to take medicines on a consistent basis. Table 5.2 lists some sample questions that can aid this inquiry.

It can help if the clinician inquires about any particular times of day that doses of medication might be forgotten or missed. Some people rush to work and forget to take their morning doses. Others fall asleep at night before taking the evening dose. Midday doses are hard to remember if the individual is tied up with school, work, child care responsibilities, lunch meetings, or other activities at that time.

To anticipate potential obstacles to adherence, it is sometimes helpful to have patients picture the usual circumstances under which they take their medicines or execute a homework assignment. What are their typical activities during the time that they generally take their medication? Where are they likely to be? Are there any other factors in their environment that may be relevant (e.g., being alone vs. with others, proximity to medication, and mealtime)? The Treatment

---

I, __(patient name)__   , plan to follow the treatment plans
listed below:

 1. Take 900 mg of Lithium CR450 at bedtime

 2. Take 4 mg of Ambien to help me sleep.

 3. See the doctor every month.

 4. Call my doctor if I think I am beginning to have more symp-
    toms or if I think a change in medication is needed. I agree to
    call before making changes to the regimen myself.

FIGURE 5.1. Compliance contract: Part I. Treatment plan.

Obstacles Worksheet in Figure 5.2 provides a format for patients to list potential obstacles.

Part II of the compliance contract lists potential obstacles to adherence (see Figure 5.3). Identifying the obstacles can be the most difficult step in the CBT approach to improved compliance. It is often necessary to use a trial-and-error method by working through initial obstacles and having patients monitor the circumstances that accompany noncompliance. Resolution of obstacles to adherence becomes the immediate goal of treatment.

Some patients who are eager to please their doctors will say that nothing will keep them from taking their medications. While this enthusiasm is usually genuine, the health care provider should not omit discussion of obstacles that although unplanned, could emerge. In these cases, it can be helpful to review past experiences where patients have had difficulty following through with treatment as it was prescribed.

The last section of the compliance contract is for making plans to avoid or overcome the obstacles listed in the second section. For each obstacle, the patient and therapist work out a plan that either reduces the likelihood that it will occur or outlines a way to cope with the obstacle should it interfere with compliance. Ask patients about strategies they have tried in the past to deal with each issue. Modify or add to coping strategies as needed and write out the plan in the third part of the contract (Figure 5.4). In the sections that follow we discuss strategies for addressing the more common obstacles to compliance with medication.

The contract can be developed by any of the health care providers

TABLE 5.1. Obstacles to Adherence

Intrapersonal variables
1. Remission in symptoms and seeing no need for further treatment.
2. Patient ran out of medication. Did not refill prescription.
3. Denial that they have a chronic illness/stigma associated with bipolar illness.
4. Forgetfulness.

Treatment variables
1. Side effects of medication.
2. Medication schedule does not conform to patient's personal schedule.
3. Patient assigned a new doctor who changes treatment plans.

Social system variables
1. Psychosocial stressors.
2. Competing medical advice.
3. Discouragement from family and friends.
4. Publicized stories of others' bad experiences with medications.

Interpersonal variables
1. Poor rapport with the therapist and/or psychiatrist.
2. Busy, uncomfortable, or otherwise unpleasant clinic environment.

Cognitive variables
1. Patient does not like the idea of having to depend on drugs.
2. Patient thinks he or she should be able to handle mood swings on his or her own.
3. Patient misattributes symptoms of bipolar illness to another source.
4. Patient is suspicious of the intentions of the psychiatrist.

working with the patient who are knowledgeable of the treatment plan. It can take up to 45 minutes initially to develop the contract. The contract should be reviewed periodically to modify the treatment goals if necessary, assess for any problems with compliance, and modify the plan for addressing treatment obstacles if needed. Sometimes patients will be more comfortable in admitting problems with adherence to clinicians other than their physicians (e.g., nurses or therapist). They try to make a good impression or fear the consequences of disappointing their doctor by admitting to noncompliance. It is not

TABLE 5.2. How to Inquire about Compliance

- "Everyone has trouble sticking with treatment. Has it ever been a problem for you?"
- "What kinds of things in the past might have kept you from taking medication regularly?"
- "What could keep you from taking your medication everyday?"

critical that the psychiatrist take part in the contract development or review. However, it is important that the treatment plan that forms the basis of the intervention is consistent with the doctor's recommendations. Asking patients to bring in their prescription bottles or speaking directly with the psychiatrist can help to avoid errors.

Reducing Obstacles to Adherence

In the sections that follow we discuss strategies we have found useful in coping with common obstacles to adherence. It should be said, however, that patients' solutions to their own treatment obstacles are often far more effective and creative than those a clinician might generate. Therefore, before launching into any CBT intervention, ask patients how they have coped previously with each obstacle. Prescribe methods that have proven successful or modify them to make them more useful and avoid strategies that have not been effective in patients' experiences.

Intrapersonal Obstacles to Adherence

Among the intrapersonal obstacles to treatment compliance are symptoms, mood, beliefs, attitudes, and fears. The severity of symptoms is an intrapersonal variable that can determine a patient's eagerness to engage in or remain in treatment. Patients with easily noticeable symptoms who desire immediate relief of discomfort are more likely to comply with treatment. If the symptoms are less noticeable and the side effects are uncomfortable, full compliance becomes more doubtful. Some symptoms of bipolar disorder, such as mental confusion, racing thoughts, poor concentration, or memory impairment, may make it difficult for patients to understand fully, recall, or organize themselves well enough to follow through with treatment.

The following are things that could possibly keep me from sticking with my treatment plan:

Practical Problems (e.g., forgetfulness, schedule changes, no money)

_____

_____

_____

Attitude Problems or Fears (e.g., *"I don't have bipolar disorder,"* *"Meds won't work"*)

_____

_____

_____

Life Stresses (family problems, job loss, family discourages medication use)

_____

_____

_____

Treatment-Related Problems (e.g., side effects, problem with doctor or clinic)

_____

_____

_____

Symptoms (e.g., mental confusion, hypomania, getting upset)

_____

_____

_____

FIGURE 5.2. Treatment Obstacles Worksheet.

I anticipate these problems in following my treatment plan:

1. If I continue to gain weight with lithium I may want to stop taking it.

2. The Ambien might stop working and I'll need something stronger.

3. I may not have time to refill my prescriptions.

4. When I get home late I'm too tired go to the kitchen to take my pills.

FIGURE 5.3.   Compliance contract: Part II. Compliance obstacles.

Symptoms of depression or mania can also affect compliance. When depressed, patients may find it difficult to motivate themselves to seek treatment, may be too tired to get up and take medication, or may not be interested in attempting a homework assignment. Feelings of hopelessness may accompany a belief that treatment is useless, so why bother? If hypomanic or euthymic, patients with bipolar disorder may see no need for further medication.

This is a time when family and friends can be particularly helpful in encouraging medication compliance or help seeking. Family members often ask whether or not they should "push" their depressed relatives to get out of bed, shower and dress, take medica-

To overcome these obstacles, I plan to do the following:

1. Join Weight Watchers. Start walking in my neighborhood.

2. Improve sleep by not drinking coffee after 4 P.M. or other caffeinated beverages.

3. Plan ahead. Mark the calendar now for when a refill should be needed.

4. Keep the evening dose at the bedside with a bottle of water.

FIGURE 5.4.   Compliance contract: Part III. Plan for reducing obstacles to adherence.

tion, or see their doctor. The answer is "yes, but gently." The recurrent nature of bipolar disorder does allow for some opportunities to plan ahead to the next episode of illness. When euthymic, patients and their family members can discuss what each should do when depression or mania recurs. For example, Edwin has begun to recover from his depression. He met with his doctor and his parents before leaving the hospital.

DOCTOR: You seem to be doing much better.

EDWIN: I think so. I didn't think I would make it this time.

MOTHER: Neither did we. We were so scared that we would come home from work one day and find him dead.

FATHER: He didn't want to go to the hospital. He didn't take his medication. He didn't want help.

DOCTOR: You started to get depressed 6 months ago, but it seemed manageable to you?

EDWIN: I was able to work up until about a month ago.

DOCTOR: I know you were initially reluctant to call me or to come to the hospital. Do you feel OK about your experience here?

EDWIN: It's OK. I feel better, but I'd rather be home.

DOCTOR: I think if we had been able to catch this episode of depression earlier, we probably could have treated you as an outpatient. If you begin to get depressed again, I wonder what we could do to get you treated more quickly.

MOTHER: I tried to get him to call you, but he refused. That's why I gave up on arguing with him and called you myself.

FATHER: We could see this coming. It was just like the last time.

DOCTOR: What did you see?

FATHER: He kept to himself. Wasn't hungry. He just sat in his room and listened to the radio. We could hear the radio sometimes at 2:00 or 3:00 in the morning. We knew he wasn't sleeping. We thought that maybe he wasn't taking his medicine.

MOTHER: He was tired. He would sleep in and be late for work sometimes and then he just stopped going. They called but what could we tell them? We just said he was sick and they assumed he had that flu that was going around.

DOCTOR: What can your parents do next time, if there is a next time, to motivate you to stay on your medicines and to get help?

EDWIN: Be supportive.

MOTHER: We are supportive!

EDWIN: You nag me every time I look a little tired. If I don't want to eat, you get upset. You always think I'm getting depressed when I'm usually just having a bad day.

DOCTOR: But you are not always "just fine." Like this time, it wasn't just work stress that made you look tired or stop eating.

EDWIN: Sometimes it is serious, but I just get tired of the nagging.

DOCTOR: What can they say when they are worried about you that would not sound like nagging?

EDWIN: (*Pauses.*) They can just say that "I'm worried about you, are you OK?" And if I say yes, they need to drop it.

MOTHER: That's what I do!

EDWIN: No, Mom, you don't believe me so you ask again and again until I get angry.

DOCTOR: Perhaps there's a solution that would get you the help you need without antagonizing you. If your parents agree to ask and then drop it when you say that you are fine, would you be willing to do a couple things?

EDWIN: Like what?

DOCTOR: Take their concerns seriously. Ask yourself if you are beginning to get depressed. You know the signs. If it is not depression, you will not have all the physical symptoms. If you are uncertain or if you think you may be having a return of symptoms, call me so we can do something about it before it gets out of control. Another thing, before you stop taking your medicines altogether, call me so I know what's going on and so we can discuss your plans.

EDWIN: I'm willing, but I'm not sure they can stop nagging.

FATHER: We'll try, but we get nervous. We want to make sure he's OK.

DOCTOR: Let's give this plan a try. If it doesn't work, we'll come up with a better plan. (*To parents*) Here is a list of symptoms of depression. If you are worried, look at the list and ask yourself if he has several symptoms at the same time. If not, it is probably nothing to be concerned about. Everyone feels down or tired from time to time, even your son.

Another type of intrapersonal obstacle to treatment compliance is misconceptions about illness and treatment. For example:

- "You only take medications when you're ill, not when you are feeling better."
- "If you take medications too long, you may become immune to them. Then, when you really need them, they won't work anymore."
- "How will I know if I still need medication if I keep taking it?"
- "When I take the medication, I feel like a pill popper. I'll become dependent on medication if I take it."
- "I resent being controlled by drugs."
- "If my depression is biological, then there is nothing that can be done about it."

The thinking errors that are typical of depressed patients can also interfere with treatment adherence. For example, *selective attention* to the negative aspects of treatment, such as potential side effects or the probability of poor response, may provide patients with more reasons not to take medications than to feel confident about their efficacy. *Overgeneralization* of prior experiences can also be a problem: "Well, I tried medication for this once, and it didn't help me. I don't see why I should take it again." *Personalizing* the bad experiences of others can also influence patients: "My mom took that, and it didn't do her any good," or "My aunt took that medication, and she had a heart attack." *Should* statements (e.g., "I shouldn't need to depend on medication" or "I shouldn't be getting sick") also keep many patients from seeking or following through with treatment.

For some patients, the continued use of medication is an uncomfortable reminder that they are different, that they are plagued with a chronic illness, and that this illness may compromise their future. Omitting the medication eliminates the reminder. In several surveys of patients who take lithium (Jamison, Gerner, & Goodwin, 1979; Johnson, 1973, 1974; Simons, Levine, Lustman, & Murphy, 1984; Vestergaard & Amdisen, 1983), one of the most common reasons that patients gave for discontinuing medication was their dislike of relying on medications to control their mood. In these cases, the obstacle to adherence is the meaning attached to taking medication. Resolution of the problem requires an examination of this special meaning, evaluation of its validity, and a redefinition of "taking medications" that is acceptable to patients and, thus, makes it comfortable for them to comply with medication treatment.

CHARLES: I hate taking these pills.

THERAPIST: What do you hate about it?

CHARLES: They make me thirsty. I've gained all this weight. It's not fair.

THERAPIST: What's not fair?

CHARLES: This stupid illness. Having to be thinking about it all the time. Not being able to do the things normal people do.

THERAPIST: What kinds of things?

CHARLES: Everything!

THERAPIST: Help me understand what you mean by "everything."

CHARLES: Life. My life isn't normal. I'm not normal and I never will be.

THERAPIST: You're right. You have an illness that makes you different from most people. Having to take medicines everyday is part of it. Are there some specific things you would like to do that you feel your illness is keeping you from doing?

CHARLES: Well, uh, I can't stay out all night with my friends like I used to. I can't drink. I'll never be able to fly planes, live free, or just have fun without worrying that I may be having too much fun, you know, losing control.

THERAPIST: Are you saying that having bipolar disorder and taking medicines is like losing your freedom?"

CHARLES: Yeah, like I'm a prisoner, restricted.

THERAPIST: Do you always feel this way?"

CHARLES: No. Most of the time I can deal with it pretty well. It's when the guys come over to watch the game and then want to go party. I have to act like my own mother and say (*sarcastically*), "No, boys. Charlie needs to stay home and take his pills."

THERAPIST: Are those the times when you stop taking your medication?

CHARLES: Yeah. I guess. But I start feeling bad after a while and I have to start taking them again.

THERAPIST: When you stop taking the pills, do you feel like you have more freedom?

CHARLES: No, not really.

THERAPIST: Then how does it [not taking pills] help you?

CHARLES: It doesn't. I'm just mad.

THERAPIST: If it is not helpful, maybe there is something else you can do when you feel like you have lost your freedom that would make you feel better.

CHARLES: Like what?

THERAPIST: Well, it sounds like you have come up with two solutions so far—total freedom, which means no medications and no illness, or total restriction, which means no fun. I wonder if there is any room for compromise?

CHARLES: I guess I could go party but come home before I turn into a werewolf. (*Chuckles*)

THERAPIST: You may be on to something. Maybe we can figure out a way for you to keep your freedom and still maintain your health. Does that sound like a good plan? This way when you begin to feel restricted, you have choices of action other than stopping your medications. What do you think?

CHARLES: OK.

In this example, the patient and therapist can remove the cognitive obstacle to medication adherence by dealing with the patient's feelings of restriction in a more effective way.

Where appropriate, clinicians may address patients' misconceptions about medication by providing them with information. Several studies have demonstrated the effectiveness of patient education in changing patients' attitudes toward the illness (Cohen, 1983; Peet & Harvey, 1991; Seltzer et al., 1980; Van Gent & Zwart, 1991), teaching social strategies for coping with symptoms (Van Gent & Zwart, 1991), and improving compliance (Altamura & Mauri, 1985; Seltzer et al., 1980; Van Gent & Zwart, 1991; Youssel, 1983). In general practice, it is best to provide verbal information to the patient and to recommend supplemental reading on the subject. A list of recommended educational materials can be found in the Appendix to this volume. Informational videotapes are available to supplement readings or verbal instruction. Patients can view these videotapes in the waiting area or in private viewing rooms if space allows.

As it is with other obstacles to compliance, prevention is the key to overcoming intrapersonal obstacles. When beginning treatment, clinicians can inquire about the patients' past experiences with treatment, medication, psychotherapy, and health care providers. Do patients have any concerns about beginning treatment again? Do patients have any concerns about the therapist? Have patients ever had difficulty adhering to treatment? Taking time to discuss this potential difficulty early in the course of treatment provides an opportunity to reduce these obstacles before they cause problems.

Social System Obstacles to Adherence

Family and friends can encourage patients to seek treatment, can provide physical care when needed, and can help patients cope with stress. Family members and friends whose beliefs about treatment are contrary to those of clinicians can negatively influence treatment adherence, however. In particular, if friends or relatives have had or have heard of others having bad experiences with medication, they may discourage patients from taking medications. Moreover, family members who believe that patients should be able to "snap out of it" alone may frown on seeking help from others. The feedback they receive can include:

- "My husband thinks psychiatry is a bunch of baloney."
- "My mom said I just need a vacation away from the kids."
- "After my roommate saw that special on television about medications, she said that, with all the risks involved, I was better off depressed."
- "My dad said only wimps take those pills."

In these cases, it can be helpful to meet with patients and their significant others to discuss these issues and provide all participants with an opportunity to voice their concerns. If patients are willing, it can be beneficial to invite family members to attend some treatment sessions, to call when they have concerns, and to become active in the treatment process. It is helpful to relabel their skepticism about the therapy and the therapist as a sign that they are interested in the patients' well-being. It is particularly important for clinicians to control their level of defensiveness and try to model open-mindedness and respect for others' opinions.

Competing medical advice is one of the most powerful social obstacles to compliance. The source of the advice can be other health care providers, television news or talk shows, newspapers, magazine articles, or the *Physicians' Desk Reference* (2003):

"When I lived in California, my therapist said I had psychological problems which stem from my dysfunctional family. He said I needed long-term psychotherapy, not medication. My family doctor says that you can get hooked on those drugs, so he never let me have them."

Clinicians take a big risk if they try to discount the words of other clinicians with whom patients may be allied. One clinician's dismissing the advice of other clinicians forces patients into the awkward position of having to choose which clinician to believe. A strategically safer position is to assume that, given the information available at the time, the recommendations may have been valid or that patients may have incorrectly recalled the views of other clinicians. Before openly disagreeing with another clinician, therapists should demonstrate an attempt to understand the competing advice. For example, the therapist may ask patients what they think about the competing advice. If they are uncertain which treatment approach is best for them, the therapist can discuss it further, refer them to readings on the subject, and/or suggest that they get another opinion.

If published materials are the source of competing medical advice, take time to discuss these materials with patients. The descriptions of potential side effects of medications listed in the Physicians' Desk Reference, for example, frequently frighten both patients and family members. It is useful to discuss with patients the probability of such problems, to weigh these effects against the potential beneficial effects of treatment, and to develop a plan for assessment of their occurrence and intervention, if necessary.

Stressors as Obstacles to Adherence

Psychosocial stressors, such as marital problems, financial strains, or unemployment, can interfere with treatment in three ways. First, people who are preoccupied with problems of daily living can forget to take medications, to complete homework assignments, or even to keep appointments. Second, stressors consume time that might otherwise be set aside for treatment-related activities (e.g., going to a support group meeting). Third, stressors exacerbate symptoms. For example, stress can keep people awake at night. The lack of sleep can, in turn, cause fatigue, lethargy, decreased motivation, or even bring on a manic episode.

Nelly had a lot on her mind. Her company had been sold, and she was afraid of losing her job soon. It had been difficult for her to find this job, and she worried that she might not be so lucky the next time. Nelly's bipolar disorder had incapacitated her for lengthy periods of time in the past 8 years. Her employment record was full of holes that were difficult to explain to potential employers. She lay awake at night thinking about these problems. When she finally fell asleep, she was restless. In the morning, she was tired and easily fatigued. Nelly knew that, without sleep, she would begin to experience the symptoms of mania before too long. Although she might be taking her medication as prescribed, it was not sufficient to prevent a breakthrough of symptoms if her sleeplessness persisted. If she recognized the emergence of symptoms, she could choose to intervene with pharmacological agents to improve her sleep, with problem-solving methods to cope with her stressors, or with behavioral techniques to facilitate sleep.

The appropriate interventions for reducing the psychosocial stressors that interfere with treatment vary according to the type of stressor. A structured problem-solving approach may be effective for problems that are under the patient's control (Chapter 10). Interpersonal problems, such as marital or family conflict, child behavior problems, or getting along with friends, may require conjoint counseling for patients and these significant others (Chapters 12). For psychosocial stressors such as unemployment, medical problems, indebtedness, or school problems for children, it may be useful to enlist the help of social service agencies. Until a stressor can be removed effectively, a compensatory plan is needed to deal with symptoms (e.g., sleeplessness) and treatment obstacles (e.g., forgetfulness).

Treatment-Related Obstacles to Adherence

Factors within the treatment regimen that make it difficult for patients to comply include complex combinations or dosages of medicines that are difficult to remember, side effects, and dosing schedules that are inconsistent with the individual's personal schedule.

> Mrs. Henry was to take her medication first thing in the morning, around lunchtime, and before bedtime. She was a late sleeper, however, and inevitably missed her morning dose. She often stayed up to watch the late movies on television and delayed taking her medication on these evenings because they made her sleepy. Sometimes, she would fall asleep during a movie before she had taken her bedtime dose of medication.

In most cases, tailoring the treatment regimen to patients' schedules and lifestyles prevents treatment-related obstacles to adherence. In practice, it may be necessary to match dosing schedules to patients' daily routines. For example, reducing the number of daily doses needed by using single-dose sustained-release formulations simplifies regimens and decreases the likelihood that patients will miss doses. The use of sustained-release lithium preparations has several advantages. Studies have shown that sustained-release formulations produce a steady serum lithium concentration more easily and reliably (Arancibia, Flores, & Pezoa, 1990; Caldwell, Westlake, Schriver, & Bumbier, 1981; Wallis, Miller, & McFadyen, 1989). There appear to be no significant differences in the total lithium bioavailability of sustained-release versus standard lithium carbonate preparations (Caldwell et al., 1981; Cooper, Simpson, Lee, & Bergner, 1978). Moreover, although somewhat controversial, there seem to be no significant differences in the side-effect profiles of the sustained-release and standard lithium formulations (Lyskowski & Nasrailah, 1981).

For antidepressants, the literature on using a once-daily versus multiple-dose regimen has concluded that, for many patients, single (generally nighttime) doses of antidepressants are as effective as a multiple-dose regimen. Specifically, patients achieve comparable medication blood levels on the two dosing regimens and patients report similar levels of treatment response. When differences do exist, it is generally in favor of the single-dose regimen. It is suggested that this is due to decreased reporting of side effects with a nighttime-only dose as side effects generally occur during the first few hours after ingestion while the patient is asleep. Single-dose schedules as opposed to multiple-dose schedules are less complicated and therefore may improve patient compliance to treatment.

In tailoring a medication regimen to patients' needs, it is helpful to consider the patient's daily activities.

> Mr. Sanders experienced a worsening of manic symptoms at the end of the day. His fast-paced and high-pressured job stimulated him. By evening, he had difficulty unwinding, turning off his thoughts about the day, and falling asleep. Because the evening activation had led to sleeplessness and eventually mania in the past, Mr. Sanders' doctor had tailored his medication regimen to this variation in symptoms. In addition, the doctor allowed Mr. Sanders to have a small amount of extra medication to help him sleep when needed.

Although the general philosophy is to minimize the number of medications prescribed, in this case, flexibility in this responsible patient helps to prevent mania.

If a regimen requires multiple daily doses of more than one medication, the dosing times can be difficult to remember for some patients. If the medication is purely prophylactic, there are no symptoms to cue individuals to take it. In this case, it can be helpful to pair pill taking with another regularly occurring event such as eating a meal, brushing one's teeth, or having a cup of coffee in the morning. Some pocket-size pill containers have alarms built into them as reminders. With time, pill taking can become part of the daily routine just like dressing or eating.

Fitting the Treatment into a Teenager's Lifestyle

Chloe came to therapy eager to learn about cognitive therapy. She was a bright 18-year-old high school senior who had been diagnosed with bipolar disorder in her freshman year. She has read all the books, attended support group meetings, and saw her doctor with regularity for medication visits. She did not seem to have much trouble with depression, but she had been hospitalized twice during manic episodes and was perpetually hypomanic. Her friends found her to be great fun. Her teachers thought her smart and creative. And the boys couldn't get enough of her. She had recently put a scare into her parents when she drove her car into the countryside presumably in search of her favorite rock star. When she ran out of gas and realized she had no money, she called her mother to ask for help. When Chloe could not tell her where she was and sounded desperate to find this music star who she thought was on location for a new video, her mother knew that Chloe was manic. Luckily, with the help of the gas station attendant, Chloe's mom was able to locate her daughter and pick her up before she encountered any danger.

At one level Chloe knew she was acting irrationally and impulsively, while at another level she didn't care. She felt caught up in the excitement of the adventure and didn't care about the consequences. On the ride home, her mother berated her for her irresponsibility and with angry words and tears, communicated to Chloe her exasperation.

"You have to take responsibility for your illness, Chloe. You can't keep doing this to us. When are you going to get it into your head that you are not like other kids? Sure, other kids do dumb things and worry their parents. But they do not end up in the middle of nowhere, run out of gas, and then don't have the presence of mind to even know where they are! What if we couldn't find you and you really flipped out!?"

Chloe didn't want to hear it, but she had to admit that she had scared herself as well. She wanted desperately to be like the other kids. The medicine she took made her dull and slow and fat. She thought she knew herself well enough to know when she needed to take it and when she didn't. But watching her mother cry made her doubt herself.

One of the challenges that teenagers diagnosed with bipolar disorder face is how to live the life of an adolescent with its pleasures and pain and cope with a chronic and debilitation illness. Periods of depression interfere with attainment of normal developmental milestones. Manic episodes witnessed by peers can cause embarrassment and social rejection. The hypersexuality and risk-taking behaviors experienced by "normal" teens are elevated in kids with bipolar disorder and add health and psychosocial problems to their burdens of coping with the illness. Attention and concentration problems can interfere with learning which, in turn, affects opportunities for the future.

The treatments aimed at preventing relapse in adolescents are not without problems. Medications can cause side effects that teens find intolerable. The recommended lifestyle alterations such as reducing overstimulation or avoiding sleep loss may not be realistic or acceptable, particularly if there are other children living at home who do not have the illness and are, therefore, not subject to these restrictions.

Getting adolescents to comply with everyday requirements at school or chores at home is a challenge for most parents. Teens resent these impositions on their time. Getting adolescents with bipolar disorder to comply with pharmacotherapy and lifestyle restrictions in addition to school and home requirements is a greater challenge and the resentment of having to be different can fuel noncompliance.

Kids, Parents, and Medication: Who's in Charge?

Monitoring and distributing medications is the responsibility of parents for young children with bipolar disorder. The ideal scenario for adolescents is that they assume responsibility for taking their own medications daily with parents monitoring the need for refills. This ideal scenario, however, is not likely to occur in any adolescent. More often parents remind, nag, cajole, or coerce their children on a daily basis. This adds to the normal developmental tug-of-war between parents and teens as the teens attempt to establish independence from their parents.

While kids do not want their parents to micromanage their medications, most lack the organizational skills to manage it consistently on their own. Parents complain about having to remind their kids to take medications, but it is unrealistic to assume that kids can comply without some assistance.

The most direct path to resolve compliance problems in bipolar teens is for therapists to facilitate a conversation between them and their parents.

THERAPIST: Thank you both for coming in today. I wanted us to have a chance to talk about how to best help Dante take his medications daily. I know this has been a stressful issue for both of you, but I think we can find a way around it.

MOTHER: I don't know why this has to be such a big deal. He knows what will happen to him if he doesn't take it. He just needs to be responsible. I take my high blood pressure medicine everyday. I told him he just needs to do what I do. Put it on the bathroom counter and take it as soon as he wakes up.

THERAPIST: Dante, have you tried following your mother's advice?

DANTE: I try to remember, but sometimes I get up late and I'm in a hurry. I tell myself to take it after I shower, but I forget.

MOTHER: I ask him about it as he's leaving the house and he always says "yes," but I look in his pillbox and they are still there. He doesn't want me to treat him like a baby, but I swear that boy would never take them if I didn't remind him.

THERAPIST: Dante, is it OK for your mom to remind you?

DANTE: I hate it when she nags me. I can do it on my own most of the time. But if I'm in a hurry I forget whether I took it or not and by the time I get home and see them in the box, it's too late.

THERAPIST: Do you think you need those morning medicines?

DANTE: Yeah, I guess so. I mean, when I don't take them for a couple of days, I can tell.

THERAPIST: What happens to you?

DANTE: I get mad. I don't want to be at school. I can't understand the teacher. I just want to get out of there.

THERAPIST: So you do better if you take the medicine every day?

DANTE: I probably do.

MOTHER: So then why do you get so mad when I tell you to take them?

DANTE: I hate being told what to do!

MOTHER: You see? I don't know what to do with him.

THERAPIST: Let's think of some solutions to the problem that work for both of you.

Therapists can lead the discussion toward a compromise where the patients get support for taking medicine rather than nagging and the parent feels less stressed or burdened. One possibility is rather than trying to get a child to conform to the prescribed dosing regimen, the regimen is changed to fit the child's lifestyle. In Dante's case it may be helpful to move his morning dose to after school or before bedtime rather than continuing to have problems taking medication as soon as he wakes up.

A second consideration is to alter the expectation of the parent. All parents would like their children to spontaneously comply with instructions without reminders, but this is not within the ability of most children. Normalizing this dynamic with parents may help them to have more realistic expectations. Once this adjustment has been made, parents can assist or remind in a neutral tone instead of with annoyance, resentment, or disappointment. If there are children in the family who are naturally more organized, mature, or compulsive, who would take responsibility for keeping up with medication, help adjust parents' expectations of the child with bipolar disorder by getting them to contrast the strengths and weaknesses of the two children, any developmental differences, and factors associated with the illness that might be relevant to compliance.

To reach a compromise between the parent and child, ask the child what his mother or father could do to be helpful. Dante asked his mom to hand him a pill and glass of water when she came into his room to wake him up each morning. Dante's mother preferred that he handle this on his own but conceded that his plan would take less of her energy than nagging him.

If a request is being made of the parent to change his or her behavior, the child should be asked what he or she would be willing to do in return. In Dante's case he agreed to take the pill right away and without argument. He also agreed to fill his pillbox each week and take the bedtime dose more consistently. The therapist helped him through the problem-solving steps to find a reminder system that worked for Dante.

Once a plan has been made for increasing adherence, a check on the new system should be made after a trial period. Both parent and child should report on their experiences and modifications made as needed.

Not all parents are organized or regimented enough to take medications themselves on a daily basis. A simple intervention that helps patients stay on track with their medications is to use divided pill containers. The advantage of divided pill containers is that they can help to reduce the conflict patients sometimes have with their family members over whether or not the former have taken their medications. Though not a foolproof method, if patients agree to leave their containers in an accessible place, family members can look at the clear plastic pill containers rather than confront patients when they suspect noncompliance.

With the advent of electronic devices such as alarm watches, personal digital assistants (PDAs), or schedule reminders on computers, there are newer methods available to cue people to take their medications.

Homework Noncompliance

Behavioral interventions assigned at therapy sessions require initiative by the patient between visits. No matter how well the homework is designed, and how supportive the therapist, execution of the assignment ultimately depends on the patient's willingness to give it a try. People can be resistant to trying new things or reinitiating activities they have avoided for some time.

Caution should be taken, however, in how the therapist approaches the discussion of homework compliance. Specifically, some patients will feel guilty for not completing an assigned task. They may be concerned about disappointing the therapist with their noncompliance. If the therapist communicates criticism or disappointment either verbally or nonverbally, patients may feel worse and the therapeutic relationship may suffer. Patients must feel like they are doing homework to help themselves, rather than to please the therapist. A therapist can do several things to reinforce this notion. First, when homework is assigned early in therapy, the therapist can emphasize that therapy sessions only last 1 hour each week. To be helpful, the majority of the work of therapy has to be done between sessions. The pace of therapy, to a great degree, depends on the amount of work patients do between sessions. Second, although guided by the therapist, homework tasks should be designed by the patient. This collaboration helps patients to "own" the homework task. Third, the therapist can ask patients to predict how they would feel talking to the therapist about being unable to complete the homework. The therapist should explore the patient's reasoning and provide corrective feedback about his or her own reaction.

Fourth, in designing a homework assignment, the therapist must consider whether the patient has the resources to carry out the task. For example, before giving a lengthy reading assignment, the therapist must consider not only whether the patient has money to purchase a book, or transportation to the library, but also whether he or she can concentrate well enough to read. The therapist should not set a patient up for failure by not taking time to consider the feasibility of homework tasks.

Fifth, the therapist should always take time to review homework at each session, preferably at the beginning of each session. This communicates that the assignment was important and worth discussion. Sixth, if the homework assignment was not completed, the therapist should reevaluate its importance, usefulness, and feasibility before it is reassigned. Maybe after more thought the patient decided it was a bad idea or maybe he or she thought of another way to approach the task. If the therapist believes that it is better not to reassign the homework, he or she should cancel the task rather than leave it uncompleted. If not withdrawn from the patient's list of things "to do," homework can become as burdensome as other uncompleted chores.

Mastering adherence with treatment is an ongoing process. Because people vary in their degree of compliance across time, the issue should be revisited periodically throughout the course of treatment. If a therapeutic environment has been established where conversations about treatment adherence are comfortable, inquiries about treatment-related behaviors and obstacles to adherence can become a routine part of medication or psychotherapy visits.

While improvements to adherence are being made, the next step in CBT for bipolar disorder can be taken—developing an early-warning system for recurrences of depression and mania. Chapter 6 covers methods for increasing surveillance of symptoms.

Key Points for the Therapist to Remember

♦ It is important to establish a precedent of discussing compliance issues at the outset of treatment. However, clinicians must first come to accept the fact that patients are not always going to follow directions, even if they are clearly explained, are in the best interest of the patient, and will greatly help the patient's condition.

♦ A person who does not understand the importance or purpose of the treatment has no reason to comply with it.

♦ Clinicians can help their patients to be knowledgeable consumers by encouraging them to ask questions and to be as active in treatment planning as they are expected to be in the execution of the regimen.

♦ The goal of CBT for bipolar disorder is to maximize adherence with pharmacotherapy and other forms of treatment over time. The emphasis on attenuation of compliance assumes that even under the best circumstances, most people will be unable to comply perfectly with treatment at all times, particularly if treatment is lifelong.

♦ Getting adolescents with bipolar disorder to comply with pharmacotherapy and lifestyle restrictions in addition to school and home requirements is a great challenge and the resentment of having to be different can fuel noncompliance.

Points to Discuss with Patients

♦ It is important to introduce the idea that full compliance can be difficult to achieve even when a person has the best intentions.

♦ It is not unusual for patients to feel apprehensive about treatment. They might agree to follow treatment recommendations while in the office but do not follow through at home. Inquiring about patients' feelings and concerns gives health care providers opportunities to address these issues before they interfere with treatment.

♦ Educating family members about bipolar disorder serves two functions. First, it helps the family members cope with their own pain and suffering and prepares them for difficult times to come. Second, it enlists them as active participants in the treatment process.

♦ It is not unusual for people with bipolar disorder to have had bad experiences with medications, particularly if their symptoms had been severe enough to require emergency treatment or hospitalization or if medicines caused severe side effects. These types of experiences may leave patients suspicious about the intentions of their psychiatrists and about the usefulness of pharmacotherapy.

♦ Everyone has trouble sticking with treatment. Has it ever been a problem for you?

♦ What kinds of things in the past might have kept you from taking medication regularly?

♦ What could keep you from taking your medication everyday?

♦ Before launching into any CBT intervention to improve adherence, ask patients how they have coped previously with each obstacle. Prescribe methods that have proven successful or modify them to make them more useful and avoid strategies that have not been effective in patients' experiences.

♦ For some patients, the continued use of medication is an uncomfortable reminder that they are different, that they are plagued with a chronic illness, and that this illness may compromise their futures. Omitting the medication eliminates the reminder.

♦ The most direct path to resolve compliance problems in bipolar teens is for therapists to facilitate a conversation between them and their parents.

CHAPTER 6

Early Detection to Prevent Relapse

As mentioned in the beginning of this book, the strength of CBT is in its potential for improving the overall course of bipolar disorder. Through early detection of recurrence or relapse, opportunities are provided to intervene before patients reach the depths of major depression or the heights of mania.

Rhonda has struggled to control her bipolar disorder over the past 15 years. She suffered through two long episodes of major depression, each lasting several years and several shorter episodes. She has only had one severe manic episode that led to a hospitalization, but has continued to have break throughs of hypomanic symptoms

To control her illness, Rhonda has tried several medications (mostly antidepressants), with limited success. She tried counseling, group therapy, and self-help groups. While these have helped in managing her stress they did not seem to keep her mood stable. Her life has centered around fighting off depression and keeping her hypomania from getting out of control while trying to work and raise her two daughters. Rhonda feels victimized by her illness. She often feels helpless to resist the biological fluctuations that tossed her about, knocking her feet out from under her, and toppling her plans.

Luckily, Rhonda has a very supportive husband who gives her encouragement when she is low and takes away her credit cards when he sees her getting too high. While she appreciates his efforts, she hates burdening him with her illness. Sometimes she fantasizes about running away from home or ending her life. A good night's sleep usually gives her new hope or changes her mood or buys her time to tell her husband about her desperate thoughts. Although it is difficult, Rhonda has found a way to stay as healthy as possible. She knows when changes are coming and heads them off with medication or by changing her behavior.

Rhonda is an example of a typical patient with bipolar disorder who has had many ups and downs and is still symptomatically unstable. To help patients like her get a handle on their mood fluctuations, it is necessary to understand which symptoms emerge first in the sequence of depression and mania, which factors might precipitate the mood shifts, and responses by the patient that either help control symptoms or cause them to worsen. Once these facts are known, the therapist can assist the patient in planning ahead for recurrences and symptom breakthroughs. Early intervention involves recognizing the earliest presentation of symptoms and making adjustments that contain their progression. Constructing a Life Chart and completing the Symptom Summary Worksheet and Mood Graphs are the CBT exercises that aid the development of an early-warning system. The Life Chart is a time line that graphically represents the onset and offset of each episode of illness, including comorbid conditions, such as periods of anxiety or substance abuse. Major life events and treatments should be added. Often there is an association between the onset of the first few episodes, either depression or mania, and major life events such as losses; physical illness and injury; or changes in jobs, family, or home (Ambelas, 1979; Glassner, Haldipur, & Dessauersmith, 1979). However, that association lessens over time as recurrences become more unpredictable.

Other common factors that precipitate recurrences of depression and mania include discontinuation of medications, periods of sleep deprivation, substance abuse, and overstimulation (Wehr, Sack, & Rosenthal, 1987; Wehr & Wirz-Justice, 1982; Brown et al., 2001). These precipitants can occur secondary to job changes, travel, childbirth, and anything else that alters the sleep/wake cycle. All these events should be documented on the life chart. Although the accuracy of the life chart is limited by the recall of the patient, it is a useful exercise for people to begin to see patterns in what might otherwise seem like random fluctuations in mood.

The Symptom Summary Worksheet sensitizes people to the affective, cognitive, behavioral, and physical changes that occur during depression, mania, and hypomania. These symptomatic states are contrasted with euthymic or normal states so that the patient can begin to distinguish illness-related changes from normal fluctuations. Identification of mild to moderate forms of symptoms is encouraged as well as experimental changes that are unique to the person and not necessarily prototypical of the illness.

Janice, for example, notices that loud noises bother her more when she is entering hypomania. Bob wants to buy new tools when he is getting high. Roxanne becomes aware that colors are brighter as her mood begins to climb. In the early stages of depression, Saul has to reread newspaper articles because his mind seems to wander. Delores wants to eat junk food rather than cook and Marta has little patience for her children's complaints about school, teachers, or friends.

While the Symptom Summary Worksheet focuses on experiences within episodes, Mood Graphs track daily fluctuations in present symptoms. Mood may not always be the best variable to monitor because cognitive, physical, or behavioral changes may be more prominent or more noticeable to the patient. In this chapter we provide a standard format for Mood Graphs, but it is more useful for patients to create their own tracking system that fits with their conceptualization of mood shifts. Directions for constructing Life Charts, Symptom Summary Worksheets, and Mood Graphs follow later in this chapter.

The Dilemma of Decreasing Hypomania

When the therapist has developed trusting relationships with patients whom he or she has seen through several episodes of depression, the therapist wants them to experience relief from their sadness so that they can improve the quality of their lives, reach their goals, or just have a break from feeling badly. When patients occasionally switch into hypomania, it is not unreasonable for the therapist to have mixed feelings about it. On the one hand the therapist is concerned that their hypomania could blossom into mania and cause them considerable grief if it were to get out of control. On the other hand, it is nice for the therapist to see patients laugh for a change. Their sense of hope returns, they see possibilities that were hidden from them during their depressions, and they seem joyful. Therapists hate to play a part in taking away their relief from misery, but the therapist would not be doing the patient a service if he or she did not share concern that the patient was becoming manic and help the patient to put the proper precautions into place.

This happened recently with a patient (MRB) I have treated for about 5 years.

Lillian is a wonderful person, a good mother, and a hard worker. She tries not to let her low moods get her down, but fighting that uphill battle takes a toll on her. She has periods of feeling exhausted and discouraged, angry and hopeless, bewildered and regretful. During those times, death seems like a reasonable alternative. Her medications have successfully kept her from becoming manic and have relieved many of the severe symptoms of depression, but I can see in her eyes the wear and tear of struggling against the tide of her sadness and fatigue. Like many people with bipolar disorder, residual depression is the norm for her life.

Lillian called me after not having seen me for several months to ask my opinion about her mood. Her husband thought she was acting "a little weird" and she had to admit that she could feel some agitation inside. She wanted to know if I thought she was manic. One look at her in the waiting room with a big smile on her usually neutral face and I knew that she was different. Hearing the hardiness of her laughter as she made a funny comment about her trip to my office reminded me of the last time she was hypomanic. She asked me to be honest with her, but it was obvious that she did not really want bad news. We tried to stay objective and reviewed her symptoms, her changes in behavior, and her improved attitude. At this early stage of hypomania, she did not have any problems. In fact, she functioned better than usual. She had new ideas for work that were creative and reasonable. She had more energy to follow through with the mounting tasks in her home that had been put off for many months. She caught up with neglected friends by telephone, joked around with her daughter more, and gave her husband more attention. Everyone was pleased but nervous.

Using CBT methods to help this patient prevent relapse had worked fairly well over the years. She avoided mania and suffered from only mild fatigue, a neutral mood, and lowered motivation that comes with residual depression. Because she and her psychiatrist found that adding antidepressants to her pharmacological regimen inevitably made her hypomanic, she compensated for her symptoms by using CBT methods and her internal fortitude to keep up with her family and work responsibilities even when she would rather stay in bed. We no longer met regularly as she and her husband and daughter were practiced in monitoring the onset of symptoms. She would call when she thought they might be returning. We would work together on helping her be more consistent with medication, discussed her reemerging anger at having the illness, and made plans for preventing her symptoms from worsening. She knew to consult her psychiatrist and would do so. We would meet weekly with sometimes a midweek telephone check-in, particularly if mania was suspected, until her symptoms remitted once again. Relapse prevention had worked.

However, when she presented recently with symptoms of hypomania, I asked how I could help her. She said she wanted me to help her stay hypomanic for a while. She knew that she could not afford to get manic and that her euphoria could quickly change to irritability and agitation, and she was worried that her hypomania might show at work. She felt in control for the time being, but she did not entirely trust the illness. It could flare up and her desire to enjoy a period without depression might make her ignore the signs and symptoms of mania.

Being highly experienced with the illness, she did not need a lecture from me on the dangers of hypomania. She knew what to do and she had to decide where to set the limit. I could only empathize with her wanting to prolong the relief from depression, encourage her to follow her own good advice about precautions, and be available if she needed me. Otherwise the ball was in her court.

CBT methods can be powerful tools in helping people with bipolar disorder to avoid relapse. But people have to decide for themselves if they want to use them. The possibility of mania can be seductive, especially for those who have euphoric manias and who have been plagued with more lows than highs in the course of their illnesses. Part of the relapse prevention methodology is helping people come to terms with the need for controls to be placed on their actions in order to maintain euthymia and avoid mania.

Examination of the advantages and disadvantages of using relapse prevention methodologies is one method of helping people decide if they are ready to take control of their illness. Rather than trying to convince them to be consistent with medications, monitor their symptoms, normalize their schedule, or give up overstimulating activities, the person must convince him- or herself that lifestyle management is worth the effort.

The Advantages and Disadvantages of Self-Control

When people with bipolar disorders come to therapy it is usually with some encouragement from doctors, therapists, or family members, all of whom have advocated self-control of some sort. When they are ready to take this step in treatment they will say, with honesty, that they will do whatever it takes to prevent relapse. However, in reality, they do not always know what this entails. Most do not know what they will have to give up in order to gain greater stability. And when they find out, they are often not very happy. Teenagers hate giving up their late nights, adults hate giving up alcohol, and no one wants to give up the highs if they have been lucky enough to have them without getting into trouble.

Cognitive therapists are trained to provide a rationale for any intervention they present to patients, and that is also true for treating those with bipolar disorder. What must come before teaching the specific interventions for relapse prevention is an acceptance of the rationale that self-control and lifestyle management can lead to fewer symptoms. To accomplish this task, the therapist must provide an overview of the rationale behind relapse prevention. This includes informing or reminding patients that their illness is chronic and recurrent and that it will need to be managed for the rest of their lives. Although people who have the illness know this, hearing it again and finding out the details of relapse prevention can stir up a lot of negative feelings about the illness and its treatment.

The element of relapse prevention that people take issue with first is the perceived restriction placed on their lifestyle. To decrease the chance of relapse, they will need to regulate their sleep/wake cycle, limit alcohol and recreational drug use, and avoid sources of overstimulation that they might otherwise find enjoyable. Some will see this as punishment for having the illness. Their displeasure with the idea may cause them to magnify their perception of the amount of restriction required and perhaps temporarily lead to resistance to or rejection of therapeutic suggestions.

To cope with these reactions, the therapist should first empathize with the patient's distress and avoid "looking at the bright side" of treatment. Socratic questions can be used to clarify the patient's perceptions of the illness, the treatment, and what he or she can do to affect the cause of the illness. Any inaccuracies can be addressed with patient education rather than using logical analysis techniques.

If the patient still has hesitations about CBT and the relapse preventions strategies or is upset about having to make lifestyle changes, a more formal thought analysis procedure may be needed. One method is to evaluate the advantages and disadvantages of making the needed changes to prevent relapse and the advantages and disadvantages of maintaining the status quo. Using a two-by-two grid, the therapist asks the patient to write down what he or she thinks or has been told are the pros and cons of making the lifestyle changes necessary to control the illness. The therapist must remember not to encourage a one-sided analysis of the options. To be convinced that change is needed, the patient must not feel pressured by anyone but him- or herself.

After completion of the four boxes, the therapist asks the patient to pick the most important items from each box. This should be limited to one or two items. Examination of the themes surrounding the most important items from each box should reveal a pattern with one compelling reason to exercise self-control, such as avoiding the stress that relapse places on the patient and family members, and one compelling reason not to, such as losing freedom or giving up the joys of life.

Stress, freedom, and joy are all fairly subjective concepts but can be addressed by operationalizing each. What does the person mean by giving up freedom or joy? Joe, a college student, said it meant never being able to go out with his friends. When they are starting their evening out, Joe would be getting ready for bed. For Barbara, it meant being unable to stay up late with her new husband, who is a night owl, and her marriage suffering as a consequence. These reactions have a flavor of catastrophizing or magnifying the negative that can be addressed with education, negotiation, and/or logical analysis methods.

Once the cognitive distortions have been identified and addressed, the final part of the task is to brainstorm with the patient on ways to maximize the advantages of self-control and lifestyle management while minimizing the disadvantages. Chapters 7 through 10 on behavioral and cognitive interventions for depression and mania provide a number of ideas for meeting this challenge. In general, some self-monitoring and limit setting are required, but complete restriction and deprivation are unnecessary.

Life Charts to Get the Big Picture

During the first few therapy sessions, patients and their therapists can work together to construct Life Charts. The process of constructing a Life Chart can be very educational for the patient, especially when medication noncompliance has predated recurrences of symptoms. The first step in constructing a Life Chart is to draw a reference line in the middle of the page that represents a euthymic or "normal" state (see Figure 6.1). Many patients report that they have never felt "normal"; therefore, the reference line must represent relative normalcy, that is, relative to the extremes of depression and mania that the person has experienced. For example:

> "Think of a time when you felt a lot better. Maybe you were able to do more, think more clearly. That will represent the middle of the graph. You have had days when you felt more depressed than that, and you have had days when you felt more hyper or manic than that."

The line represents the passage of time from the beginning of your illness to present. Use the sample episodes from Figure 6.2 to draw out your pattern of depression and mania over time.

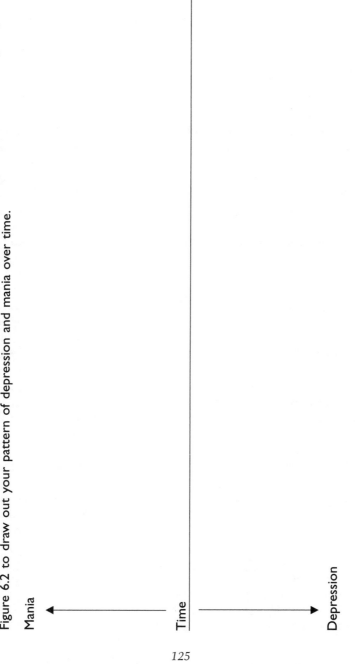

Mania

Time

Depression

FIGURE 6.1. Life Chart.

The second step is to draw the episodes of depression, mania, and mixed states on the time line. Points below the reference line represent depression; points above the line indicate mania. Figure 6.2 provides examples of how these episodes might be represented. The greater the distance from the reference line, the more severe the symptoms. The width of each episode on the time line reflects the relative length of the episode. The onset of the illness should be on the far left end of the chart, the patient's current mood state on the far right end. The Life Chart shows the evolution of the illness from its beginning to the present. Figure 6.3 is a sample Life Chart.

In most instances, patients can draw their own Life Charts. Begin by explaining how the chart works. Draw a reference life for patients and explain how depressions and manias are depicted. Ask how they are feeling now and mark the far right side of the line as is shown in Figure 6.1. Next, ask when they believe the current symptoms began. Another way to think about it is to ask them to recall when they last felt well, asymptomatic, or "normal." Make a mark on the line, note the approximate date, and ask them to draw how the symptoms evolved from the start point to the present time. The next step is to draw the first episode together. Give the patient a pencil and the chart and ask him or her to draw in the remaining episodes.

If an individual has had numerous episodes of illness, the construction of a Life Chart may be difficult. In other cases, the course of bipolar disorder does not begin with an easily defined, distinct episode of depression or mania. There may have been problems at school, at home, or on the job, or there may have been some difficulty in getting along with others. It is usually easiest to start with the most recent episode and work backward in time. It can also be helpful for the patient to try to recall hospitalizations or emergency room visits and use these events as reference points for episodes. Reviewing medical records or talking with family members can also help flesh out the patient's course of illness for a Life Chart.

The next step is to fill in the types and dates of treatments received. The medical record may be particularly helpful in completing this task. Although a clinician may have prescribed medications over distinct periods of time, it is possible and even likely that the patient did not always take them. This part of Life Chart construction provides the clinician with an opportunity to introduce the topic of medication compliance by simply conveying that many people have difficulty taking medications regularly, especially if they are feeling better or are having uncomfortable side effects. Does the patient recall taking medications regularly prior to each episode of illness? When appropriate, write in "stopped medication."

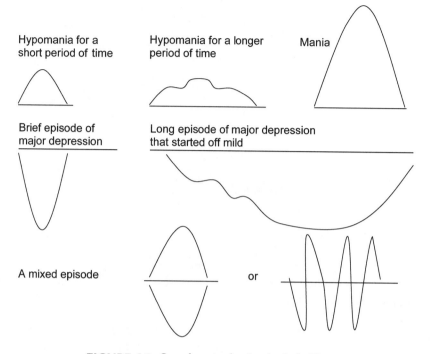

FIGURE 6.2. Sample episodes for the Life Chart.

Developing an Early-Warning System

Everyone has fluctuations in mood in reaction to factors in the environment such as stress, good news, disappointments, or internal events such as humor, hormone shifts, fatigue, worry, and affection. In fact, within a single day it is not unusual for a person to experience several different mood states. Because it is normal for people to react emotionally to both internal (e.g., recollections and fears) and external (e.g., football and television commercials) stimuli, patients with bipolar disorder will have "normal" mood shifts and "abnormal" or symptomatic mood shifts. The challenge for clinicians, patients, and their family members is to differentiate the two.

Normal mood fluctuations are transient and/or tied to specific stimulus events. When the stimulus event has passed, the mood slowly returns to normal. Some stressful events, such as divorce, will have an enduring impact and are not considered abnormal. The stresses involved are not discrete events that end when the person goes to sleep; each day may present new problems or powerful reminders of

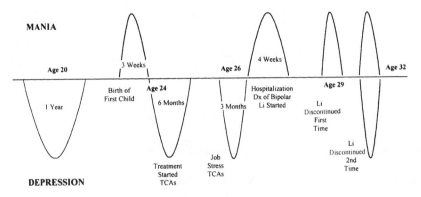

FIGURE 6.3. Sample Life Chart.

the old. Other events (e.g., death in the family) may be discrete, but the emotional reaction may persist for some time. As a general rule, once a stressor has ceased, a person's mood should begin to improve. A persistent or gradual worsening of mood rather than improvement may indicate that the initial reaction may be evolving into a clinically significant depression.

The mood state alone may not provide enough information to determine whether a reaction is normal or abnormal. The concomitant cognitive, behavioral, and physiological changes may be more informative. To distinguish normal from abnormal mood shifts, the patient and the clinician need a reference point against which to gauge symptomatic changes.

Early Detection through Self-Awareness

The ideal scenario for relapse prevention is prophylactic pharmacotherapy that is 100% effective and patient adherence to treatment that is 100% consistent. Of course, it would also be critical that stress stay at a minimal level; sleep is never lost due to travel, schedule changes, or overstimulation; and alcohol and recreational drug use, pregnancy, and general medical conditions are avoided altogether.

Because the ideal is not often possible or desired, the next best situation is to be as consistent as possible with sleep, medication, and stress control and to be watchful of the return of symptoms of depression or mania. Early detection provides an opportunity for early intervention and containment.

The trouble is that most people are unaware that they are beginning to relapse until symptoms are many and fairly severe. To aid in the development of an early-warning system, self-awareness of symptoms must be heightened and refined. Tables 6.1 and 6.2 present the mild, moderate, and severe forms of common manic and depressive symptoms. The goal would be for people with bipolar disorder to become aware of the mild form of symptoms they experience and make adjustments as needed to avoid sleep loss, monitor medications more closely to avoid missed doses, limit stimulants such as caffeine or noise, and take measures to reduce stress. Small preventive actions may be all that is needed to regain stability.

If these measures are insufficient and symptoms persist or worsen into moderately severe forms, more direct pharmacological and/or nonpharmacological interventions may be needed. Consultation with the treating psychiatrist and/or therapist should be sought as soon as possible either by phone or in the office.

The presentation of the common symptoms of depression and mania in Tables 6.1 and 6.2 can also be used as part of the patient education process, particularly for those who are newly diagnosed with bipolar disorder. Provide patients with a copy of each list and ask them to circle the ones they have experienced. If they circle the severe or moderate and not the mild form of a symptom inquire about their feelings prior to the onset of the episode. New patients may not be able to recall the mild forms, especially if recovering from mania. Family members or close friends who may have had the opportunity observe the patient as the episode evolved can assist with the education process by reviewing the list and telling patients and health care providers what they observed. This can be accomplished through conjoint therapy sessions with significant others or, if not practical, as a homework assignment for the patient to take the lists of symptoms to those whom they trust and ask them to circle the symptoms they observed. This exercise helps the clinician to know what symptoms to watch for and to prepare the patient to create his or her unique symptom summary list, which is described in the next section.

Symptom Summary Worksheet

While the Life Chart provides a global view of a person's course of illness, the Symptom Summary Worksheet focuses more closely on the specific symptoms that occur during episodes of depression and mania. As shown in Figure 6.4, the Symptom Summary Worksheet is one way of beginning to differentiate normal from abnormal mood states and symptoms. The worksheet summarizes the major symptoms of depression and mania for a given patient and contrasts those symptoms with the person's normal or euthymic state. This provides the patient and the clinician with guidelines against which to compare mood and

TABLE 6.1. Common Symptoms of Mania

Mild form of symptom	Moderate form of symptom	Severe form of symptom
Everything seems like a hassle; impatience or anxiety	More easily angered	Irritability
Happier than usual, positive outlook	Increased laughter and joking	Euphoric mood, on top of the world
More talkative; better sense of humor	In the mood to socialize and talk with others	Pressured or rapid speech
More thoughts; mentally sharp, quick; lose focus	Disorganized thinking; poor concentration	Racing thoughts
More self-confident than usual; less pessimistic	Feeling smart; not afraid to try; overly optimistic	Grandiosity—delusions of grandeur
Creative ideas; new interests; change sounds good.	Plan to make changes; disorganized in actions; drinking or smoking more	Disorganized activity; starting more things than finishing
Fidgety, nervous behaviors like nail biting	Restless; preferring movement over sedentary activities	Psychomotor agitation; cannot sit still
Not as effective at work; having trouble keeping mind on tasks	Not completing tasks; late for work; annoying others	Cannot complete usual work or home activities
Uncomfortable with other people	Suspicious	Paranoia
More sexually interested	Sexual dreams; seeking out or noticing sexual stimulation	Increased sex drive— seeking out sexual activity; more promiscuous
Notice sounds and annoying people; lose train of thought	Noises seem louder; colors seem brighter; mind wanders easily; need quieter environment to focus thoughts	Distractibility—have to work hard to focus thoughts or cannot focus thoughts at all

symptom fluctuations. If some of the symptoms listed on the worksheet under depression or mania accompany mood fluctuations, these are more than "normal" reactions to stressors and should be monitored closely. Figure 6.5 is a Symptom Summary Worksheet for a 35-year-old man with a history of bipolar disorder.

To begin the symptom summary, the clinician may ask patients to

TABLE 6.2. Common Symptoms of Depression

Mild form of symptom	Moderate form of symptom	Severe form of symptom
Blue, down, or neutral mood	Cry more easily	Severe sadness
Not in the mood to socialize	Less involved with others	Lack of interest in usual activities
Usual activities are not as fun as expected	Have fun until activity is over	Decreased pleasure
Blame self more readily when things go wrong; see own faults	Self-critical	Excessive and inappropriate guilt
Not as hungry as usual; can skip meals occasionally and not feel hungry	Eating brings less pleasure	Decreased appetite
Clothes fit slightly looser, no big weight loss (e.g., 1–3 pounds)	Noticeable weight loss	Significant weight loss
Sleep seems less restful; ruminating at bed time; falling asleep takes a little longer	Takes much longer to fall asleep; wake up briefly during the night	Insomnia—cannot fall asleep easily, wake up during the night and stay awake
Lose interest in tasks such as reading; get frustrated with tasks that are lengthy	Must reread text; thoughts cannot be focused well	Impaired concentration
Feel as if moving slowly; not mentally sharp	Slowness in movement is noticeable others; long pauses before answering questions	Psychomotor retardation
Wish pain would go away; thoughts of running away; pessimistic	Thoughts that life may not be worth living; hopeless; can't imagine feeling better	Suicidal ideas or attempts; not caring if they died
Self-doubt; some self-criticism	Low self-esteem, dislike appearance, feel like a loser	Feelings of worthlessness

describe what they are like when in a "normal," nonsymptomatic state. This can be difficult at first, especially if patients have been symptomatic more often than not in the past few years. Probing for a description of their personality, style, typical behavior, likes and dislikes, temperament, sense of humor, and daily habits and routines can help. A running list of these descriptors can be kept on the Symptom Summary Worksheet in the column labeled "When feeling OK." Input

Category	When manic	When depressed	When feeling OK
Mood			
Attitude toward self			
Self-confidence			
Usual activities			
Social activity			
Sleep habits			
Appetite/eating habits			
Concentration			
Speed of thought			
Creativity			
Interest in having fun			
Restlessness			
Sense of humor			
Energy level			
How noise affects you			
Outlook on the future			
Speech patterns			
Decision-making ability			
Concern for others			
Thoughts about death			
Ability to function			
Other areas:			

FIGURE 6.4. Symptom Summary Worksheet.

Category	When manic	When depressed	When feeling OK
Mood	Irritable	Sad	Content
Attitude toward self	I'm the only one with a brain	I hate myself	I'm OK
Self-confidence	Very self-confident	No confidence	I think I am capable of a lot
Usual activities	Starting but not finishing tasks	Lay in bed or watch TV	Work. Clean house. Exercise
Social activity	Can't stand to be around people	I don't want anyone to see me	Visit with friends and family
Sleep habits	4 hours each night	Sleep all the time	7–8 hours of sleep
Appetite/eating habits	I forget to eat	I'm not hungry	I like to eat
Concentration	Can't hold on to thoughts	Stare at a page, but can't read	Pretty good. I can read the paper
Speed of thought	Fast and disorganized	My mind is slow and sluggish	I'm usually a quick thinker
Creativity	Very creative until I reach my peak	No creative thoughts	Can be creative at home
Restlessness	Very hard to sit still	I don't want to move off couch	I like to be busy and keep moving
Sense of humor	More sarcastic	Nothing is funny	Like to tell jokes
Energy level	High. Nervous energy	None	Enough to get things done
How noise affects you	Noises get on my nerves	I don't hear what's going on around me	It doesn't usually bother me
Outlook on the future	Anything is possible	There is no future	I'm not certain what tomorrow will bring
Speech patterns	Talk fast and incessantly	Have difficulty forming words or will not talk	Talkative, but do not interrupt others

cont.

FIGURE 6.5. Sample Symptom Summary Worksheet.

Decision-making ability	Decisions are made impulsively	Cannot make decisions	Can make good decisions
Concern for others	Not worried about others	Concerned about what others think of me	Considerate of others
Thoughts about death	I think more about God	Others would be better off without me	I don't think about it
Ability to function	At my best for a while	Can function with a lot of effort	Function normally
Other areas: Sex drive	Can't stop thinking about sex	No interest	Rarely interested

FIGURE 6.5. *cont.*

from family members and friends can be particularly useful for this exercise, because they can often recall what the patient was like before the illness began.

Separately for episodes of depression and episodes of mania, the patient lists the symptoms that he or she most commonly experiences. If uncertain, the clinician can review the symptoms identified at the time of a past diagnostic evaluation. For each symptom, the clinician asks how it differs in the other states. For example, if insomnia is a symptom of depression, the clinician may ask how the person's sleep habits are different when hypomanic or manic and when euthymic. Each symptom is listed in the appropriate column on the worksheet. (The symptoms of hypomania are added to the mania column of the worksheet.) If symptoms of both depression and mania commonly occur within a single episode, the clinician marks on the summary worksheet that the symptoms in two columns occur simultaneously. Probing questions that help patients to recall symptoms include the following:

- "How does your life change when you are depressed or when you are manic?"

- "How, if at all, do your views of yourself, others, and the future change when you are depressed, when you are manic, and when you are feeling fine?"

- "What do other people notice during symptomatic times?"
- "What kinds of comments do you hear from others?"

The responses to each of these questions can be included on the Symptom Summary Worksheet.

When completed, the worksheet provides a fairly detailed description of the patient in depressed, manic, and asymptomatic states. A copy of the Symptom Summary Worksheet is given to the patient and another copy kept in the chart for reference. If family members or friends are participating in the session, it may be helpful to provide them with a copy of the worksheet as well. More information can be added as it becomes available.

Like the Life Chart, the Symptom Summary Worksheet allows the clinician and the patient to look for larger patterns of symptoms across the history of the illness. With prevention of relapses and recurrences of depression and mania as the goal, this information provides a reference point against which the patient can check fluctuations in symptoms. When these fluctuations seem transient and minimally distressing, the patient can learn to note them but not worry. When they persist and begin to resemble the descriptions of depression and/or mania on the Symptom Summary Worksheet, it is time to intervene to circumvent a relapse or recurrence.

Making Use of the Symptom Summary Worksheet

Communication

Among the uses for the Symptom Summary Worksheet is to facilitate communication among the patient, various health care providers, and family members and/or significant others. If all parties are aware of how mania and depression present in a given patient, communication about concerns and the need for intervention can be more complete and precise. For example, if a patient's wife calls his therapist to express concern over changes in sleep patterns or activity changes, the Symptom Summary Worksheet can help the wife to explain which symptoms are being observed. If when the therapist meets with the patient it becomes clear that he lacks awareness of symptoms, the worksheet can be reviewed and the observations of the wife discussed.

In another scenario, if the patient presents with symptoms to her therapist and requests that the therapist help her explain to the psychiatrist what is happening, the Symptom Summary Worksheet helps the therapist and psychiatrist to share a common understanding of the symptom presentation of that patient.

> Maria came to her evening therapy session complaining about her mother. It was clear to the therapist that Maria was more irritable than usual and was speaking more rapidly than was typical of her. When the therapist inquired about symptoms of mania, Maria took offense and quickly blamed her mother for recent conflict that had kept her up all night feeling angry. Maria trusted her therapist and was willing to calm down and listen to the therapist voice her concerns. They decided together that she could not afford to have another sleepless night, but Maria wasn't sure what to do about it. Together they called Maria's psychiatrist to ask for advice. Because the psychiatrist also had a copy of Maria's Symptom Summary Worksheet, he understood the therapist's concerns and suggested a medication option that would help Maria to sleep. The symptom list facilitated communication between providers that expedited the decision-making process.

Relapse Detection

When people who have bipolar disorder suffer the normal ups and downs of life they experience the same kinds of stress and its many manifestations as do people who do not have the illness. Therefore, it is not always clear if they are becoming depressed or just feeling stressed or distressed as might be expected when troublesome events occur.

The Symptom Summary Worksheet helps people to distinguish between symptomatic relapse and normal fluctuations in emotions. By reviewing the worksheet, the patient can tally up the number of symptoms he or she is experiencing. If unclear, a question mark can be placed next to the symptom and it can be assessed again the next day. If depression or mania were reemerging, it would be expected that a number of symptoms would develop simultaneously. If it is merely a reaction to psychosocial events, positive or negative, then only one or two symptoms would be present and only in their mild or moderate form.

Patients who have achieved symptom stability and are no longer in regular contact with a therapist might call in to ask for assistance in determining if relapse is imminent. If both the therapist and the patient have copies of the Symptom Summary Worksheet, they can quickly review it by phone to determine if a visit is necessary. If used as a screening tool during the earliest phases of episode development, relapse can often be caught quickly and resolved.

If relapse is not occurring, any mild symptoms that were present often resolve themselves before the patient makes it to a follow-up visit.

Ending Family Disputes

When Prudence and her husband Walter argue about the kids or about money, Walter will sometimes question Prudence about whether she has taken her medication. He implies with this question that he thinks Prudence is getting sick. Prudence hears this as Walter's way of pushing away blame for the problem they are discussing. He indirectly communicates that he does not think her argument is valid and that he will not take her concerns seriously. This always infuriates Prudence, so she argues back more adamantly. Her increased volume and negative statements about Walter's behavior further convince him that she is overreacting and has probably neglected to take her lithium as has occurred in the past.

Unfortunately, this type of confrontation plays itself out in the homes of many people diagnosed with bipolar disorder. Family members, particularly spouses or parents, believe that they are only trying to be helpful. The problem is their choice of timing. The questioning about symptoms or medications is introduced in response to a challenge. Therefore, it functions as a defensive statement rather than a genuine show of concern.

To settle an argument about whether the patient is upset because of a real family problem or is irritable and negative because mania or depression is returning, the Symptom Summary Worksheet can be reviewed. If it is the illness, several symptoms should be present not just during the argument but throughout the past few days. If it is not the illness but a family or marital problem, the only symptoms would be those expressed during the interaction, such as anger, irritation, negative statements, or more rapid speech.

If it is the illness (i.e., if several symptoms are present), the patient will need to take the necessary precautions but revisit the problem under discussion at a time when emotional expression is not being fueled by the illness.

If symptoms are not present, the discussion should be resumed and the problem resolved. Because arguments can increase irritation and interfere with sleep, it would serve the patient well to monitor his or her mood more closely to be certain that the conflict does not cause a worsening of symptoms.

The therapist can help negotiate an agreement between the family and the patient. Whenever there is a question about symptoms, the patient will take the concern seriously and will review the Symptom Summary Worksheet. In exchange, the family member will try to be objective about the presence of symptoms but will review the Symptom Summary Worksheet as well and not use it as a fighting strategy. The therapist must clearly explain how symptoms evolve and how to tell the difference between a negative reaction and a relapse.

Communication problems unrelated to bipolar disorder are common in couples or families that are having difficulty getting along. Therapists can be helpful by functioning as referees during family visits, making sure that all parties have a chance to speak their minds and be heard without interruption. Chapter 12 covers interpersonal problems in bipolar disorder and includes guidelines for helping people to become better communicators.

Evaluating Manic Ideas

At times it can be a clinical challenge to distinguish manic ideas from creative ideas. Just because a person is feeling creative does not necessarily mean that he or she is getting manic. However, the increased energy and fluidity of thought that comes with mild hypomania can facilitate creative thinking and stimulate problem-solving actions. Excitement over new ideas and possibilities can brighten a person's mood and put a bounce back in his or her step. These changes can easily be mistaken for symptoms of mania, especially in those who have been through a lengthy bout of depression.

The Symptom Summary Worksheet can help the person and his or her doctor or therapist to evaluate these situations. Most people would prefer not to get manic and want to know if concern is warranted. Reviewing the list of manic symptoms can reassure the patient that he or she is merely happy and not hypomanic; thus, any new ideas do not have to be suspect. If a review shows that several symptoms are present, even if only to a mild degree, it would be best to monitor them closely and avoid taking action on any new plans until the patient was certain that he or she was not being influenced by mania.

Evaluating Depressive Ideas

Similar to the process of differentiating a good mood from a hypomanic mood, the Symptom Summary Worksheet can also help a person distinguish negative thinking associated with depression from negative reactions to normal life events.

> Cheryl is fed up with her boss. She has taken all the criticism she can tolerate and is ready to quit. As she was typing up a draft of her letter of resignation she thought to herself, "are you sure you are not just depressed?" Doubt entered her mind. She had every reason to be angry with her boss. Anyone would be angry. But changing jobs, right now, might not be the best thing either. She could not afford to make the mistake of quitting in haste and regretting it later when her depression lifted.
>
> To help her make a decision, Cheryl made an appointment with her therapist to review her symptoms and resume treatment if needed. Although symptom presentations can vary slightly from one episode of depression to the next, the depression items on the Symptom Summary Worksheet provide a point of reference for the patient and therapist. If symptoms are emerging, Cheryl should be experiencing several symptoms from the list. If she is merely stressed, she should not have more than a few such as a low mood and perhaps some sleep disturbance.

When in doubt, it is best to monitor symptoms closely and delay making major life-changing decisions until it is certain that the negative outlook common to depression is not influencing the choices. It can also be helpful to use cognitive restructuring methods to evaluate the evidence surrounding negative perceptions, as with her job in Cheryl's case.

Monitoring Progress

Another use of the Symptom Summary Worksheet is to monitor progress toward symptom remission. While standardized assessment measures might provide normative scores of symptom severity, a personalized list allows the patient and his or her health care providers to monitor changes in symptoms specific to each patient. If treatment is effective or as episodes of illness naturally remit, the number of symptoms experienced from those on the list should decrease, as should their severity.

Mood Graphs

Mood Graphs can be used to narrow the focus from the broad groupings of symptoms during typical episodes to daily changes in mood, cognition, and behavior. It is this level of monitoring that is required to identify subsyndromal symptoms that precede episodes of mania and depression. The Mood Graph can be used to rate affective changes such as sadness or euphoria but is most helpful when used to track symptoms that are the earliest signs of symptom worsening for a given individual. Some people are most sensitive to changes in their outlook on life (more optimistic or pessimistic) or their views of themselves (more confident or more self-critical). Others notice changes in energy (increased or decreased) or activity (more active or more socially withdrawn). The Symptom Summary Worksheet can help the clinician and patient decide which symptoms will be most useful to monitor.

The anchor row in the middle of the graph shown in Figure 6.6 represents euthymia. The points above the anchor row, from 0 to +5, represent levels of mania; the highest points on the graph indicate manic episodes. The points below the anchor row, from 0 to –5, represent levels of depression, with the lowest points indicating major depressive episodes. Normal variations in mood vary from –1 to +1. Ratings of +2 to –2 alert patients to begin monitoring their symptoms a little more closely. A score of –3 or +3 indicates that it is time to intervene to keep the symptoms from worsening. For example, at a rating of +3 or –3, it is time to call the doctor if the patient does not have an appointment scheduled within the next few days.

This simple Mood Graph may be sufficient for some patients. However, it is better to tailor a Mood Graph to the special needs of each patient. For example, those who have several shifts in mood during a day may need a Mood Graph designed for separate ratings at different times of the day (e.g., morning, afternoon, and evening). Information about the circumstances surrounding mood shifts can be noted on the graph. This information can help clinicians to design interventions that prevent worsening of moods. For example, patients may find that their mood shifts when they leave home and go to work, when their children return from school, when they see their spouses, or when they are hungry. These mood shifts do not necessarily require a pharmacological intervention, but may be addressed with CBT techniques.

The amount of alcohol consumed, money spent, and medications needed can also be monitored on a graph. Similarly, symptom shifts, such as sleep changes, can be tracked. Because the selection of symptoms to be monitored depends on the special symptom presentations of the patient, it is wise to work with each patient in developing a personalized monitoring system. The clinician should encourage each

Mood Graph

Name: _____

Week of: _____

Manic		Plan	Sun	Mon	Tues	Wed	Thur	Fri	Sat
+5	Not sleeping, psychotic	Go to the hospital	•	•	•	•	•	•	•
+4	Manic, poor judgment		•	•	•	•	•	•	•
+3	Hypomanic	Call doctor	•	•	•	•	•	•	•
+2	Energized	Take action	•	•	•	•	•	•	•
+1	Hyper, happy	Monitor closely	•	•	•	•	•	•	•
0	Normal		•	•	•	•	•	•	•
-1	Low, down	Monitor closely	•	•	•	•	•	•	•
-2	Sad	Take action	•	•	•	•	•	•	•
-3	Depressed	Call the doctor	•	•	•	•	•	•	•
-4	Immobilized		•	•	•	•	•	•	•
-5	Suicidal	Go to the hospital	•	•	•	•	•	•	•
Depressed									

What caused the mood shift?

FIGURE 6.6. Mood Graph.

patient to be creative in developing a graph that will provide as much useful information as possible.

Connecting the Dots

Mood Graphs and the Symptom Summary Worksheet are tools for helping patients become more sensitive to the onset of symptoms. They are also intended to help people draw connections between their changes in mood and other internal or external events. In doing so, the person with bipolar disorder can come to know the situations or events that could precipitate symptom exacerbations as well as being more tuned into the subtle changes in thoughts, feelings, or actions that occur early in episodes of depression and mania.

It is not unusual for people with this illness to attribute symptoms to the wrong source. Common errors include blaming external noise for depression-related insomnia or family problems for mood swings. If symptoms are dismissed as normal responses to stress, change, or external events, opportunities for early intervention may be missed.

In the converse, there are stimuli other than the illness that can produce subjective experiences similar to symptoms. For example, changes in work schedule that reduce sleep can cause tiredness or fatigue. Premenstrual hormone changes can cause moodiness and weight gain. Being alone or listening to sad songs can make a person feel blue. And unpleasant people at work can lower motivation to be there. These circumstances are all within the normal range of human experience and do not necessarily indicate depression.

Similarly, good news can make a person feel happy and perhaps even euphoric for a while depending on the type of event. Talking with interesting people or seeing new places can stimulate new ideas. Anticipation of pleasant or exciting events can make it difficult to fall asleep at night. Finding a new romantic partner can stimulate the libido. While these could be symptoms of mania, if they are transient and do not occur concurrently, they are probably normal positive responses to good things in life.

If Mood Graphs are used to monitor both symptom changes and the circumstance surrounding those shifts, connections can be drawn between the two that help the patient and clinician better understand the nature of mood fluctuations. Patterns can usually be found between symptom changes and stressors, incomplete compliance, sleep loss, or hormone cycles.

Knowing the precipitants to symptomatic mood changes can help the person plan ahead for exacerbations.

Estelle, for example, always has symptoms of depression premenstrually. She is more tearful, very sensitive to criticism, and sometimes irritable. She becomes preoccupied with her sad feelings, which she usually attributes to external events such as being ignored by her boyfriend. After keeping Mood Graphs for several months, the pattern became clear. After that point, Estelle could plan ahead for these time periods making special efforts to nurture herself and to avoid overreacting to perceived rejection. She also began working with her gynecologist to control her hormonal problems.

Stan has difficulty controlling his mood during football season. His wife has been telling him for years that he gets overly excited about the sport and shouldn't watch. Stan thinks she is imagining this. To test her theory, Stan agreed to keep a Mood Graph during football season. There was an increase in irritability and sleep loss after Monday Night football. Games ran late. Stan had to be at work by 8:00 A.M. so he got less sleep on Monday nights. Sleep loss made him irritable. Thursday night games were not a problem because he was off on Fridays and could sleep in. When the pattern repeated itself each week, Stan could not deny the connection.

Lifestyle Management

Each time a person has a mood swing, symptoms breakthrough, or recurrence of depression or mania, he or she has an opportunity to learn more about the factors that increase vulnerability to relapse. With that knowledge, adjustments can be made to avoid or cope with these circumstances. The most common factors that precipitate mood swings or symptom breakthroughs for those who have bipolar disorder are inconsistent adherence to pharmacotherapy regimens, sleep loss, stress, and overstimulation of various sorts.

To avoid recurrence of symptoms, it is possible to plan ahead for times of the year that seem to bring about symptoms such as springtime mania or holiday depressions. This might include altering medication regimens, monitoring symptoms more closely, setting limits on activities, or learning new ways to manage common stressors.

Julia increases her lithium a little beginning in early March. That's when she is prone to mania. Harriett gets stressed during the summer when her children are off of school for several months. It is easy for her to get overextended, exhausted, and irritable. By September, when the kids are back in school she is already depressed. Harriett could make use of the behavioral interventions covered in the following chapters to control her stress and thereby reduce her risk of relapse.

If certain life events seem to precipitate relapse such as job changes, childbirth, relationships ending, or the loss of a loved one to death, it may be possible to plan ahead for self-protection when these events are anticipated. This is where psychotherapy can be particularly useful. The therapist can help the person cope with loss, maintain healthy habits, avoid obstacles that interfere with medication adherence, and replace ineffective coping strategies with those that solve problems and prevent relapse.

Key Points for the Therapist to Remember

♦ To help them get a handle on their mood fluctuations, it will be necessary to understand which symptoms emerge first in the sequence of depression and mania, factors that might precipitate the mood shifts, and responses by the patient that either help control symptoms or cause them to worsen. With this information in hand, the therapist can assist the patient in planning ahead for recurrences and breakthroughs.

♦ Examination of the pros and cons of compliance should reveal a pattern with at least one compelling reason to exercise self-control, such as avoiding the stress that relapse places on the patient and family members, and at least one compelling reason not to, such as losing their freedom or giving up the joys of their life.

♦ Most people are unaware that they are beginning to relapse until symptoms are many and fairly severe. To aid the development of an early warning system, self-awareness of symptoms must be heightened and refined.

♦ Each time a person has a mood swing, symptoms breakthrough, or recurrence of depression or mania, he or she has an opportunity to learn more about the factors that increase vulnerability to relapse. With that knowledge, adjustments can be made to avoid or cope with these circumstances.

Points to Discuss with Patients

♦ CBT methods can be powerful tools in helping people with bipolar disorder to avoid relapse. But people have to decide for themselves if they want to use them.

◆ Rather than trying to convince them to be consistent with medications, monitor their symptoms, normalize their schedule, or give up overstimulating activities, the person must convince him- or herself that lifestyle management is worth the effort.

◆ Most don't know what they will have to give up in order to gain greater stability. And when they find out, they are often not very happy.

◆ Therapists must provide an overview of the rationale behind relapse prevention. This includes informing or reminding patients that their illness is chronic and recurrent and that it will need to be managed for the rest of their lives. Although people who have the illness know this, hearing it again and finding out the details of relapse prevention can stir up a lot of negative feelings about the illness and its treatment.

◆ The best scenario is for patients to be as consistent as possible with sleep, medication, and stress control and to be watchful of the return of symptoms of depression or mania. Early detection provides an opportunity for early intervention and containment.

◆ It is not unusual for people with this illness to misattribute symptoms to the wrong source. Common errors include blaming external noise for depression-related insomnia or family problems for mood swings. If symptoms are dismissed as normal responses to stress, change, or external events, opportunities for early intervention may be missed.

CHAPTER 7

Management of Behavioral Symptoms

TRIGGER CONTROL AND INCREASING POSITIVES

In the earlier chapters of this book, we have mentioned or suggested several behavior management strategies. In this chapter, we elaborate on those strategies. In many cases, the behavioral interventions that are helpful in controlling the increased or poorly organized behavior of mania can also be used to overcome behavioral deficits in depression. Variations for each exercise are discussed, but the full procedures for each intervention are only presented once.

Two rules of thumb for addressing behavioral problems in bipolar disorder are as follows:

1. It is easier to add positive behaviors than to stop negative behaviors.

2. Before trying to make things better, first try to get patients to avoid making things worse.

Behavioral Control of Symptom Triggers in Depression

Although there are considerable variations from person to person, some commonalities in symptom triggers exist across people who suffer from depression. We describe those common patterns later. However, it is best to inquire for each individual patient about those factors that seem to predictably worsen his or her depression. One category to consider is avoidance or withholding of positive reinforcers such as contact with caring people or engaging in pleasurable activities. Positive stimuli can distract people from their problems and provide a more balanced view of reality that includes positives as well as negatives. The absence of positives leaves the individual to experience only distress and negativity. The cognitive model of depression proposed by Beck, Rush, Shaw, and Emery (1979) suggests that people need to feel a sense of accomplishment or mastery as well as a sense of pleasure to maintain a euthymic state. The low energy and motivation and hopeless outlook that characterize depression often keep people from engaging in or completing tasks that would provide a sense of mastery over their world. Hence, they lack feelings of satisfaction. Also, when mood is severely dysphoric, and nonreactive to positive stimuli, engagement in positive activities will not easily produce feelings of pleasure or joy. When this is the case, people who are depressed shy away from opportunities that might bring even a minimal amount of gratification and therefore cannot accumulate positive experiences to offset the misery of depression.

Another category to consider when inquiring about factors that can worsen an individual's depression is exposure to negative stimuli. Negative or stressful experiences worsen depression, especially when a person temporarily lacks the ability to solve problems or organize their thinking well enough to overcome obstacles in life. Common negative stimuli are conflict with others, television news that emphasizes the disasters in the world, sad music or movies, other depressed people, complaints from others, a disorganized or messy environment, financial troubles, and mean-spirited people. Excessive exposure to these negative stimuli can increase sadness, irritability, and anxiety and can affect people's outlook on themselves and on life. In the face of adversity they will feel more hopeless about the future and helpless to overcome strife, and in turn will see themselves as worthless. Also, when they are unable to cope, they will miss opportunities to feel positive reinforcement for their efforts.

A third category of factors that can worsen depression is avoidance behaviors. When people are depressed and faced with problems often they evade stress rather than cope with it. Because avoidance works to reduce stress, according to learning theory, the avoidance behavior is negatively reinforced. That is, it turns off the stress, if only temporarily. Therefore, the depressed person is more likely the next time to use avoidance as a tactic rather than to confront problems. It turns off unpleasantness faster and takes less effort than resolution of the problem. Avoidance behaviors include procrastination, withdrawing from others, or engaging in an alternative behavior as a distraction from difficulties. Unfortunately, hiding from the world only makes matters worse for the person who is trying to overcome depression. While the depressed person understands this logically, the quick reduction of stress that comes from avoidance is a powerful reinforcer and difficult to resist.

The intervention is to ask patients what they know they could do that would make their depression worse. Ask them to write down this list in session. If they have had some experience with depression, they will know the things in the past that have made them feel worse rather than better. Getting overwhelmed, isolating from others, getting into angry conflicts, recalling past losses, reviewing regrets, and talking to people who are also depressed are among the things that make depression worse. Once these items are listed, patients are instructed to avoid these negatives until they are feeling stronger. To fill the time that would be otherwise taken up by these negative events, add positive activities that are not any more energy consuming and that could distract the person from these negatives until new coping skills can be taught. The patient might find it helpful to share this intervention with family members or friends and elicit their insights into what seems to make the patient's depression worse.

Behavioral Control
of Symptom Triggers in Mania

People who have been through manic episodes in the past usually know what can make manic symptoms worsen. Given the high likelihood that hypomania will turn into mania (Gelenberg et al., 1989), those who have had negative experiences with mania will be motivated to control the symptoms while they are mild. Some may have learned from experience that there are several factors that can drive hypomania into mania. The benefit of that experience is that they know what to avoid. Not all people who have experienced mania will know what made their symptoms worsen and will require guidance from the therapist or psychiatrist to monitor behaviors that carry potential consequences for exacerbating hypomania.

The most common factors that contribute to the development or worsening of mania are medication noncompliance, sleep deprivation, overstimulation, and use of alcohol and drugs of abuse. Chapters 4 and

5 covered strategies for prevention and remediation of adherence problem. In this chapter we cover behavioral methods for coping with sleep loss and overstimulation.

When asked what could worsen their hypomania, those with experience list examples of overstimulating situations and people, nighttime activities that interfere with a good night's sleep, attempting to extend the high with alcohol or drugs, making sudden changes or taking on new activities, and engaging in activities that provide too much excitement, such as socializing, shopping, or driving fast. The dilemma for people who suffer from bipolar disorder is that while they know these behaviors can make matters worse, they are also highly reinforcing, seductive, and not problematic for their friends or family members with whom they socialize. Contributing to the urge to engage in potentially dangerous behaviors is the increased flow of ideas characteristic of hypomania and mania. Add to that impairment in judgment, increased distractibility, and an inability to perceive risks and the result is behavior that exacerbates manic symptomatology. Therefore, although it is critical that people who are beginning a new episode of mania contain behaviors that can exacerbate the situation, the desire to do so is mixed with the desire to have pleasurable experiences, particularly if the individual has recently recovered from a lengthy bout of depression.

Many people with bipolar disorder prefer evening activity to morning activity. Late-night chats with others in person, on the phone, or online are pleasurable and stimulating. Such contact is so enjoyable that the hypomanic person does not always realize how late it has gotten. Once the conversations are over it can take some time to slow down and stop thinking about the discussion and, therefore, sleep is further delayed. If the person must wake up early to attend to work, school, or family responsibilities, he or she may be able to get only a limited amount of sleep. Sleep loss exacerbates mania. However, asking someone in this situation to forego evening activities in order to sleep is problematic for several reasons. If they agree to do so, they may still have difficulty in falling asleep. If going to bed early is viewed as deprivation or restriction, it may be met with resistance and resentment. And if the need to reduce stimulation and sleep normally is realized and accepted, it can also remind the person with bipolar disorder that he or she is not like everyone else. This can stir up thoughts of being strange, weird, or abnormal and feelings of anger or sadness.

A therapist's sensitivity to these issues is critical to resolving them with the patient. It is important to empathize with the person for the restrictions placed on him or her in order to control the illness. At the same time, the therapist must allow the person to make his or her own decisions about taking preventive actions. We frequently say to patients, "You know what you need to do and only you can make the decision to do so. You understand the consequences of your actions, and only you can choose to set limits on yourself or go with your urges and take your chances. I cannot tell you what to do. I can only give you guidance. The decision each day whether to set limits is entirely up to you."

A therapist can help to educate patients about the actions they can take to reduce the risk of relapsing into mania, especially if they are not aware of the contributing factors. If patients are willing to take action, they can generate lists of potentially problematic situations, such as sleep loss or late-night activities, during therapy sessions and avoid these stimulating factors while improving adherence with treatment or seeking augmentations to their medication regimens. Table 7.1 provides an example of one patient's list of things that could make her mania worse.

Adding Positives

Just as people can predict what will make their depression or mania worse, they are usually pretty good at identifying healthy habits to add to their daily routine. As mentioned at the beginning of this chapter, it is much easier to add positive behaviors than it is to eliminate negative behaviors. Time taken for developing or resuming healthy habits means less time available for engaging in ineffective or self-defeating behaviors. Therefore, before engaging in elaborate behavioral interventions, simply ask patients about the positive habits they know they should develop or resume but have neglected. The most common ones will surround healthy eating, controlling alcohol and caffeine use, keeping a daily routine, taking medications regularly, and exercise. Some report procrastination as a problem and express the desire to

TABLE 7.1. "Things That Could Make My Mania Worse"

- Watching TV until 3:00 A.M. and getting up at 6:30 for work
- Going out to a club with my friends—loud music, out late, too much alcohol
- Skipping my medication because I think I am fine
- Arguing with my mother late at night
- Giving in to my urge to shop, too much time in the mall, getting caught up in sales, spending

take action on tasks they had been actively avoiding such as house-keeping chores, paying bills, or filing their taxes.

Adding a Positive and Stopping a Negative

A simple method for helping people to make positive changes is to have them first select a healthy habit to improve. Examples include having a healthier diet, more regular exercise, paying bills on time, or drinking less coffee. The second step is to ask patients to start one new behavior that might lead them closer to their goal. The final step is to have them select one problematic behavior they would like to stop. If healthy eating is the habit they select, they might choose to stop eating late at night, for example after 8:00 P.M., and to start eating breakfast in the morning. While this is only one step in the process, it is simple and if successful will motivate the patient to go further.

> Jim has had a problem of accumulating paper in his office. He has piles of mail, newspapers, magazines, old advertisements, print-outs from Internet sites, files, office supplies, food wrappers, and other trash that has not been discarded. Jim knows this is a prob-lem, but he doesn't have the desire to take it on, has no time to get organized, or finds other things he would rather do than sort through the piles. He knows that he needs to have better organi-zational habits and that the disarray in his office keeps him from being productive and efficient. And because he keeps his office at home, he sees the clutter spilling over into other areas of his house. Jim decided to begin taking on this problem by starting to open his mail when it arrives and discarding the unneeded pieces of paper such as envelopes or advertisements. This will not help him deal with the piles in his office, but it will keep him from contributing to the piles. The habit he chose to stop was printing information off Internet sites. He chose instead to save the files on his computer in a special folder for things of interest he might need at a later date. Similarly, this stops the accumulation but does not help Jim clean out his office. However, behavior changes that are improvements will increase a person's confidence to han-dle other difficulties and in turn produce a small amount of emo-tional relief from the stress caused by the problem. Jim's initial behavioral intervention that stopped the accumulation of paper made him feel more in control of his environment rather than a victim of it. This increased his motivation to take on the cleanup task in small increments and convinced him that to solve a prob-lem it would not be necessary to take it on all at one time, a pros-pect that had stopped him taking action on many occasions.

Some people who are unemployed have lost the ability to keep a daily routine without the structure of a work schedule. They may stay awake at night and sleep during the day, eat meals at unusual times, and keep no regular social, educational, recreational, or housekeeping commitments. These same people complain of feeling lost, alone, out of sorts, out of touch with the world, and disorganized. They know that they need structure but have no external controls to provide it. People in this group might choose to add structure, such as trying to go to bed and wake up at a set time each day and stop the habit of napping during the day. This type of schedule switch is difficult for some to accomplish and may require incremental changes over time.

Figure 7.1 provides a structure for helping patients to take stock of their current behavior and identify healthy habits they wish to initiate or resume.

Sleep Enhancement

As suggested in the previous example, maintaining consistency in the sleep–wake cycle can be a critical part of maintaining stability in bipolar disorder. Sleep loss has been found to precipitate mania (Wehr et al., 1987; Wehr & Wirz-Justice, 1982), while restabilizing sleep is a key to controlling symptoms. There are some preventive measures patients can take to increase the likelihood that they will have a good night's sleep. However, because sleep disruption is a key symptom of both depression and mania, its occurrence should signal the need for a medication consult and possibly augmentation or adjustment in pharmacological treatment.

Figure 7. 2 provides a summary of suggestions for sleep improvement that can be passed on to patients. In general, they emphasize stimulus control to enhance sleep. In less behavioral terms this means maintaining consistency in sleep schedule, avoiding behaviors that can interfere with sleep, and creating an environment that facilitates sleep.

In a hypomanic or manic phase, the patient may find it easy to fall asleep but wakes earlier than usual and does not feel a need for more sleep. Four or 5 hours of sleep may feel sufficient, when 7 or 8 is more normal. In these cases, the individual may not feel motivated to improve the duration or quality of sleep and may instead view insomnia as an opportunity to engage in new activities, take on new projects, or accomplish neglected tasks, each of which is overstimulating and can further impair sleep. Although a little insomnia seems harmless at first, it will undoubtedly lead to increased irritability and agita-

List below some of your healthy habits and those you would like to develop or strengthen. Include better ways to manage your symptoms, organize your life, and get more enjoyment out of life.

Healthy habits I regularly practice:

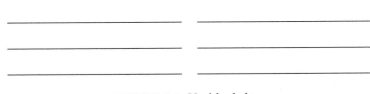

Healthy habits I need to strengthen:

New healthy habits I would like to develop:

FIGURE 7.1. Healthy habits.

tion, greater impairment in concentration, and eventual decompensation. If the patient has had enough experience with mania to know this, he or she will be motivated to take action to control sleep.

Insomnia during the depressed phase is quite different. The person does not feel refreshed but is left exhausted. The prospect of sleep is met with anxiety and dread and, as the sleepless hours pass, some people begin to panic. When sleep occurs but is interrupted only a few hours later, it is difficult for the patient not to feel frustrated or annoyed, and these negative feelings only arouse the patient further.

There are also behavioral strategies that can be implemented when insomnia occurs that can facilitate sleep. Figure 7.3 lists them in a form that can be shared with patients. They consist of efforts to relax the mind and body, limit forms of overstimulation late at night, and avoid panic over insomnia. In addition to these methods, standard relaxation exercises can be used.

Setting the stage for a good night's sleep

Be consistent. Try to go to sleep and wake up at about the same time each day, even on the weekends.

It's a nighttime thing. Avoid sleeping during the day and staying awake late at night. If your sleep cycle is already switched around, work with your doctor on a plan for getting your sleep back to normal.

Keep your bed a place for sleep. Make it a habit to watch TV, eat, read, or pay your bills in another room, at a table, or on a couch. Teach your body to associate going to bed with falling asleep.

Get comfortable. Make your sleep area comfortable by picking pillows, blankets, and clothing that make you feel good.

Gear down for the night. Start preparing to sleep at least an hour ahead of time by quieting your environment and quieting your mind.

Avoid stimulants that might keep you awake. A hot cup of cocoa or coffee, a few cigarettes, or some dessert might sound good at night time, but for those who are sensitive to caffeine, nicotine, or sugar, they will only make it harder to fall asleep. If you have any digestive problems, late dinners or spicy meals might trouble your stomach and keep you awake.

FIGURE 7.2. Suggestions for sleep improvement.

Encouraging Contact with Others

When people become depressed they feel inclined to withdraw from others. There are many reasons for this inclination. Some say that they lack the energy it takes to interact, especially if they do not want to confide their distress to others and feel the need to act as if everything is fine. Some stop caring if they see people, lose interest in social inter-action, and in general do not want to be bothered by others. They fail to see any positive reasons for the interaction. Others isolate them-selves because they want to avoid confrontations. They anticipate questions about their behavior or think they will be put on the spot to perform a social or family task. They do not want to say no, so they avoid contact altogether. Depression can affect a person's appearance by contributing to weight gain and lowering the motivation to keep up personal hygiene.

Emma hates to have to leave her home, in part because her isola-tion from others has led to her feeling anxious about the outside

What if I can't fall asleep?

Don't panic. Anxiety and sleep are not a good mix. If you start to worry or even panic about your inability to sleep, it will only make it harder to fall asleep. Sleep happens automatically. It is not a thing you can easily will your body to do, so the harder you work at convincing yourself to fall asleep, the longer it can take.

Calm your body. Your body and your mind work together to help you fall asleep. If your mind is too busy to settle down, you can help the process along by trying to relax your body. Start with your toes and work toward your head. Focus on letting go of tensions in each muscle and getting your body into a comfortable position.

Too alert to fall asleep? If you are too wide awake to fall asleep, you would be better off getting out of bed and doing something else that is relaxing like watching television, reading a book or any other activity that usually calms you or tires your mind.

Things *not to do* when you are having trouble sleeping

Caffeine. Don't make yourself a pot of coffee. The caffeine can keep you awake. If you enjoy a hot cup of coffee on a cold night, buy some decaffeinated coffee for evening and nighttime use.

Internet. Avoid getting out of bed to surf the Internet. Instead of getting sleepy, you will most likely stimulate your brain, getting excited or intrigued rather than getting sleepy.

TV and books. If you are going to watch TV or read a book, choose something that is not likely to keep you up. A good boring book will do the trick or a television rerun. Avoid shows with people arguing, cliffhangers, or real-life docudramas.

Chores. Don't get up and clean your house. Although unfinished chores may be on your mind, the process of doing physical labor in the middle of the night will tense your muscles rather than relax them. To be mentally alert enough to do chores you have stay awake. This defeats the purpose of getting a good night's sleep.

Exercise. It is probably not a good idea to get out of bed to exercise even if you know that exercise can wear you out. Any physical activity like this will overstimulate your mind and body. If exercise is usually a good idea for you, schedule time before you go to bed for a workout.

FIGURE 7.3. Coping with insomnia.

world, but also because going out of her home means that she has to shower, groom her hair, go through the frustrating task of finding something to wear that still fits, and deal with the hassle of applying make-up. Very few out-of-home activities are worth the effort.

However, avoidance of human contact also deprives the depressed person of positive interactions that would provide support, assistance with coping, a chance to laugh and experience joy, and opportunities to receive validation, love, and caring from others. These are normal human interactions that give us strength in difficult times, increase hopefulness about the future, and make us feel good about ourselves. Their absence leaves the depressed person to do all these things for him- or herself, a task that is not easily achieved.

Too much time alone can be dangerous for the person in a depressed phase of bipolar disorder. It provides too much time to think. Depression leads to distortions in information processing that will be thoroughly covered in the next chapter. In short, depression makes it easy to think about all that is wrong and difficult to recall anything that is right. This makes people review their lives and make mental lists of regrets, focus intensely on negative events, taking them out of context and magnifying their severity or impact on others. Isolation can mean no disruptions in rumination so that there is plenty of time to contemplate losses, failures, and reasons to end their lives. Isolation not only prevents people from gaining needed positive interactions but also can be quite dangerous in the hands of a depressed person.

If the initial goal of therapy is to increase positives rather than eliminate negatives, a good candidate for this exercise is social interaction. Increased interaction with other people whether family, friends, or strangers, provides the depressed person with potential opportunities to receive encouragement, distracts them temporarily from rumination about their personal problems, and may give them new reasons to live. If a social network is in place, the patient can be encouraged to return phone calls from friends, accept invitations to visit with family members, or contact neighbors or other acquaintances. If they previously belonged to a support group, resuming attendance can be encouraged. This could include group therapy, Alcoholics Anonymous meetings, faith-based support groups, or the local gardening club. Those who lack support systems might be encouraged to seek out others, such as the Depression and Bipolar Support Alliance (www.dbsalliance.org), the National Alliance for the Mentally Ill (www.nami.org), or one of the many other depression and bipolar support groups available online. Contact time with others in person, on the phone, or online detracts from time alone and rumination about problems.

All Work and No Play

Many patients suffering from depression complain of a life consumed with work and problems. They see no way out of the daily grind. When they are not depressed, they still have problems, but they balance these problems with positive events. When they are depressed, they no longer engage in pleasurable activities because they lack the energy to plan and initiate them, as well as the ability to enjoy them.

When problems and demands dominate patients' lives, it can be helpful to restore balance by "prescribing" fun. The goal of the intervention is to improve dysphoria by prescribing tasks that are pleasurable to the patients, may lift their spirits, or change their view of life as all work and no fun. If successful, the patients may experience some relief from the depression and feel more competent to cope with existing stressors.

It is best to start this intervention with pleasurable activities that take little effort to arrange and execute. Patients can begin by making a list of things that they would enjoy doing. If they are unable to generate a list, the clinician can ask them what activities they enjoyed before the depression began. A pleasurable activities list may include such activities as the following:

- Going to a movie
- Reading the comics on Sunday morning
- Watching a television show
- Reading a good book
- Taking the kids out for ice cream

Patients can choose one or two activities from the list to try before the next session. The activities chosen should have a high probability of success; that is, they should be activities for which patients are likely to have sufficient time, energy, and resources.

Initiating pleasurable activities may be stressful for some patients. If they are uncomfortable in social situations, for example, they may associate "fun" with potential scrutiny by others. If they suffer from panic attacks and/or agoraphobia, leaving the house to have fun can place them in anxiety-arousing situations. If they are critical of themselves for their shortcomings or their inability to cope when depressed, any failure of their plans for fun may give them further confirmation of their ineptitude or worthlessness. For these reasons, caution is necessary in assigning fun activities. Patients should not attempt pleasurable activities that place them at risk for experiencing rejection, anxiety, or a sense of failure.

There are two common problems with prescribing fun activities for depressed individuals. One is that they may not be able to derive pleasure from the experience. The second problem is that even if they can derive pleasure, their negative thinking may cause them to overlook any positive aspects and focus instead on the negative (e.g., my hair looked bad, the sound in the theater was poor, we sat next to a loud party in the restaurant).

In the first scenario, patients sometimes say they knew intellectually that they were engaging in a positive activity but they did not feel pleasure. The therapist should be persistent in assiging of fun while they work on other aspects of the depression. Use the compliance model discussed in Chapters 4 and 5 to identify the obstacles to enjoyment of positive activities.

In the second scenario, where the positive experience is viewed through a mental filter that only allows the negative aspects into awareness, it is essential that efforts be made to reduce the filter and evaluate events more objectively. Once an activity has been selected, ask patients to predict how they believe the event will go; this provides an opportunity to discuss ahead of time any concerns and to alter the plan accordingly. Some patients find it difficult to imagine themselves having fun. They may be skeptical that small pleasures can have any effect on their depression. The homework can be conceptualized as an experiment that tests patients' predictions about pleasurable events and more objectively tests the effect of fun on mood, energy level, and overall view of life. If effective, improvements in at least one of these three areas should be noticeable. If no changes are noted, exploring the aspects of the experience that seemed to sustain, or possibly worsen, the person's mood and outlook on life may help the patient to better understand his or her depression, can reveal underlying schemas that mediate responses to positive events, and can help in future activity planning. For example, a depressed patient who is attempting to repay debt accrued during a manic episode spending spree was assigned pleasurable tasks. He did not receive enjoyment from these activities. Exploration of the circumstances revealed tremendous guilt and a belief that he did not deserve to experience pleasure until his debt was paid. Taking time to play meant time away from work that could help pay his debt.

The Activity Rating Scale shown in Figure 7.4 aids in the evaluation of pleasurable activities. Just before attempting an activity, ratings are made for mood, energy level, and view of life on a 1–7 scale. A score of 1 means extremely low or negative and 7 means extremely high or positive. After completing the activity these are rerated using the same scale. At the next therapy session this information can be used to evaluate the accuracy of patients' predictions about their ability to experience pleasure. If ratings are made immediately preceding and following the event, it increases the chance that the event will be viewed without the interference of a negative filter. This will help patients to better evaluate their experiences between sessions and their mood without having to rely on the distortions of memory. If negative predictions were correct, the clinician and the patient can carefully review the event to determine what interfered with the plan's success, develop a new plan that takes into account the experiences on the first attempt, and discuss new predictions for the upcoming events, as well as any fears or concerns that the patient may have. If the prediction for the new assignment is a negative one, it is helpful to use the "evidence for/evidence against" procedure to help patients examine their prediction (see Chapter 9). If there is convincing evidence that the event will turn out badly, the plan should be altered. If the prediction is based on emotional reasoning and has little or no objective basis, the event can be reframed as an experiment to test the prediction.

When people enter therapy they are eager to solve problems, decrease distress, and learn new methods for coping. They might be initially inpatient with a positive approach unless this strategy is placed in the overall context of managing their illness. The therapist should explain the advantages of increasing positives as outlined throughout this chapter, including how it improves both mood and attitude. If there are negative habits that require immediate attention, pair one of the exercises from this chapter with one of the exercises for decreasing negatives covered in the next chapter. Be mindful not to overload the patient with interventions despite his or her enthusiasm for learning. It is better to do a few interventions well than to try to address too many problems at one time and risk overwhelming the patient further.

Key Points for the Therapist to Remember

♦ Two general rules of thumb for addressing behavioral problems in bipolar disorder are: (1) it is easier to add positive behaviors than to

Activity Schedule: Sunday–Tuesday

Time	Sun Date:	Mon	Tues
9:00 A.M.	☐	☐	☐
10:00	☐	☐	☐
11:00	☐	☐	☐
12:00 P.M.	☐	☐	☐
1:00	☐	☐	☐
2:00	☐	☐	☐
3:00	☐	☐	☐
4:00	☐	☐	☐
5:00	☐	☐	☐
6:00	☐	☐	☐
7:00	☐	☐	☐
8:00	☐	☐	☐
9:00	☐	☐	☐

Put an "X" in the box after you have completed each task

FIGURE 7.4. Activity Rating Scale.

Activity Schedule: Wednesday–Saturday

Time	Wed Date:	Thur	Fri	Sat
9:00 A.M.	☐	☐	☐	☐
10:00	☐	☐	☐	☐
11:00	☐	☐	☐	☐
12:00 P.M.	☐	☐	☐	☐
1:00	☐	☐	☐	☐
2:00	☐	☐	☐	☐
3:00	☐	☐	☐	☐
4:00	☐	☐	☐	☐
5:00	☐	☐	☐	☐
6:00	☐	☐	☐	☐
7:00	☐	☐	☐	☐
8:00	☐	☐	☐	☐
9:00	☐	☐	☐	☐

Put an "X" in the box after you have completed each task

FIGURE 7.4. *cont.*

stop negative behaviors and (2) before trying to make things better, first try to get patients to not make things worse.

♦ People need to feel a sense of accomplishment or mastery as well as a sense of pleasure to maintain a euthymic state.

♦ It is important to empathize with the restrictions placed on the person in order to control the illness. At the same time, the therapist must allow the person to make his or her own decisions whether or not to take preventive actions.

Points to Discuss with Patients

♦ The absence of positive stimuli leaves the individual to experience distress from depression without activities to distract him or her from problems or provide a more balanced view of reality that includes positives as well as negatives.

♦ Avoidance turns off the stress, if only temporarily. Therefore, the depressed person is more likely the next time to use avoidance as a tactic rather than confrontation of problems. It turns off unpleasantness faster and takes less effort than resolution of the problem.

♦ The most common factors that contribute to the development and/or worsening of mania are medication noncompliance, sleep deprivation, overstimulation, and use of alcohol and drugs of abuse.

♦ When people become depressed they feel inclined to withdraw from others. However, avoidance of human contact also deprives the depressed person of positive interactions such as support, assistance with coping, a chance to laugh and experience joy, and possible opportunities to receive validation, love, and caring from others. These are normal human interactions that give us strength in difficult times, increase hopefulness about the future, and make us feel good about ourselves.

CHAPTER 8

Management of Behavioral Symptoms

CONTROLLING NEGATIVES

Eliminating Negatives

If preliminary steps have been taken to avoid factors that make depression and mania worse and efforts have been made to increase positive behaviors, the next step is to help patients cope with symptoms and problems. In the sections that follow, behavioral intervention strategies are described that will help the patient to cope more effectively with the symptoms of depression and the symptoms of mania. In most cases, the interventions provided can be used with either depressive or manic symptoms. In general, behavioral interventions can be useful for controlling, decreasing, or containing behavior in mania and for increasing behavioral deficits in depression. For example, the next section covers interventions for feeling overwhelmed. When people are depressed they are often overwhelmed with too much to do and too little energy and motivation. In mania, people can feel overwhelmed also because they have too many thoughts to track or their thinking is too disorganized to guide their actions. In either case, the suggested behavioral coping strategy should be helpful.

Feeling Overwhelmed

Life is overwhelming for people when they are depressed for several reasons. Coping ability is diminished; the responsibilities neglected due to low energy and motivation accumulate; and self-doubt, poor concentration, indecisiveness, and low self-confidence interfere with resolution of problems. As a result, small problems, such as not writing a check to pay rent, can become big problems, like getting evicted. Bigger problems are harder to resolve and are therefore avoided more actively. Early in the depression the patient's confidence may have been only moderately diminished, but energy and motivation were too low to take action. By the time the depressive episode has evolved, so have the troubles. But confidence to undertake their resolution may be all but gone. Feeling overwhelmed with accumulated difficulties is one of the more common exacerbating factors in depression.

Often, feeling overwhelmed stems from a person's conceptualization of a problem. That is, problems are viewed as overwhelming and unsolvable if they are complicated or if the person lacks the decisiveness or problem-solving skill to resolve them. The issue or issues may not, in fact, be unsolvable, but the way that they are construed magnifies their size and complexity. And the way a depressed person views his or her coping strength only minimizes confidence to confront problems. When problems are avoided and they accumulate, they can become more overwhelming.

Another cognitive process that makes life seem overwhelming is the mental aggregation of tasks, chores, responsibilities, desires, and problems into one big cluster or mass of difficulties. The person loses the ability to compartmentalize tasks, set goals for each individual activity, and take on one problem at a time. The behavioral intervention for coping with overwhelming tasks or responsibility is called graded task assignment.

Graded Task Assignment

The goal of graded task assignment (GTA) is to take large, overwhelming tasks and break them down into smaller, more manageable pieces. This changes the conceptualization of the tasks from one large overwhelming cluster to a series of small and more easily accomplished exercises.

To get started, patients list all the tasks that require their attention. This would include problems to be solved, chores, responsibilities, neglected social contacts, and any other task that requires the patient's attention. After a patient has made a project list, it is necessary to divide the tasks into smaller, more easily accomplished steps and to devise a plan to guide the patient from one task to the next, avoiding the pitfalls that have contributed to inertia in the past. The degree to which the person is overwhelmed and his or her level of inertia and energy determine the size of each subtask. The greater the inertia and the lower the energy, interest, and motivation, the smaller each step should be made. For example, listing "clean the kitchen" may be sufficient for those patients who have enough energy to complete all the steps involved in this chore. For others, however, it will be necessary to divide this chore into each of the subtasks required, such as (1) wash the dishes, (2) put the dishes away, (3) sweep the floor, (4) empty the garbage, and (5) clean off the countertops.

It can be helpful to prioritize tasks on the project list by importance or urgency and approach them in that order. However, it may be better for the patient to attempt the easiest tasks first to gain some sense of control and accomplishment. Another strategy is to have the patient select the tasks whose completion will give the greatest amount of subjective relief.

> Tom feels overwhelmed as soon as he walks into his apartment because his living room is such a mess. He can head home feeling better after spending time with friends or attending an AA meeting but feel instantly depressed as soon as he walks through his apartment door. Knowing this, he sometimes finds things to do outside of his home to avoid feeling to bad. When initiating GTA, Tom chose to take on cleaning his living room first. Because he was a "packrat" by nature (he had accumulated a number of worthless items and a great deal of paper that was sitting on the floor of his living room), it was necessary to divide this chore into small parts. For example, his first task was to throw away junk mail and old newspapers that had accumulated. His second step was to put away the clothes that had been left on the couch and chairs. The third was to put away the tools that had been taken out while he was repairing a chair. The fourth was to take dirty dishes to the kitchen, and so on. During therapy sessions the tasks are assigned as homework and reviewed at the following session.

Usually, it is only necessary to assign the first few parts and the sense of accomplishment experienced by the patient motivates him or her to continue on. The therapists should follow up on the progress of the GTA. This will provide an opportunity to positively reinforce patients' efforts with praise and to inquire about the effect of the activity on self-confidence, mood, and motivation, which reinforces the CBT model.

To maximize the impact of this behavioral intervention, ask patients to predict their likelihood of attempting each GTA step. If they believe they are very likely to attempt the task, ask why they believe it is so. Remember that in the past it has been extremely difficult to initiate activities. What is different now? This may be an opportunity to illustrate how positive expectations can increase motivation. If the prediction of success is low, the therapist has an opportunity to explore the logic of this prediction. Ideas such as "I'm too lazy," "I can't handle stress anymore," and "If I try anything today, I'll just feel worse," can be evaluated with cognitive restructuring techniques (see Chapter 9).

Guilt Associated with Inertia

It is common for patients to feel considerable guilt for their decreased interest, motivation, and activity that comes with depression. Their personal explanations for their inertia may include character flaws, such as laziness, incompetence, or weakness. These self-denigrating thoughts worsen mood, which can, in turn, maintain the inertia. If the patient is unaware that low energy and motivation are symptoms of depression, an explanation like the following can be provided:

> "Each person has a certain amount of energy available each day. Generally, people have a sufficient amount of energy to accomplish the tasks required for a given day. There are times, however, when the amount of energy needed to complete activities exceeds the amount of energy that the person possesses that day. For example, a person who has 10 units of energy but has 15 units of work to do runs out of energy before the tasks are completed.
>
> "There are ways to acquire more energy, such as by refueling the energy system (e.g., by sleeping or eating) or by obtaining units of energy from someone else (e.g., by getting assistance from a family member). It is also possible to reduce the number of activities to match the level of energy available. When people are depressed, they have fewer units of energy available to them than they would normally possess. If they attempt to accomplish the same number of tasks that they did when they were well, they will run out of energy before they run out of work. The trick is to attempt the number of tasks equivalent to the amount of energy available."

Providing an explanation of this nature can help patients to understand inertia as a symptom of depression rather than as a sign of procrastination or laziness. This reframing of the problem often reduces guilt and anxiety associated with feeling overwhelmed by tasks.

Some patients intellectually understand that they are not capable of the same level of activity when depressed as when well (asymptomatic), yet they feel pressured to perform at the same level. For these patients, depression is an explanation but not an excuse. If they misattribute the problem to a character flaw in themselves or to the behavior of others, it may be helpful to examine the evidence for and against their assumptions before generating alternative explanations. Helping patients to evaluate the validity of their own assumptions or explanations can be a more powerful intervention than attempting to convince them that the illness explanation is more valid. If patients do not themselves suggest that their inertia is a result of their depression, the clinician may find it useful to educate them about the symptoms of depression. For patients who readily accept or endorse this explanation but discount it as an excuse for their own inertia, it is important to discuss and evaluate this line of reasoning objectively.

Overstimulation

Antonio had manic episodes 3 years in a row all beginning in early March and all ending only after hospitalizations. The first time Antonio had no idea what was happening to him. He was 25 years old, a graduate student, going to class, and making friends when "suddenly" he felt "out of control." People said he was "acting strange" and "drinking up a storm." He thought he was "losing his grip on reality." His roommate convinced him to go to the emergency room after he cut his hand while preparing a meal. Another friend thought that Antonio had "mental problems" and needed to see a doctor. The hand injury provided an opportunity to have a doctor examine him. After tending to his hand, the doctor called Antonio's family and a decision was made to admit him to the psychiatric unit. Antonio's parents and friend were relieved.

Not convinced that his own personal "March madness" was a problem that could repeat itself, Antonio discontinued the mood stabilizer he had been given in the hospital once his manic symptoms seemed to have subsided. He did well through the rest of that year and through the holiday season, but in mid-February the mania returned. It took several weeks before Antonio admitted to himself that he was changing. His denial still intact, he thought the changes he felt were just from relief that the cold winter months were over and basketball season was well on its way. After several days of sleep loss, Antonio listened to his mother and called his psychiatrist. Antonio was admitted to the hospital for a short stay to reinitiate his medication treatment.

When the third springtime episode of mania came around, Antonio knew it. Determined not to "lose it," he called his doctor for help. Medication treatment was resumed and Antonio did his part to not make matters worse by avoiding giving in to what his doctor had called stimulation seeking. During Antonio's prior two manic episodes he had felt "bored" with his life as a student. He realized that, like many people who have had manic episodes, during such times he was not only sensitive to the effects of overstimulation but also craved it. He had great difficulty sitting in a quiet library, reading through piles of materials, and focusing his thoughts. He believed the problem was that he needed more excitement in his life. The solitude of study got to him, making him more and more anxious until he felt he had to get out of the library before he crawled out of his skin. He craved people, pleasure, and movement, Antonio found a club near campus with live music and plenty of girls. He started spending more time there and less time with his books. He wasn't worried about school. He felt increasingly confident in his ability to succeed without study. It wasn't long before Antonio became overstimulated and could no longer tolerate the noise, confusion, and crowds in the club, even with the numbing effect of alcohol.

Antonio's doctor helped him to remember what had happened during his first two manic episodes and explained how overstimulation from cognitive changes in mania and from his environment had escalated his mania in the past and could do so again. This time, Antonio admitted that his doctor was right. Antonio had been trying to convince himself that he didn't really have a mental illness. After three years in a row of mania he was ready to listen to the doctor and take the precautions necessary to control this illness. Although in the back of his mind he had hoped it would go away, he knew that continuing to ignore the problem was not going to make that happen.

Increased speed of thought can cause a person to perceive activity around him or her as slow or boring; thus, he or she may seek more stimulation. The problem is that too much stimulation appears to drive mania by increasing activity, disrupting sleep, escalating racing thoughts, and encouraging risky behaviors. Prevention or control of mania must include self-monitoring of the need for stimulation and stimulation-seeking behaviors, as well as the feelings associated with overstimulation such as anxiety and irritability.

Table 8.1 lists examples of overstimulation coming from within the individual. Some are common symptoms of mania. Others result from the mental activity generated by symptoms. Table 8.1 also lists examples of overstimulation stemming from the environment. The symptoms of mania can lead a person to seek out some of these environmental stimulants and they may feel good when symptoms are rela-

TABLE 8.1. Sources of Stimulation

Internal sources of overstimulation	External sources of overstimulation
• Racing thoughts	• Noise
• New ideas	• Clutter
• Making plans	• Confusion
• Being creative	• Too many people
• Starting new projects	• Traffic on the road
• Talking about your problems	• Loud laughter
• Reminiscing about the past	• Loud music
	• Phones ringing
	• Children playing
	• Group therapy

tively mild. Unwanted sources of stimulation, however, can cause irritation, annoyance, or anger.

Lifestyle management to prevent relapse includes limiting stimulation, particularly when the individual is vulnerable to recurrence of hypomania or mania.

> Sandra made it a habit to turn off the television by 9:00 P.M. during the spring and summer when she was more vulnerable to mania. She spent the rest of the evening reading or talking with her husband. When she thought she might have difficulty getting to sleep, she tried to relax. She had tried yoga in the evenings but found it too difficult. Instead she found that listening to peaceful music, taking a warm bath, or listening to an audiotape made by her therapist that helped her relax her muscles from head to toe worked best.

Contact with others can also be overstimulating and can interfere with sleep. This includes talking about family problems at night after the children have gone to bed or having an enjoyable conversation on the phone or online with friends that lasts into the early morning hours. Sexual activities can be overstimulating for some and may be better in the morning or early evening hours. Arguments at the end of the day are certainly overstimulating and should be avoided when possible.

> Sandra's mother was in the habit of calling Sandra late in the evening when she had something on her mind. Sandra didn't want to

be rude or appear uncaring, but listening to her mother complain almost always upset her. Usually, the complaints were about other family members. When Sandra tried to end these conversations her mother would say something like, "You're the only one I can talk to. No one else cares." The truth was that others wouldn't listen to her mother's complaints because her mother never listened to advice or accepted assistance. Sandra explained to her mother that evening phone calls were bad for her mental health. Although she said that she understood, Sandra's mother would call back a few evenings later. To solve this problem Sandra had to be self-disciplined and allow the answering machine to pick up her mother's evening calls. Although Sandra's fear was that one of these evenings her mother might really need her, Sandra's husband helped her remember that her mother was a resourceful person and would be able to get through to the other family members and several of her friends in case of real difficulty.

New ideas can also be considered a source of overstimulation. Before cognitive processes become disorganized or incoherent, there is often a period when thoughts are especially clear and creative. People make new connections between ideas, have moments of insight, solve problems in new and effective ways, or come up with unique and ingenious plans. While these are all very positive experiences, the actions, including planning and execution of new projects, can themselves be overstimulating. This is particularly true if they occur late at night and, thereby, interfere with sleep or lead to risky behaviors.

It would not be well received for a therapist to discourage creativity and insight. But attention and concern are warranted if a patient's new ideas are accompanied by the other symptoms of mania. To help patients make good use of their creative thoughts without risking overstimulation, inquire about any precautions being taken. If the patient is unaware of what is needed, review rules of sleep hygiene, consistency in medication adherence, and the importance of safeguards from overstimulation. This can be a sensitive area of discussion, as some patients will perceive this as discounting their great ideas, overpathologizing their creativity, or otherwise putting a damper on their enthusiasm as significant others may also do. Following is an example of such a conversation:

TEDDY: I am so excited. I think I have finally come up with an idea that is going to change my life.

THERAPIST: Really. What is it? [Thought: I hope he's not getting manic.]

TEDDY: [Thought: She doesn't believe me.] You probably would think it's stupid.

THERAPIST: I'd love to hear about it. [Thought: I need more information before I can tell if this is mania.]

TEDDY: [Thought: She's testing me.] I'm thinking about starting a small business out of my home.

THERAPIST: What kind of business?

TEDDY: Income tax preparation.

THERAPIST: Tell me more.

TEDDY: I help my neighbor a little each tax season. She does this at home and she said she would help me get started.

THERAPIST: That sounds interesting. [Thought: So far it sounds reasonable. He's good in math and I've heard him mention the neighbor before.]

TEDDY: I'm going to get my brother-in-law to send me his clients. He's a lawyer and he knows a lot of people. My aunt will help me too. She's a college financial aid counselor and I bet she'd send some of those students to me. Their taxes are pretty simple.

THERAPIST: What about your regular job? [Thought: Sounds a little grandiose.]

TEDDY: I would do this after work. I usually get off at 4:30 P.M. That will give me a lot of time before bed. [Thought: She thinks I'm going to stay up all night and get manic.]

THERAPIST: That sounds like a real possibility and I can see how the extra money could help pay off some debt. But you know me; I'm a little concerned that a second job would be too much for you. [Thought: I need to make him aware that hypomania is a possibility but not discourage his attempt to solve problems.]

TEDDY: (*angrily*) I knew it! Every time I come up with a new idea you think I'm manic!

THERAPIST: I do have to admit that I get concerned. Do you know why that is?

TEDDY: You're like all the others. You want to hold me back.

THERAPIST: Do you really think that's true?

TEDDY: (*Sighs and pauses.*) No. I know it's not true. I just don't want to be told that I'm crazy or my idea is crazy, or that I can't handle it.

THERAPIST: You're right. I did say I had concern about you being able to handle it. I'm sorry if I insulted you.

TEDDY: It's all right.

THERAPIST: One of the reasons you come to see me is to help you stay well and to help you watch for the signs that mania or depression are returning so we can do something to stop them.

TEDDY: I know.

THERAPIST: So while I am listening to you, I can appreciate your excitement over this plan but the cautious part of my brain can't help but listen for signs of trouble. I'd like your plan to succeed and I would hate for hypomania or mania to keep you from pulling it off.

TEDDY: Me too.

THERAPIST: So what do you need to do to be successful at this without mania spoiling it?

TEDDY: Keep taking my medicine, watch for signs of getting hyper, and try not to lose sleep over it. I'll start small and see where it goes. I have to take some classes first. I like the idea of starting with student tax returns. They don't usually have much, so there's not a lot of paperwork involved.

THERAPIST: Great? How can I help you be successful and not go overboard?

TEDDY: Be honest with me if you think I'm getting manic even when I don't want to hear it.

THERAPIST: That I can do.

During times when activity has the potential to overstimulate the patient, it can be useful to have the patient keep a Mood Graph. On a daily basis patients can monitor mood or more salient symptoms such as concentration, sleep pattern, or activity level. When they see shifts they should make note of their likely cause and make adjustments in behavior as needed.

Overstimulation in Depression

Overstimulation can be distressing for people during depressive episodes as well. Internal sources of stimulation such as racing thoughts or a flood of new ideas are not usually a problem unless the person is experiencing a mixed episode. However, external sources of stimulation such as loud noises, excessive movement, bright lights, confusion, or a messy home environment can leave the depressed person feeling overwhelmed or anxious.

Being faced with numerous responsibilities when energy is low can also overstimulate and cause irritability and agitation. The temptation is often to escape the "noise" by avoiding tasks and withdrawing from others. While avoidance is usually considered counterproductive, it can give temporary relief by lessening stress. Time away from overstimulation helps patients to regroup before returning to face their world.

Increased Interests, Ideas, and Activity

Perhaps one of the most enjoyable aspects of mania is the grandiosity. When manic, some patients with bipolar disorder believe they can do anything:

> "I don't mean to sound conceited, but I am the smartest person in the world. I didn't get past the tenth grade, but I have had training on the job in science and engineering. I know enough to get a PhD right now. Honest, I have so many ideas that I can hardly tell you about them."

The proliferation of new ideas and projects, coupled with the overconfidence inspired by mania, creates a cycle of activity that can itself perpetuate and escalate the mania. Not all patients with bipolar disorder experience this symptom of mania. It is necessary to review each patient's history to determine if past episodes of mania included increased ideas or activity.

Because it usually begins slowly and builds over the course of the episode, the increased activity associated with mania can serve as a marker of the onset of mania. The patient's Mood Graph can be used to track the progression of increased ideas into increased activity and overstimulation. The first step is to help the patient draw a connection between changes in interest or activity level and changes in mood. As an example, the clinician may ask the patient to note on the previous week's Mood Graph his or her activity level for the past few days, using the same scale (e.g., -1 to +1 for the normal range). The clinician and the patient can then review the graph together to determine if there is an association between mood and interest or activity changes. Figure 8.1 shows an example of such a Mood Graph.

This patient began the week with more activity than usual and an

Mood Graph

Name: _____

Week of: _____

Manic		Plan	Sun	Mon	Tues	Wed	Thur	Fri	Sat
+5	Not sleeping, psychotic	Go to the hospital	•	•	•	•	•	•	•
+4	Manic, poor judgment		•	•	•	•	•	•	•
+3	Hypomanic	Call doctor	A	A	A	•	•	•	•
+2	Energized	Take action	•	•	•	•	•	•	•
+1	Hyper, happy	Monitor closely	•	•	•	A	A	A	A
0	Normal		•	•	•	•	•	•	•
-1	Low, down	Monitor closely	•	•	•	•	•	•	•
-2	Sad	Take action	•	•	•	•	•	•	•
-3	Depressed	Call the doctor	•	•	•	•	•	•	•
-4	Immobilized		•	•	•	•	•	•	•
-5	Suicidal	Go to the hospital	•	•	•	•	•	•	•

Depressed

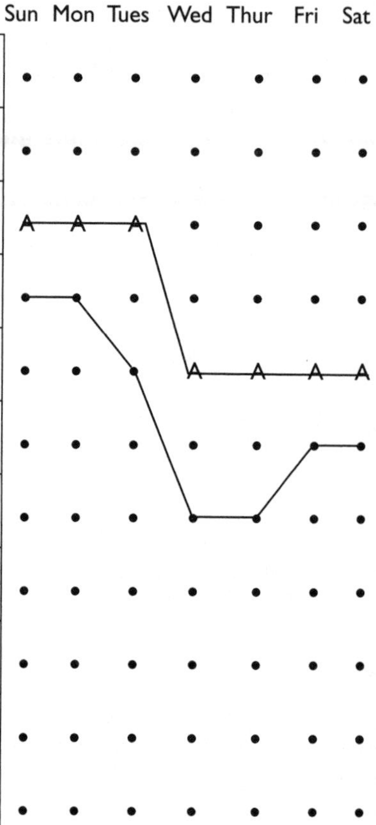

What caused the mood shift?

FIGURE 8.1. Mood graph.

elevation in mood. She had begun an exciting new project early in the week and she felt somewhat elated. She had been relatively inactive for several weeks and welcomed the opportunity to do something new. After a few days of feeling "a little too good," she began to watch herself more carefully. By Tuesday she had made the decision to decrease her activity. She had found herself taking control of the new project, assuming more responsibility than necessary. This was a familiar pattern for her and one that often left her feeling out of control.

For a few days after pulling back from the project, her mood dropped into mild dysphoria. She hated the fact that she could not handle the work without "getting sick," and she missed her friends on the job. After a few days of what she called "feeling sorry for herself," her mood began to improve.

The time to begin tracking interest and activity levels on the Mood Graph is when hypomania is suspected. Patients who know the time of year that they are most likely to experience mania can begin mood and activity graphing at least a month before this vulnerable time. This approach makes it possible to identify the changes in mood (affect), activity level (behavior), and interest (cognition) that are the precursors to mania. If these changes can be identified before they reach manic proportions, the increased stimulation can be contained to some degree and pharmacological interventions can be strengthened.

The objective of the intervention at this point is to help patients who are becoming manic choose a limited number of activities from their plethora of ideas and pursue those that have the highest probability of success and the lowest probability of negative consequences. To teach patients how to organize and set limits on their interests and activities, the clinician begins with an examination of their current activities. Using the first column of the Goal-Setting Worksheet shown in Figure 8.2, the patient lists current activities, responsibilities, and interests, as well as future plans, in any order. The list should include daily home and work responsibilities, school requirements, regularly scheduled activities outside the home (e.g., church activities and bowling club), obligations to extended family members or friends, social activities, personal interests that are currently being pursued or planned (e.g., diets and reading), and new interests or ideas. In the second column, the patient lists the anticipated date of the activity or deadline, as applicable. If an activity is ongoing, the patient should note this fact in the date column also.

The next step is to organize the activities so that the patient focuses his or her efforts on the tasks with the highest priority. To accomplish this, the patient must attach a priority ranking to each of the activities. Therefore, in the third column of the Goal-Setting

Current activities, responsibilities, and interests	Priority			Rank order
	High	Medium	Low	
_____	H	M	L	_____
_____	H	M	L	_____
_____	H	M	L	_____
_____	H	M	L	_____
_____	H	M	L	_____
_____	H	M	L	_____
_____	H	M	L	_____
_____	H	M	L	_____
_____	H	M	L	_____
_____	H	M	L	_____
_____	H	M	L	_____
_____	H	M	L	_____
_____	H	M	L	_____
_____	H	M	L	_____
_____	H	M	L	_____
_____	H	M	L	_____
_____	H	M	L	_____
_____	H	M	L	_____
_____	H	M	L	_____

FIGURE 8.2. Goal-Setting Worksheet.

Worksheet, the patient rates each activity as a high priority (H), moderate priority (M), or low priority (L). The therapist can ask questions or make observations that may facilitate this process, but the priority ratings must come from the patient. Once this task is complete, the patient assigns numerical rankings to assign priorities within each group of activities.

Finally, the patient selects a reasonable number of tasks to attempt in the following week. The grandiosity that accompanies hypomania may leave patients feeling that they can accomplish all the tasks on their list and, in fact, their extra energy and their decreased need for sleep may make it possible for them to do so. To make activity scheduling more effective, it is essential to include sleep on the plan for the week. With the help of the therapist, the patient sketches a rough outline of the time activities will occur and the time they will stop so the patient can prepare for sleep. The clinician must make it clear, however, that the overstimulation caused by the increased activity can actually worsen symptoms. Patients may lose their concentration, become more and more disorganized, and be unable to complete tasks successfully. Setting limits on activity can help to contain the progression of mania.

Patients with bipolar disorder commonly report that, when manic, they start several projects but rarely complete them. They become increasingly excited with each new idea and are anxious to begin the next project right away. With activity planning and prioritizing, the patient must agree to complete each task before attempting the next.

As new ideas are formulated, they can be added to the Goal-Setting Worksheet and prioritized accordingly. The purpose of this process is to create a cushion of time that allows patients to think through their new ideas and plans before they act. If the process does not slow activity, more aggressive pharmacological interventions are probably necessary.

"A" List and "B" List

A big challenge for people with bipolar disorder is to take care of themselves, in part by protecting themselves from feeling overextended, overwhelmed, or overstimulated, but still be able to effectively cope with life. Responsibilities, challenges, and difficulties cannot be ignored altogether even when the person lacks energy, hope, motivation, or internal fortitude due to the illness. Getting through a day without succumbing to thoughts of suicide can be challenging enough without the burdens of work, family, or loneliness. Unsuccessful attempts to cope with normal life stresses and strains can escalate sadness and irritability, further weaken self-esteem, and make ending their lives seem like a reasonable alternative to continued frustration and ineffectiveness.

Part of the problem is that people with bipolar disorder expect themselves to function as well as those without mental illnesses.

Another part is that society does not easily accommodate people with difficulties or disabilities.

> "It's hard to be me," says Lynn. "I know what to do and how to do it, but there are days when I can't think straight, can't organize myself. It's so frustrating. I'm tired, but that's no excuse. My bills still need to get paid. My apartment still needs to be cleaned. My dog still needs to be walked. My mother still needs help. It doesn't matter that I'm depressed or hyper or hopeless or disorganized."
>
> Lynn's bipolar disorder interferes with her functioning, and her resulting inefficiency or lack of productivity makes her feel worse. To get something accomplished would boost her confidence, even if it took her longer than she would prefer. For people like Lynn, the "A" list/"B" list exercise can help.

This behavioral intervention formalizes a mental activity that most people do without much effort. It involves identifying a limited number of high-priority tasks that can be accomplished in a day and completing them before doing anything else. In depression, this combats the inertia caused by being overwhelmed with too much to do. In mania, this exercise limits activity, particularly if people can follow the instructions to finish the high-priority items on which have been placed on the "A" list before starting the lower-priority tasks selected for the "B" list. Consciously deciding to limit the number of tasks to only a few of the most important makes it easier to resist the manic urge to start many tasks and finish few. In depression, decision making can be impaired. Creating a short "A" list of tasks that must be done the next day and a short "B" list of tasks the person would like to do if time and energy allow eliminate the distress people can face each morning when they know there is much to do, but do not know where to start.

Figure 8.3 provides an example of a typical series of "A" lists and "B" lists a patient might create to help him get through a difficult week.

Priorities will change from day to day, so the items on the "A" list will vary by demand. When depression is a problem it is best to make plans in the evening for the next day. At other times some people prefer making their lists each morning as a way of getting organized for the day. What is not completed one day can be added to the next. When organization and decision making have improved, this intervention can be discontinued.

Some people are natural list makers and always keep a running tally of tasks to do. While this may seem second nature to them, the review of long lists of tasks can be overwhelming and inhibit progress.

	"A" list	"B" List
Day 1 Monday	Pay rent Go to work Buy groceries for dinner	Do a load of laundry Return sister's phone call
Day 2 Tuesday	Pay electric bill Go to work Fold and put away laundry	Go to DBSA meeting
Day 3 Wednesday	Pay credit card bill Go to work	Go to mom's for dinner
Day 4 Thursday	Make a plan for weekend Go to work Make an appointment to see doctor	Visit with neighbor Sort through the week's mail
Day 5 Friday	Go to work	Go to movies with a friend
Day 6 Saturday	Clean the living room Wash two loads of laundry	Clean bathroom Spend time outdoors at the park or in the yard
Day 7 Sunday	Call mom Finish cleaning bathroom Put away clean laundry	Buy groceries for the week Read the newspaper

FIGURE 8.3. "A" list/"B" list examples.

Some people can keep a "master list" of activities and pick some daily for their "A" and "B" lists. For others, it is best to substitute the master list for the simplified version until symptoms improve. Those who are accustomed to keeping daily calendars can schedule tasks ahead by assigning them to a specific day. This is more helpful than simply noting deadlines.

This chapter and the previous one on controlling triggers and adding positives have been more behavioral in nature. They constitute the "B" in CBT. Behavioral problems, including faulty coping skills, increased and disorganized activity, taking risks, and procrastination or lethargy, are all fueled by cognitive processes. According to the cognitive model, how people think greatly influences their choices of action. In Chapters 9 and 10 we discuss the content and the process changes in cognition that occur in depression and mania, which includes not only what people think about when they are symptomatic but also the quality of their cognitive processing when they are ill. To be most effective, symptom control in bipolar disorder requires the use of both cognitive and the behavioral interventions.

Key Points for the Therapist to Remember

♦ Often problems are viewed as overwhelming and unsolvable if they are complicated or if the person lacks the decisiveness or problem-solving skill to resolve them. The issue or issues may not, in fact, be unsolvable, but the way that they are construed magnifies their size and complexity.

♦ It would not be well received for a therapist to discourage creativity and insight. But attention and concern are warranted if these new ideas are accompanied by the other symptoms of mania.

Points to Discuss with Patients

♦ It is common for patients to feel guilty for their lack of interest, motivation, and activity, so they call themselves lazy, incompetent, or weak. These self-denigrating thoughts worsen mood, which can, in turn, maintain the inertia.

♦ Too much internal and external stimulation appears to drive mania by increasing activity, disrupting sleep, escalating racing thoughts, and encouraging risky behaviors.

♦ External sources of stimulation such as loud noises, excessive movement, bright lights, confusion, or a messy home environment can leave the depressed person feeling overwhelmed or anxious.

♦ People make new connections between ideas, have moments of insight, solve problems in new and effective ways, or come up with unique and/or ingenious plans. While these are all very positive experiences, the actions, including planning and execution of new projects, can themselves be overstimulating.

♦ A big challenge for people with bipolar disorder is to take care of themselves, in part by protecting themselves from feeling overextended, overwhelmed, or overstimulated, but still be able to effectively cope with life.

CHAPTER 9

Management
of Cognitive Symptoms
CONTENT CHANGES

As described in Chapter 2, the cognitive-behavioral model of bipolar disorder illustrated in Figure 2.1 (p. 24) emphasizes stopping the evolving course of the illness by intervening at any place in the cycle. In this chapter, we are discussing methods for breaking the cycle at the level of cognitive changes. Controlling cognitive decline should help to prevent problematic behavioral changes that can cause a decline in functioning and the development of psychosocial problems.

The cognitive symptoms of depression and mania include both content changes, the types of things that people think about, and process changes, including the way information is processed and the amount and quality of thoughts. This chapter focuses on methods for dealing with these changes during manic and depressive episodes. In this chapter we cover content changes and interventions that can be helpful to reduce their influence on actions. In Chapter 10 we discuss cognitive process changes and appropriate interventions for containing these symptoms. Table 9.1 summarizes common content and process changes in depression and mania.

Content Changes in Cognitions

The cognitive errors made popular in the writings of Aaron Beck (Beck et al., 1979) and David Burns (1980) fall into four general cate-

TABLE 9.1. Content and Process Changes in Depression and Mania

Depression	Mania
State-dependent content changes	

• Cognitive errors
  – Tunnel vision
  – Making guesses
  – Absolutes
  – Misperceptions
• Suicidal ideation
• Low self-esteem
• Negative attitudes
	• Grandiosity/increased optimism
	• Risks overlooked
	• Paranoia/suspiciousness
	• Increased self-confidence
	• Urge to make changes

State-dependent process changes	
• Slowed thinking • Impaired decision making • Difficulty concentrating • Impaired problem solving • Easily overwhelmed • Rumination	• Increased fluency of ideas • Distractibility • Difficulty concentrating • Sounds seem louder and color brighter • Racing thoughts • Disorganized thinking • Impaired judgment

gories, and Table 9.2 provides examples of their occurrence in depression and mania.

In general, these four categories reflect how emotional states affect the way information is processed. In "tunnel vision," the individual focuses on a limited amount of information that is consistent with current mood and ideas and ignores or does not attend to contradictory information. This narrowing of focus causes conclusions to be drawn without the benefit of all available data. The typical depressed person, for example, can easily enumerate his or her faults and failures but does not consider strengths and successes. In mania, the person may see benefits and ignore risks. When "making guesses," the individual is responding to gaps in information by filling in the blanks with ideas that are consistent with his mood and attitude. If it is unclear what someone else is thinking, the person in a depressed state will assume the worst, that others are critical, while in a manic state he might assume that others think well of or admire him or, if he is anxious, that others are trying to do him harm.

"Absolutes" are rigid ideas that are often polarized as good or bad.

Global labels such as "failure," "lazy," and "unlovable" are examples of absolutes a person might use during depression to describe herself. Absolutes can also include rigid rules about how a person "should" act or think as well as judgmental comments about others. Suicidal ideation can become rigid and inflexible if the person believes her situation to be hopeless or the misery to be unbearable. These terms, "hopeless" and "unbearable", are absolute in nature and prevent the depressed person from seeing any room for negotiation (i.e., no shades of gray in his or her circumstances).

In mania, the absolutes are evident in single-minded thinking. New ideas are seen as flawless and urgent. Waiting before taking action is unacceptable because the patient feels absolute certainty about the likely success of a plan. The opinions of others are viewed as

TABLE 9.2. Examples of Common Thinking Errors

Category	Examples in depression	Examples in mania	Interventions
Tunnel vision	• Listing failures • Seeing what is going wrong, ignoring what is going right	• Risks overlooked	• Examine the evidence • Perspective of others • Get the big picture
Making guesses	• Taking things personally • Catastrophizing • Jumping to conclusions	• Paranoia • Suspiciousness • Projection	• Examine the evidence • Alternative explanations
Misperceptions	• Magnify problems • Dismiss compliments	• Gradiosity • Increased confidence • Discounting negative input	• Get feedback • Recognize symptoms • Monitor symptoms
Absolutes	• Black-and-white thinking • Suicidal ideation	• Change is urgent • Single-mindedness	• Cognitive continuum • Advantages/disadvantages[a] • Problem-solving[a] • Reasons to live • Reasons to have hope

[a]Interventions for these are covered in the next chapter.

unnecessary and, if contrary, unenlightened. Even the desire for change itself can be an example of absolute thinking if the change is perceived as mandatory or critical and the urge compelling.

In the case of absolutes, the patient categorizes information as black or white (as a success or failure), sees others as "with me" or "against me," or sees the future as either hopeless or hopeful. Information that is in the "gray zone" between these extreme views is either restated to make it fit into one of the two categories or rejected as useless, irrelevant, or occurring only by chance.

"Misperceptions" describe information that the patient distorts by magnification or minimization. In depression, negative events or information are magnified and positives are minimized. For example, a suggestion from an employer to improve work performance may be perceived as a hurtful criticism, a rejection, or a significant embarrassment. A compliment about work effort given as part of the feedback might be minimized by comparison, rejected as insincere, or missed altogether.

During hypomania or mania, the value of new ideas or projects may be magnified. Good ideas become great ideas. Wishes become mandates. Risks, in turn, are minimized, or viewed as worth taking, given the potential gains. Self-confidence may also be magnified and weaknesses dismissed.

Distortions in cognitions can lead a person to draw incorrect conclusions. This is problematic in that an incorrect conclusion, either overly negative or overly optimistic, not only dictates a person's emotional reaction to events but also influences his choice of actions. Overly positive estimates coupled with misperception of risks might lead a person in a manic state to go on shopping sprees, engage in promiscuous behaviors, or engage in other impulsive actions. An overly negative conclusion may immobilize the person in a depressed state so that he or she does not resolve problems or neglects responsibilities. These actions usually exacerbate difficulties or add unwanted complexities to the person's life.

To disrupt the evolution of depression and mania by controlling cognitive symptoms, the patient must be able to recognize or "catch" cognitions that could be distorted by depression or mania. Recognizing these thoughts as they arise would allow the patient to "control" the potentially negative influence of these cognitions on mood and actions. With this knowledge, patients can "correct" or compensate for the distortions (see Table 9.3). Having a more accurate perception of reality will increase the chance that any actions patients take will be helpful and not hurtful to them. Methods for catching, controlling, and correcting distorted cognitions are discussed in the sections that follow.

TABLE 9.3. Coping with Content Changes

1. *Catch* depressive cognitions.

2. *Control* their influence on choice of action.

3. *Correct* any distortions.

Catching Distorted Cognitions

Before it is possible to control and correct distorted cognitions they must be captured. For some this is a difficult task, because these thoughts, often referred to as automatic thoughts, occur rapidly, sometimes outside conscious awareness. Frequently, they come in a string, such as when a person is flooded with new ideas or when listing one's failings.

The therapist can introduce the concept of automatic thoughts by first sensitizing patients to negative automatic thoughts that may have occurred when they were in bad moods. There are several useful strategies. It is most common to inquire about recent stressful events that might have stimulated a change in mood. Generally, people can recall with some detail what occurred but may have more difficulty pinpointing ideas or thoughts that accompanied upset feelings. To get at those automatic thoughts, the therapist should ask patients what it was about the event that made them feel upset. It may also be helpful to inquire along the lines of the cognitive triad—that is, thoughts about self, others, and the future as they apply to the situation. For example, Gilbert told his therapist about an argument he had had with his older brother the previous week. The brother, Paul, was giving Gilbert instructions on how to grout a bathtub they were installing in their mother's house.

> "He treats me like I'm a child. I'm 40 years old. He thinks he knows everything. I hate working with him." When the therapist probed further, he heard the following automatic thoughts: "No one thinks I can do anything," "I shouldn't have to work for my brother. I should be running a business," "I'm such a loser, no wonder he thinks he has to hold my hand," and "Things are never going to change."

The therapist was able to feed back this information to the patient and explain that these are examples of automatic thoughts.

Another strategy is to ask patients to recall the last time they felt depressed or down and the type of attitude they might have had toward self, others, the world in general, and the future during that time. Many patients will immediately identify negative automatic thoughts prominent during depression. A more difficult challenge is to get patients to recall how their automatic thoughts might have been different during hypomanic or manic periods, unless they are currently in one. To facilitate their recall, ask patients to compare the automatic negative thoughts to how they might view themselves, others, or the future when their mood was more positive or more irritable.

Some patients may find it difficult to identify specific automatic thoughts when they flood their minds more rapidly than can be verbalized, or their thoughts may consist more of general impressions and visual images than specific words. In either case, ask patients to describe their general impressions or images until they are able to identify the themes, beliefs, or underlying concerns. To elicit thoughts, ask patients to imagine themselves in the stressful situation and describe the picture they see in as much detail as possible. Who is present? What are they doing or saying? What is the emotional tone of the image? How is the patient feeling? What does he or she think will go wrong? What are the consequences?

Automatic Thought Records

To analyze the validity of any automatic thoughts associated with mood shifts, the patient must be able to identify mood shifts, the events that precipitated them, the associated automatic thoughts, and the actions that followed. One method traditionally used to monitor the occurrence of negative automatic thoughts is a patient diary. There are many forms and names for the thought diary, the most common of which is the Automatic Thought Record. Figure 9.1 provides an example.

The instructions for completing the Automatic Thought Record are as follows:

1. When a mood shift occurs, describe in the first column the circumstances under which the change occurred. Only a few words are necessary as a reminder of the stimulus for the mood shift.

2. In the "Thoughts" column, list the thoughts that were associated with the event. To identify these thoughts, it is helpful for the clinician to ask what it was about the event that made the patient's mood change; for example, "What was it about your mother's criticism that made you feel guilty?" "What was it about that situation that made you angry?" "What made you feel like crying?" Using a 0–100%

FIGURE 9.1. Automatic Thought Record.

Date	Event	Feeling	Intensity (0–100%)			Automatic Thoughts	% Believed (0–100%)		
			Time 1	Time 2	Time 3		Time 1	Time 2	Time 3

scale, where 0% means a total lack of belief and 100% means absolute certainty, rate the intensity with which the automatic thought was believed at the time of the event.

3. Indicate in the third column the types of emotions that occurred (e.g., sadness, anger, and anxiety). If several emotions are experienced simultaneously, list each separately. Use a 0–100% scale to rate the approximate intensity of these emotions as they were experienced at the time of the event. In this scale, 0% is the absence of that emotion and 100% is the greatest intensity of that emotion ever experienced.

4. In the fourth column, list the actions taken in reaction to the event. This would include taking no action at all.

An assessment of the intensity of the emotion experienced and the intensity of belief in each of the negative automatic thoughts provides a baseline against which to compare any changes that cognitive restructuring subsequently produces. Because patients often complete the Automatic Thought Record long after the precipitating events, the intensity of the emotion and belief may have changed. If so, it suggests that some intervening event (either internal or external) caused that change. Therefore, the record includes three columns to rate intensity (1) at the time of the event, (2) at the time that the form is completed, and (3) after an intervention with CBT. If the intensity changed (increased or decreased), determining the reason for the change may be helpful in identifying existing strategies for coping with strong emotional shifts.

For example, if an event that elicited anxiety occurred (e.g., worker received a memo that the boss is calling a meeting), there is usually a cognitive response ("Oh no! This isn't good"). With time, however, the person could have ruminated over the event and heightened the emotional reaction by contemplating the catastrophic potential of the event ("I bet the company is going under and we'll all lose our jobs"). Others could reconsider the same event and minimize the catastrophic feeling of the initial reaction ("It's probably about that memo that went out last week"), putting it into perspective, thereby decreasing the intensity of the emotion. In either case, it is helpful for the therapist to know what cognitive process occurred that created the change. Cognitive strategies that decrease emotion can be applied to new events that arouse negative emotions. Cognitive strategies that increase emotion will give clues about how a person responds to stressful events. This information will help therapist in selecting interventions appropriate for a given patient.

Controlling Distorted Cognitions

Once patients understand that automatic thoughts can be distorted and, therefore, can lead them to draw incorrect conclusions, they are in a position to control these ideas from negatively influencing their choice of actions. The Symptom Summary Worksheet described in Chapter 6 can help patients to identify typical automatic thoughts that herald the onset of depression or mania. Examples include a patient's thinking that the future is hopeless when he is depressed or thinking he is the smartest person on the earth when he is in a manic state. If these types of automatic thoughts can be caught when they recur, they can signal the need to take precautions to avoid inappropriate actions that might fuel recurrences of illness. A general rule of thumb for this type of prevention is that negative automatic thoughts should be taken with a grain of salt as they typically appear during depression and lessen during remission. And positive or euphoric automatic thoughts should not be entirely trusted if they encourage a dramatic change in actions or risk taking. Instead, a pause must be inserted until the thought can be verified and a plan of action more thoroughly reviewed.

There are several ways to control the effects of automatic thoughts on actions. In hypomania and mania where there is a desire to increase activity or engage in potentially risky behavior, the 24-hour rule is useful. In this case, the patient agrees to wait 24 hours before initiating a potentially problematic behavior, longer if it seems appropriate. The logic is that if a person is having a good idea and not a manic idea, it will still be a good idea tomorrow or next week or next month when manic symptoms are not influencing mood or actions. Some specific examples provided by patients include freezing credit cards in a large container of water so that they must be defrosted in order to use them for a shopping spree. Another is to disconnect the telephone or screen calls with an answering machine to avoid speaking to annoying callers when patients are feeling irritable. Some people make themselves get more information about new ideas before putting plans into action, such as asking the opinions of family members or friends, reading more on a topic, or asking for a professional consultation.

In depressive episodes, it is easier to keep automatic thoughts from affecting actions because the desire is usually to avoid activity or to do less rather than to do more. Negative automatic thoughts that interfere with action include catastrophizing about the possible outcomes, not believing that there are any prospects for change, and viewing oneself as incompetent or lazy. These depressogenic thoughts will inhibit activity. Anxious thoughts will encourage avoidance as well, especially when stress is relieved when the individual evades the situation he or she fears, as described previously in Chapter 7. To control negative automatic thoughts, it will be necessary to take the next step and evaluate and correct any distortions that inhibit activity.

Correcting Distorted Cognitions

Often, the automatic thoughts associated with clinically significant upward or downward shifts in mood are either partially or completely invalid or inaccurate. Because the bias in automatic thoughts generally elicits or exacerbates mood shifts, one of the goals of CBT is to teach patients how to evaluate the validity of their own automatic thoughts and correct any distortions. One technique is to collect and examine the evidence that supports the validity of their thoughts and the evidence that contradicts or refutes the validity of their thoughts. This technique helps patients to focus on the facts that support their view instead of the "gut-level" feelings that can influence their thinking. This is more effective than trying to change peoples' views by dismissing them (e.g., "Don't worry about it"), discounting their validity (e.g., "Oh, that's ridiculous"), or otherwise attempting to convince others that their views are false (e.g., "You don't really believe that, do you?" and "Don't think that way").

The first step in the process is to refer to the Automatic Thought Record and select the automatic thought associated with the greatest amount of emotion or the one that troubles the patient the most. The Evaluating Your Thoughts Worksheet shown in Figure 9.2 can be used for this exercise. After providing a rationale for this intervention, ask patients to list all the facts that support or validate the automatic thought (evidence for) and all the facts that refute or invalidate the thought (evidence against). It is usually more difficult for people to generate evidence against negative automatic thoughts because their idea "feels right" and they may never have considered the possibility that their first impressions could be wrong. In this exercise, the clinician does not lead the patient by suggesting evidence against the thought. Instead, the clinician may pose facilitating questions, such as:

- "Is there anything else that makes you think this idea is true?"
- "Is there anything else that makes you think it is false?"

FIGURE 9.2. Evaluating Your Thoughts Worksheet.

My thought is:

What evidence do I have that my thought is true?	What evidence do I have that my thought is not true?	What would someone else say in this situation? What is another explanation?	My conclusions and my plan for what to do next.

- "Does anyone say or do things to you that make you think this idea is true/false?"

- "Have you had any experiences that suggest this idea is true/false?"

By not attempting to refute any of the evidence for or against the automatic thought, even if it seems silly or illogical, the clinician tries to provide a neutral response. Only when the two columns of evidence have been completed is there an attempt to evaluate the quality of the evidence. The patient weighs the evidence for and against the automatic thought and draws a conclusion about its validity. An informal review of the two columns may be sufficient, but it is important to remember that the column with the greatest number of entries is not necessarily the one that is more accurate or the one that carries the most weight. Some pieces of evidence may carry less weight than others or may have a greater influence on the conclusion drawn.

There are three possible outcomes in the evaluation of distorted automatic thoughts. First, the individual may conclude that his or her automatic thought was false. In this case, the clinician encourages the patient to replace the thought with a more valid statement. For example, if the automatic thought was, "I can't do anything right" and this was found to be incorrect, a more valid statement may be, "I do some things well, but there are other things I'm not very good at, such as keeping the house clean."

Second, the patient and the therapist may conclude that the automatic thought is true. If the clinician believes that there is some validity to a patient's negative evaluation (e.g., "I ruined my marriage"), it is not helpful to attempt to revise or replace the negative automatic thought with a more positive thought (e.g., "This frees me up to find someone better"). Instead, the content of the negative automatic thought can become a specific target for change in CBT—for example, mending the relationship, coping with the separation. Third, the patient may find that the evidence for or against the automatic thought is inconclusive. Table 9.4 summarizes these steps.

If it is unclear whether the automatic thought is true or false, more information is necessary to complete the evaluation. An experiment can be set up to gather more data. Experiments are activities that allow a person to observe him- or herself while testing contrary automatic thoughts. For example, if the patient's negative thought is that she cannot handle stress, the patient would put herself into a stressful situation, perhaps after learning some stress management methods,

TABLE 9.4. Evaluating Negative Automatic Thoughts

1. Choose an automatic thought to evaluate. Choose one listed in the Automatic Thought Record for the week. A thought or belief associated with a significant amount of negative emotion should be selected and listed at the top of the Logical Analysis of Automatic Thoughts worksheet.

2. Explain that the task is to first generate evidence to support and refute the automatic thought and then to objectively review the evidence. Ask the patient to list all evidence supporting and refuting the automatic thought in the appropriate columns.

3. After examining the evidence for and against the thought, the patient may conclude that the thought is invalid, that the evidence is inconclusive, or that the thought is indeed valid. Use your clinical judgment and decide what intervention(s) should be implemented even the results of the logical analysis. Some suggestions are:

   a. Invalid thoughts: Revise the original automatic thought to make it more accurate.

   b. Valid thoughts: Ask the patient what the consequences are given that the negative thought is valid and what the probability is of these consequences occurring. If the probability is high and the consequences are significant, take a problem-solving approach to generate a plan for decreasing the probability of negative consequences.

   c. Inclusive evidence: Find out what kind of evidence would be needed to confirm or disconfirm the thought. Generate a plan for accumulating more evidence.

and observe her actual ability to "handle it." Another example is testing the idea that people "don't like me and won't want to talk to me" by conducting a social experiment in which a patient picks someone to talk to in a social setting and observes the response received. The actual experience is compared to the patient's original prediction for the event. This process usually clarifies whether a negative thought is valid and, if so, what must be done to solve the problem. For example, if the person finds that she cannot handle stress well, therapy can focus on improving skills in this area.

Gaining Emotional Distance

Taking a different perspective regarding an upsetting event often allows patients to look at a situation more objectively and, thus, to draw more objective conclusions. To accomplish this, clinicians may ask patients to evaluate the situation as if it were happening to someone else, such as a friend, relative, or even a stranger. This method allows patients to examine a stimulus problem without the emotion that may be distorting their perceptions, as they are less likely to make the same negative interpretations of situations from the perspective of others that they make from their own perspective.

When the less personal perspective generated is different from the individual's initial assessment of the problem, the clinician may ask him or her to examine and explain the discrepancy. For example, the clinician may ask, "How is it that, when you focused on your experience with your husband, you concluded that he doesn't care, but when you looked at it from a friend's perspective, it seemed to be the wife's fault as much as the husband's? How is your situation different from your friend's? How might you apply this new observation to your own situation?" The goal of this technique is for logic to override emotional reasoning. In hypomania, a patient proposing a risky venture, for example, can be asked if he would advise his child or spouse to do to the activity he proposes. If he says "no," inquire about the double standard.

Alternative Explanations

Like taking another individual's perspective, exploring alternative explanations for events listed in the Automatic Thought Record can elicit additional, more objective evaluations of these events. These evaluations are sometimes referred to as rational responses. In this intervention, the clinician asks patients to generate alternative explanations for their own behavior and experiences (see Figure 9.2). For example, if the automatic thought is "I am incompetent," the list of alternative explanations may include "I'm not very good at this task," "I didn't have time," "Someone tried to make it difficult for me," "I was having a bad day," "I had too much on my mind," or "I've never been trained to do this particular task." When the lists are complete, the patient examines and evaluates the listed items. After eliminating unlikely explanations, the patient considers the remainder to determine if any apply to the circumstance under evaluation. The patient can then choose the alternative explanation for the event that is most appropriate. If in a hypomanic episode a patient thinks he received a negative employee evaluation because his boss is out to get him, the alternative explanations for the encounter might be that the boss is in a bad mood, that the hypomania is interfering with his job performance, or that the evaluation, while not perfect, was an improvement over the previous one.

The final step is to gather evidence to determine the validity of that alternative explanation. Some clinicians prefer to use the evidence for/evidence against technique; others ask the patient to monitor new experiences to determine whether the alternative explanation is correct. For example, if an alternative explanation for "incompetence" is a lack of skill in a specific area, the patient can evaluate his or her competence and skill in executing a similar task on the next attempt. If further examination shows this alternative explanation to be valid, it can become a treatment goal for the patient (e.g., to gain more training in that particular work-related area). In the aforementioned job evaluation example, the employee can elicit additional feedback from the boss or others to determine if there is validity to the negative marks on his evaluation. If that does not feel appropriate, improvements can be made in job performance and additional feedback requested to determine if the boss is more satisfied.

Prediction of Automatic Thoughts

After learning to catch, control, and correct automatic thoughts, patients can learn to predict their occurrence before they become a problem. It is helpful first to identify situations that typically elicit emotion and negative thoughts. In many patients' lives, there are typical situations that arouse strong emotions, positive ones and negative ones. Such situations may predictably elicit anxiety, anger, sadness, or guilt on the negative side, or excitement, arousal, glee, or a sense of urgency on the positive side. Rather than waiting for events or biologically driven mood swings to stimulate automatic thoughts, patients can reflect on past experiences and analyze their cognitions in a more dispassionate manner. This reanalysis of their automatic thoughts can provide patients with alternative responses to them. For example, if sometime in the past, the breakup of a relationship led a person to think she was a loser, she could reevaluate the situation after gaining some emotional distance to determine if being a loser was the only explanation for the breakup. Perhaps if all contributing factors could be identified, there would less self-doubt about initiating relationships in the future. In prior experiences of hypomania or mania people might recall feeling an irresistible urge to make changes in their life, in their routines, or in their relationships. A retrospective assessment of those experiences conducted when the person is no longer hypomanic or manic may allow him or her to see how mood and symptom changes might have caused an overestimate of the urgency of change and a minimization of the risks involved. With this information, the person can be better prepared to handle new ideas that emerge along with other symptoms of hypomania or mania.

Thoughts about Death and Suicide

Suicidal ideation is common in people who suffer from bipolar disorder, and it is estimated that up to half attempt suicide at some point in their lives (Chen & Dilsalver, 1996; Goodwin & Jamison, 1990). The number of suicide completers is approximately 15 times greater in people who have bipolar disorder than in the population at large (Goodwin & Jamison, 1990). This means that any suicidal ideation must be taken seriously even when clinicians doubt its sincerity.

There are several different forms that suicidal ideation can take. In general, they fall into two categories: desires to die, escape, or avoid psychic pain and repetitive thoughts that are more obsessional in nature. The former usually accompany hopelessness and distress. The latter seem more like habitual thoughts that pop into people's minds not when they are contemplating their misery but at other times. When these obsessional thoughts occur, they may be mistaken as indicators of distress. Therefore, the person begins to feel down. They may actually indicate anxiety, or they may be completely unrelated to mood. When they are more like obsessional thoughts they can be addressed with thought stopping coupled with distraction as might be done in obsessive–compulsive disorder. When they are mood congruent and indicate a lack of hope and exasperation with life, analysis of thoughts and cognitive restructuring are more appropriate.

Reframing Methods

Thoughts about suicide, whether specific desires to be dead or general wishes that suffering could end, usually result from believing there is no other solution to intense distress. Suicide appeals to some because it is within their realm of control when so many other things are not and because it is a definite solution when they have been unable to figure out any other solutions to their myriad problems. Knowing there is a way out can be comforting.

A direct cognitive intervention for suicidal thoughts is to reframe the problem as a desire to stop hurting rather than a desire to be dead. If the person can agree that what he or she would ideally desire is to stop hurting, then problem solving becomes an option. Problem-solving ability usually declines in depression and mania as cognitive processes become impaired. That is usually why people feel there is no other way out but death, because they no longer have the ability to generate alternative solutions.

There is often one problem more distressing than the others to the suicidal person. It is there that therapeutic efforts should be focused. The following questions are examples of how a therapist might help a patient identify that critical issue. "If you could solve one problem right now, which one would make you feel better?" "If solving a specific problem today would make you feel more hopeful about the future and more confident in your ability to survive, what would that problem be?" "If we could make your stress smaller by taking away one problem that is troubling you, which would it be?"

Once the issue has been identified, the therapist should inquire about what types of attempts the patient has made to cope with it. It is not uncommon for prior attempts at problem solving to have been incomplete or ineffective. At times a sustained effort was needed, but the person gave up before the problem was solved. Or fear of failure has kept a person from implementing a reasonable solution she has already identified. When energy and motivation are low because of depression, the patient may not have the strength to implement a solution. The therapist's job is to evaluate the possible solutions and help the patient to select a strategy that has some potential for relief, preferably immediate relief. This may not mean the actual problem is immediately solved but that a concrete step is taken that the patient can see as leading to a resolution, and because of this enough hope is restored to keep the patient alive until things get better.

Because of slowed cognitive processing in the patient, the therapist must take a more active role in problem solving than might be the case when the patient is less distressed. This does not mean, however, that the therapist selects a solution and prescribes it for the patient. Instead, he or she works more actively to identify solutions the patient has considered, might have used in the past, or would be consistent with the patient's usual approach to problem solving. The "correct" solution will become obvious through discussion with the patient.

Getting Help from Others

When people reach the point that suicide feels like the only real option available to them they are also usually feeling quite alone in the world. There may be people in their environment, but they have emotionally or physically detached themselves from those people, either because they find their attention overwhelming or irritating or because they do not wish to burden others with their troubles. People who are suicidal try to convince themselves that all others would be better off without them or that they will not be missed. They withdraw from others as part of their effort to gain the strength to kill themselves. Other people are deterrents. Avoidance of others means they can emotionally disengage from them and feel less guilty about the act.

When problems have gotten so overwhelming that death seems to be the only answer and no solutions seem viable, the patient needs others for assistance and support. While they may not have the solution to their problems, others might have ideas. Finding those people to provide support can make the patient feel resolution is possible, hope may not be completely lost, and, most important, they are not alone in their distress.

Reasons to Live

Another strategy for combating suicidal ideation is to break through the tunnel vision typical of this process and help the patient to call to mind reasons to live. Suicidal thought makes people focus on reasons not to live. This is the tunnel vision. The patient will find it easy to list all the things that would be resolved by his or her disappearance, but will have a more difficult time generating reasons to the contrary. The worksheet provided in Figure 9.3 can help prompt the patient to consider reasons to live. Completion of this exercise can take quite a bit of time given the patient's mental status, but it is time worth spending in therapy. It should be started in the office and sent home as homework. If the patient is in an inpatient facility, the therapist can start the exercise, and other health care providers can follow up throughout the day to check on the patient's progress and to assist in its completion. Negative thinking is a powerful force that can block access to positive thoughts. Therefore, the patient will usually need some prompting, such as in the categories listed on the worksheet.

Reasons to Have Hope

A variation on the previous exercise is to control black-and-white thinking that all is hopeless by inquiring about factors that might suggest there is some reason to be hopeful that things will improve. Signs of hope can include an early response to medication that although not complete, does show potential for working, or past experiences when treatment was helpful or successful. Table 9.5 presents several Socratic questions a therapist might pose to a patient to identify reasons for hope. If the patient initially answers each question in the negative, the therapist can offer examples from observations of the patient that might be reasons for hope overlooked by the patient. Remember that

Reasons to Live

Make a list of reasons to continue living. When you begin to have dark thoughts about life, look over the list to remind yourself of reasons to hold on another day.

Reasons why I shouldn't leave:

People to live for:

Things I would miss:

Experiences I have not yet had:

Things that matter to me:

FIGURE 9.3. Reasons to Live Worksheet.

when a patient is locked into the idea that all is hopeless, he or she will resist evidence to the contrary. Probe further or try different questioning strategies, but refrain from debating with the patient about the presence of hope and do not generate the list for the patient. The power of the exercise is in the patient's ability to break out of his absolutistic view of hopelessness and consider the possibility that it might be worth living a little longer to find out if things can get better.

If after completion of these exercises the patient is still significantly hopeless, another strategy is for the clinician to tell the patient his or her reasons to be hopeful that things will change, including faith

TABLE 9.5. Socratic Questions to Elicit Reasons for Hope.

- "Are you doing anything differently now that might suggest there is hope for improvement?"
- "Are the problems that bring you down likely to be temporary? Will they resolve themselves with time?"
- "Why do other people believe that there is hope for the future?"
- "Is it possible that you have not yet given it all your effort?"
- "Have you been through times like this before? Have things usually gotten better with time, effort, or patience?"

in medications and other treatments. For example, "I know things are seeming pretty dark right now and you are barely hanging on. It is taking a lot of your energy to stay alive, but I feel strongly that there is reason to be hopeful. You have responded to medication and therapy in the past, and I think you will beat this depression again. I have seen many people recover from severe depression, and for that reason I have hope. Why don't I lend you some of my hope for now until yours kicks back in? Would that be OK?"

Remarkably, reaching out to a person by sharing reasons to be hopeful can be a powerful intervention. The trick is not to offer it until the patient has had a chance to summon his or her own feelings of hope. Any of these interventions should be used along with other risk management methods usually prescribed.

This chapter has focused on how the content of thoughts change during periods of depression and mania. In the next chapter, the focus turns to changes that occur in thought processing such as the speed and clarity of ideas. If it is difficult for patients to identify specific automatic thoughts in need of restructuring, it may be that improvements are needed first in slowing, focusing, and structuring thoughts. Chapter 10 provides methods for accomplishing these goals.

Key Points for the Therapist to Remember

◆ Collecting and examining the evidence that supports the validity of automatic thoughts and the evidence that contradicts or refutes the validity of their thoughts is more effective than trying to change peoples' views by dismissing them, discounting their validity, or otherwise attempting to convince others that their views are false

◆ Suicidal ideation can take several different forms: desires to die, escape, or avoidance of psychic pain and repetitive thoughts that are more obsessional in nature. The former usually accompany hopelessness and distress. The latter seem more like habitual thoughts that pop into people's minds, not when they are contemplating their misery but at other times.

♦ Thoughts about suicide, whether specific desires to be dead or general wishes that suffering could end, usually result from believing that there is no other solution to intense distress.

♦ Problem-solving ability usually declines in depression and mania as cognitive processes slow. That is usually why people feel that there is no other way out but death, because they no longer have the ability to generate alternative solutions.

♦ It is not uncommon for prior attempts at problem solving to be incomplete or ineffective. At times a sustained effort is needed and the person gave up before the problem was solved. Or fear of failure has kept a person from implementing a reasonable solution they have already identified. When energy and motivation are low because of depression, the patient may not have the strength to implement a solution. The therapist's job is to evaluate the possible solutions and help the patient to select a strategy that has some potential for relief, preferable immediate relief.

Points to Discuss with Patients

♦ Distortions in cognitions can lead a person to draw incorrect conclusions. This is problematic in that an incorrect conclusion, either overly negative or overly optimistic, not only dictates a person's emotional reaction to events but also influences his or her choice of actions.

♦ Having a more accurate perception of reality will increase the chance that any actions taken will be helpful and not hurtful to the patient.

♦ Negative automatic thoughts should be taken with a grain of salt as they typically appear during depression and lessen during remission. And positive or euphoric automatic thoughts should not be entirely trusted if they encourage a dramatic change in actions or risk taking.

♦ Often, the automatic thoughts associated with clinically significant upward or downward shifts in mood are either partially or completely invalid or inaccurate. Because the bias in automatic thoughts generally elicits or exacerbates mood shifts, one of the goals of CBT is to teach patients how to evaluate the validity of their own automatic thoughts and correct any distortions.

♦ A retrospective assessment of those experiences conducted when the person is no longer hypomanic or manic may allow him or her to see how mood and symptom changes might have caused an overestimate of the urgency of change and a minimization of the risks involved.

♦ People who are suicidal try to convince themselves that all others would be better off without them or that they will not be missed. They withdraw from others as part of their effort to gain the strength to kill themselves.

♦ When problems have gotten so overwhelming that death seems to be the only answer and no solutions seem viable, the patient needs others for assistance and support. Although others may not have the solution to the patient's problems, they might have ideas.

CHAPTER 10

Management
of Cognitive Symptoms
PROCESS CHANGES

Cognitive processing is also altered during episodes of depression and mania. Speed, clarity, logic, organization, perception, and decision-making ability are compromised. These deficits can have a negative effect on a person's ability to cope with daily hassles and major life difficulties and, in fact, can cause new psychosocial stressors. Improvements in cognitive processing can, therefore, break the evolving cycle of depression and mania at the point of behavior change, impairment in psychosocial functioning, or when psychosocial problems develop as indicated in Figure 2.1 (p. 24).

Cognitive processing can be compromised in a variety of ways. Table 10.1 provides some examples of common cognitive difficulties in depression and mania.

Responses to Stimulation

Some patients in manic or hypomanic episodes may note early in its evolution that they are experiencing perceptual changes. They may report a heightened awareness of or sensitivity to colors, smells, sounds, or touch. For example, the leaves on the trees appear far more intensely green than usual or the colors on the television set or in a magazine advertisement appear brighter than usual. In depression, stimulation, both internal and external, can be overwhelming. In contrast to mild or moderate

TABLE 10.1. Examples of Cognitive Processing Problems

Category of cognitive processing	Examples in depression	Examples in Mania
Response to stimulation	• Easily overwhelmed	• Distracted easily • Sounds seem louder • Colors seem brighter
Speed in thinking	• Slowed thinking • Production of ideas is impaired	• Racing thoughts • Increased fluency of ideas
Organization	• Cannot compartmentalize problems and selectively address them	• Difficulty grasping and organizing thoughts
Concentration	• Cannot hold focus without mind wandering	• Too many thoughts to process • Distracted and loses train of thought
Decision making	• Self-doubt interferes with decision making • Problem solving is abandoned	• Cannot prioritize • Impaired judgment • Problems with follow-through

mania, where stimuli engage, distract, or inspire an individual, too much stimulation blocks cognitive processing in depression and interferes with taking action. At the peak of mania people experience this type of overwhelming effect from external and internal stimulation and their functioning can become equally impaired.

Speed and Fluency of Thought

Speed of thought may also increase during a hypomanic or manic episode. Patients describe their thoughts as racing through their head, sometimes more rapidly than can be spoken. Some say that they can follow several trains of thought simultaneously. As one patient put it, "It's like watching several television programs simultaneously and understanding all of them." Unfortunately, as speed continues to increase, clarity lessens and confusion increases. With increased speed and fluency comes a wealth of new ideas, interests, and plans. The world seems full of possibilities just waiting for the right person with the intelligence and drive to make them happen. For example, when entering into a manic episode, people with bipolar disorder may begin to think of new business ventures that they view as virtually guaranteed of success. Some of these ideas may, in fact, be ingenious and potentially successful. The natural intelligence, creativity, and adventurousness of some people with bipolar disorder can sometimes lead to financial successes. Unfortunately, during mania a person's ability to distinguish between good ideas and grandiose delusions is compromised.

In depression, thought processes slow. Imelda describes her experience with this symptom.

"It's like when a machine that used to work at a normal speed starts to run more slowly, like playing a tape on a tape recorder whose batteries are running low. You can still make out the voices, but they are slow and groggy sounding. That's what my thoughts are like when I try to pay bills or plan a meal. I used to be able to think and figure out what to do pretty easily. I can still do it, but it takes ten times longer."

Mental Organization

As symptoms of mania worsen, thinking becomes more disorganized and more difficult for patients to control. People who have experienced this disorganization note a decreased ability to synthesize information into organized groups. That is, they cannot pull ideas together to form a complete picture of a particular problem or task. Their thinking becomes muddled.

Thinking may become so disorganized that logic, information, and the patient's own experiences no longer carry any significant weight in making judgments or evaluating ideas. Some are aware of their inability to synthesize ideas and are eager to try methods that help impose structure on their thinking. However, in mania, although usually apparent to others, the person may not realize the degree to which his or her ideas are disorganized.

Concentration

It's not unusual for people with bipolar disorder to complain of memory and concentration problems. This is because in order to retrieve information from memory it must first be stored. And the limited attention span and poor concentration can prevent a person from holding on to thoughts long enough to store them into memory.

Concentration in depression can be possible for short periods, but the person usually finds his or her mind wandering off to other subjects. Some find that they have to reread the same paragraph over and over until they can understand the information or follow the story. Holding facts in short-term memory while they try to complete a larger task can be a struggle as well.

In mania, concentration is derailed by distractions. Other fleeting thoughts and environmental stimuli take focus away from a task or idea. Rather than try to refocus or force attention back to the task, the person in a manic or hypomanic state is more likely to follow the distraction and lose sight of the original idea or activity.

Decision Making

Although impaired in both depression and mania, the disruption in decision-making ability is qualitatively different in each type of episode. As the cognitive symptoms of depression worsen, self-doubt tends to increase. People do not trust their decisions, fearing failure or disapproval if the "wrong" choice is made. Mental slowing and tunnel vision make it difficult to generate new solutions to problems. And as anxiety increases, it becomes easier to imagine the worst-case scenario for any solutions considered. The magnitude of problems is perceived as great and the consequences overwhelming, and as a result, there is often a paralysis in decision making.

> Carmen is a 35-year–old homemaker and mother of two young sons. She describes her decision-making problems as fueling her depression. "I have to make decisions every day and each one feels like a burden and a new chance to mess things up. My husband questions my judgment even when I'm feeling fine, so when I'm depressed, I'm afraid that one more mistake and he'll walk out on me and the boys. So I let things stack up. I haven't unpacked the boxes since we moved in six months ago because I can't decide where to put things. I haven't bought the boys any new school clothes because I'm not sure where to shop. I need to start exercising, but I don't know if it would be best to join the YMCA or a private gym or sign up for a class at the community center. I want to find a place where I fit in and that won't cost too much. My husband wants me to start walking around the neighborhood with him, but then I have to find someone to watch the kids at night or early in the morning. I

get so overwhelmed with trying to make it work that I just give up and tell myself that I'll deal with it later."

Impaired judgment, grandiosity, and impulsivity can all affect the decisions made during hypomanic and manic episodes. As described previously, magnification of positives and minimization of negatives can interfere by providing an unbalanced view of the risks and benefits of any plan. It is not unusual for people in a manic phase to act on impulsive urges without pausing to consider alternative actions or solutions. Poor judgment is not always an indicator of impaired decision making. Actions taken in poor judgment can result from a failure to slow down long enough to attempt problem solving.

Coping with Cognitive Process Changes in Depression and Mania

While cognitive processing changes are symptoms of depression and mania, they can also cause new problems for people, impair functioning further, and exacerbate episodes. A strategy for addressing cognitive processing problems is first to slow thoughts enough to allow the patient to compensate for them. The second step is to focus attention on one problem at a time. And finally, the third step is to impose some type of structure on cognitive processing to allow problems to be solved or decisions to be made (see Table 10.2). If the patient can accomplish these three steps, there is a chance to prevent impulsive actions, to decrease avoidance of responsibilities, and to more effectively deal with or prevent life hassles and difficulties. Table 10.3 summarizes the cognitive-behavioral methods used to accomplish these goals.

How to Slow It Down

As summarized in the previous section, the cognitive process changes in depression and mania affect the speed, organization, and clarity of

---

TABLE 10.2. Coping with Process Changes

1. *Slow It* by slowing the body and mind.

2. *Focus It* one idea at a time.

3. *Structure It* by using decision-making exercises

TABLE 10.3. Methods for Coping with Process Changes

Slow It	Focus It	Structure It
• Relaxation exercises	• Prioritize—goal setting	• Exercises
• Decrease stimulation	• Pick one thing at a time	– Reduce the mental list
– Internal thoughts	• A list/B list	– Problem solving
– External noise		– Decision making
		– Advantages/disadvantages
		– Feedback from others
		– 24-hour rule

thought as well as how people respond to stimulation. The notion of slowing down the thought process in depressive states may, at first, seem illogical because complaints are usually of slowed thinking. However, despite feeling slow when depressed, people continue to try to think, to reason through difficulties, and to make decisions. Being easily overwhelmed, the depressed person will have trouble focusing on one problem long enough to see it though to resolution. Worries flood the mind, and short attention spans coupled with low energy leave problems unresolved and tasks incomplete. Slowing the thought process in depression as in mania facilitates improvement in focus. Two key methods for slowing down thought processes are relaxation and decreasing stimulation.

Relaxation Training

Relaxation training is a behavioral intervention that is commonly used in the management of anxiety, but it also appears to be helpful in controlling racing thoughts and excessive worry in bipolar disorder. In Chapter 11 we cover relaxation training in more depth when we discuss stress management. For now, note that there are many methods to achieve physical and mental relaxation. Formal methods include traditional muscle tension and relaxation methods such as the Jacobsonian techniques, yoga, meditation, and deep muscle massage. Informal strategies include reading, listening to music, taking a walk, sitting outdoors, taking a warm bath, or simply sitting in a quiet place. Some people find playing solitaire on the computer to be relaxing as it helps them tune out unpleasant thoughts and slow their thinking. When using relaxation training to control cognitive symptoms of depression or mania it is not necessary to force the mind to be still. In fact, it is easier for people with bipolar disorder to focus on a single new thought rather than to force racing thoughts to stop. Focus exercises can take many forms. Repetitive statements such as chants or prayers, self-hypnosis exercises that include a preplanned relaxing image, and distraction techniques can all focus thoughts on something new while the body relaxes. This technique slows the body and mind and, in turn, slows racing, overwhelming, and disorganized thoughts. Relaxation methods are intended for temporary use to calm the mind long enough enable the patient to focus his thoughts on a specific problem to solve. Because anxiety and tension are also relieved by formal and informal relaxation exercises, it is tempting to stay in a relaxed state rather than taking the chance of disrupting a peaceful moment to work on problems. The intent is not to aid avoidance behaviors but, rather, to put the patient in a better position to solve problems, organize thoughts, or deal with worries. Therefore, when relaxation exercises are prescribed by the therapist, they should be monitored to ensure that the patient is using the interventions to resolve rather than avoid difficulties.

Reducing Stimulation

In Chapter 8 we discussed overstimulation as something that can negatively affect behavior. Decreasing external or environmental stimulation can also help to control cognitive process changes such as racing thoughts. External or environmental sources of stimulation tend to fuel cognitive processes changes. Noise, movement, and bright lights as found in shopping malls, family gatherings, restaurants, or amusement parks can all become overwhelming even if they occur during an event intended to be enjoyable or pleasant. Arguments, messy households, piles of unopened mail, and news broadcasts are negative stimuli that are equally overwhelming. When exposed to these sources of stimulation, people often lose their concentration, begin to feel irritable or anxious, and can no longer focus on one task or activity at a time. There is usually an urge to escape the situation, but escape is not always practical or possible. Enduring overstimulating situations can elicit or worsen cognitive processing problems and arouse negative emotions.

The intervention for controlling overstimulation is part planning and part self-control. Environmental stimulation is not always intolerable. Many people can enjoy a fun and noisy activity when they are in the right mood. The trick is to recognize mood states that make a person vulnerable to the negative effects of overstimulation. When people come to therapy and complain about a family or social event that turned out to be an awful experience, they will usually say that they had already been in a bad mood before it started and the activity just made matters worse.

RHONDA:There was too much noise. Kids were running around screaming. I wanted to scream after a while. I shouldn't have gone. I knew it was going to be a bad day.

THERAPIST: How did you know?

RHONDA:Before I even left he house, people were getting on my nerves. My mother was calling to remind not to forget this and that. I know she is trying to be helpful, but she acts like I can't think for myself. Then the car was really low on gas, so I was going to have to stop along the way and I didn't have very much money on me. That ticked me off. My brother borrowed the car the night before and didn't bother to put gas in it.

THERAPIST: I can see how you would have been uptight before you even got to the party. Why did you go?

RHONDA:I didn't have a choice. It was my niece's first birthday and my sister was making a big fuss. As if the kid has any idea what's going on.

THERAPIST: Would it have been better for you not to go?

RHONDA:It would have been better until my mother jumped my case for it. Then it wouldn't have been worth it.

If a person can recognize the vulnerability to become overstimulated, then precautions can be made or methods employed to control the situation. Vulnerability can come from feeling irritable or anxious, from sleep loss that causes fatigue or limits patience, from being with people who can be annoying even under the best circumstances, or from having to participate in an activity that the person does not enjoy. In any of these scenarios, the patient can become overwhelmed by too much environmental stimulation.

Planning ahead for such situations might include choosing not to participate at all, limiting the amount of participation, or taking a time out from the situation when beginning to feel overwhelmed. Feeling a sense of control over a potentially upsetting situation may be all that is needed to avoid becoming overstimulated. That is, if the person goes to a social event but drives separately from others, the option to leave early is always open. Even if it is not necessary to escape, knowing that it is possible can reduce anxiety over the event.

Taking short breaks from stimulating experiences is also an option. Perhaps excusing oneself to step outside, take time in the bathroom, go out the car, or have a cigarette break can be all that is needed to regain one's composure, relax for a moment, and prevent internal overstimuation from occurring. Planning ahead allows the person to consider his or her options for limiting stimulation. In Rhonda's case, it probably would have been better for her to take time to calm down before she went to the party. If she was not feeling as irritable and angry, the stimulation of the party may not have affected her as much.

Self-control becomes part of the plan when a person is becoming overstimulated but does not necessarily want to leave the situation. For example, if a late-night conversation is getting him or her "wound up" and overly excited to the point that sleep may become impossible, there has to be enough self-control to end the conversation. If at a party and having a great time, he or she may feel the mania building but enjoy the feeling and not want it to end. In this case, overstimulation may feel good in the short run and cause problems in the long run. Leaving early can be a difficult choice to make. If planned ahead, the person might know that he or she is about to have a great time and must limit the length of time spent at the event. Some call this the "Cinderella plan," where they tell themselves they can have all the fun they want but they have to leave the festivities by midnight. This method takes a great deal of self-control and it is not unusual for people to consciously decide to take the risk and enjoy themselves longer. Sometimes they get overstimulated and are sorry for it, but sometimes things go fine. The latter events are what they remember and what sway their decision to push the limits. Therapists might prefer that their patients set limits and exercise control but must also respect patients' rights to choose to put themselves at risk.

How to Focus on One Idea at a Time

The increased number of thoughts and ideas in hypomania and mania can lead to an increase in activity. The activity driven by hypomanic thoughts can be overstimulating, thereby fueling cognitive process changes. The goal is to contain activity by organizing ideas and setting limits. The goal-setting exercise presented in Chapter 8 can help people to focus their thoughts and set priorities. The graded task assignment intervention described in Chapter 8 can also be used to organize thinking and activity. The simplified version, "A" list/"B" list, may be easier and more practical when patients are symptomatic. The list of ideas, plans, and interests are reduced to a daily or weekly activity plan. Higher-priority activities for the week are put on the "A" list, lower priority tasks on the "B" list. If hypomanic, patients try to put too many activities on the lists. In a depressed phase, people become easily overwhelmed if too many items are on the lists. Planning for the week's activities must include time for usual home, work, and social responsibilities. The items on the "A" and "B" lists are added to patients' schedules. To contain activity, patients must complete the "A" list items before going on to the "B" list items. An inability to suppress urges to skip ahead or add more activities is an indication that symptoms are worsening and that pharmacological interventions should be more aggressively applied. The key to success in this type of intervention is completion of tasks before beginning new ones. The Goal-Setting Worksheet (see Figure 8.2 at p. 177) can be used as a continuous log of new ideas so that the person does not have to worry about forgetting creative ideas.

How to Pick One Thing at a Time

When a person is flooded with thoughts that include responsibilities, failures, regrets, incomplete tasks, and unaccomplished goals, all of which feel equally pressing, it can be difficult for him or her to choose a direction and make a plan. Selecting one task and ignoring the others is often uncomfortable if the person feels that he or she *should* accomplish them all or *should* stay on top of tasks at all times. Therapists sometimes have to give patients permission to do one thing at a time. If patients resist the notion of doing one thing at a time, the clinician might use Socratic questions to inquire about the efficacy of their strategy of trying to keep up with all tasks at all times and what they stand to lose by trying a different strategy.

A common scenario in therapy for people who are overwhelmed with responsibilities, regardless of their mood state, is to begin talking about one problem and digress to numerous others. The following is an example:

> "My parents are on my case about finding an apartment. They want me to live near them and I don't want to. I found a place I like, but I'm not sure I can qualify for it myself since I haven't worked that much. I'm waiting to hear on that. They make me so mad. They offer to help me, but then they want to control everything. They even opened my mail that came to their house. They looked at my bank statements. Can you believe that? I am so

angry. Then I had to get a lecture on money management. If they would only give me access to the money my grandmother left for me I wouldn't have money management problems. Then they jumped my case because a warrant came in the mail for some old speeding tickets. I know I have to take care of them. I don't need a lecture about it. Then my mom gets all into my face about drinking and driving. She thinks I'm going to kill someone. I don't drive when I'm drinking. I stay with friends. I've told her that before. And I want to sign up for some classes to get that certificate that I was thinking about, but my parents want me to do it right now. I'm not going to do it right how just because they told me to do it. I'm not a little kid. And I'm waiting to hear on that new job so I can't sign up until I know my schedule. They have a class starting in two weeks, but I got to go to court on the day it starts for one of my tickets. I'm not even sure what I have to do. My lawyer hasn't returned my call. Do you know what's going to happen?"

A therapist cannot possibly help a person resolve all these problems in one therapy session. While patients logically knows this, they may still resist picking only one item to work on. To structure the therapy session and to help them focus on one problem at a time, therapists can make running lists of problems as patients verbalize them. Share the list with them and suggest a strategy for their resolution, which involves focusing on problems that are pressing and that are within their control. First, have them review the list and cross off any items that are past events. In the foregoing example, his parents opened his mail without first asking. Give the rationale that at least for now nothing can be done about past events. Second, have them cross off any items that are beyond their control. In the example provided, the patient cannot make people return his phone calls faster. The third step is to omit any items that do not require an immediate resolution. Although in the patient's mind all the items mentioned feel interrelated and pressing, they are actually separate items that vary in urgency. For example, when inquiring further, it was clear that although the patient wanted to find an apartment immediately, his current lease would not be up for another month and a half. After eliminating the nonurgent items it became clearer that the most pressing matters were preparing for going to court in 1 week and finding a job. Once patients have focused their attention on a specific goal, they can go on to the next step, problem solving and decision making.

How to Structure Decision Making and Other Thought Processes

Before discussion of the more elaborate methods for problem resolution and decision-making, consider the *slow it, focus it, structure it* method of intervention could be applied to the problem of rumination. While rumination can occur at any time during the day, it often occurs at bedtime. As people begin to relax their bodies to fall asleep, it is not unusual for their minds to begin to wander over the events of the day, conversations with other people, or unresolved problems. This type of mental activity in the person who suffers from insomnia can make it even more difficult to fall asleep. Some people are more prone to worry than others, and for those who inevitably use bedtime to review their days, the following behavioral exercise can help to control the process and prevent it from prolonging sleep onset. The first step is to schedule a time at the end of the day, preferably after dinner and at least 1 hour before bedtime, to review the day. The hour can be adjusted as needed to ensure enough time to mentally disengage from the process before going to sleep. This exercise should not take place in bed but, rather, at a table or other area that makes it easy to take notes.

The second step is to have the patient mentally review the day and take notes on any events that were troublesome or that require additional attention. These are the events that would normally cross the person's mind when trying to fall asleep. Typical categories would include things to do the next day, tasks left uncompleted, conversations with others that aroused emotion, disappointments, and worries. For each troublesome item, the patient should make a note of what needs to be done the next day to rectify the issue. In some cases, nothing can be done, so the intervention might be to let it go and spend no more time worrying about it. In other cases, action must be taken. The person can decide if action must be taken the next day or if it can wait. Perhaps the plan will be to gather more information on how to solve a problem as a next step. At times the worry is about an interaction with another person that still weighs heavy on the patient's mind and requires an additional response. While the person may not be able to plan what to say to the other person the next day, the interim plan may be to schedule some time the next day to consider the possibilities and talk to others about them. It is rarely possible to solve a problem all at once. Instead of forcing a solution before bedtime, it is better to make a plan to set aside time the next day other than bedtime to work on it.

The third step is used if at bedtime rumination begins again. The patient should remind him- or herself that the day has already been reviewed and a plan for tomorrow has already been made. The person must be convinced that further rumination or worry will not lead to better solutions. It will only lead to sleeplessness. If this self-talk is ineffective, the patient can use standard thought-stopping techniques like those often used for control of obsessional thoughts in obsessive–compulsive disorder.

Problem Solving

Most people engage in problem solving every day. It occurs automatically for many of the small decisions needed to navigate through each day's activities. For example, "Should I get up now, or can I sleep 10 minutes longer?" Quickly, the possible choices and the relative risks and benefits of obeying the alarm clock or sleeping later come to mind. More sophisticated problems are as easily addressed. For example, "I have three tasks that need to be completed by the end of the week. How am I going to get them all accomplished?" After considering the possible strategies, one is chosen and implemented. If it proves ineffective, an alternative strategy is implemented. People who can define problems, consider options, make choices, and implement a plan have all the basic skills required for effective problem solving. Reminding patients that they can make decisions may increase their confidence in their ability to handle more complex difficulties.

Even when patients have the necessary skills, obstacles to effective coping can impede problem solving. In these cases, a more formal step-by-step procedure for defining problems and for generating and implementing solutions can be useful. Table 10.4 shows step-by-step procedures for helping patients and their family members to solve problems. These procedures are fairly generic and can be applied to many different scenarios.

Problem Definition

The most difficult step in resolving psychosocial problems is identifying and defining the problem in a way that facilitates its resolution. Because the definition must be as objective and specific as possible, the problem should be described in terms of observable phenomena rather than subjective feelings.

Mr. Washaw's complaint that he "can't cope" is too general. To define the problem more precisely, it is necessary to specify the situations in which he has difficulty coping (e.g., disciplining the

TABLE 10.4. Problem-Solving Steps

Step 1. Problem identification and definition	• State the problem as clearly as possible. Be specific about the behavior, situation, timing, and/or circumstances that make it a problem (e.g., "I need to pay the phone and credit card bills, and I don't have enough money to cover both this month"). • If the problem is a personal hurt, state the specific action that caused the hurt feeling (e.g., "You hurt my feelings when you said I couldn't handle the money").
Step 2. Generation of potential solutions	• List all possible solutions without evaluating their quality or feasibility. Try to list at least 10. Be creative. Do not worry about the quality of the solution. • Eliminate less desirable or unreasonable solutions • Order the remaining solutions in terms of preference. • Evaluate the remaining solutions in terms of their pros and cons. • Specify who will take action. • Specify how and when the solution will be implemented.
Step 3. Implement solution	• Implement the solution as planned • Evaluate the effectiveness of the solution • Decide whether a revision of the existing plan or a new plan is needed to address the problem better. • If needed, return to step 2 to select a new solution, and repeat remaining steps or return to step 2 to revise the existing solution, and repeat remaining steps.

kids). Is it always a problem in this particular situation? [No.] If not, when is it more or less a problem? [It is more a problem with his son than with his daughter.] What has happened when he has tried to address the problem? [He gets very angry, says things that he does not mean, and later regrets what he said.] A more specific definition of Mr. Washaw's complaint, therefore, is that he gets too angry and overreacts when he disciplines his son. The situation is defined in observable, operational terms. That is, outsiders would understand "I have difficulty in disciplining my son" more easily than they would understand the meaning of "I can't cope."

To facilitate problem definition, therapists can ask the following questions:

- "What is the problem?"
- "When is it most likely to occur?"

- "Are other people involved?"

- "How do they help or make the problem worse?"

- "How would the therapist know if the problem were occurring?"

- "Would anyone else notice?"

- "In what way does it cause a problem?"

- "What are the consequences?"

- "How often does the problem occur?"

- "Are there circumstances that make it better or worse?"

- "In general, what, when, where, how, and with whom is it a problem?"

If the problems involve other people, it is very likely that each participant has a somewhat different view of the situation.

> Mrs. Fujitsu complained that her husband could not be trusted to pay the bills properly, making it necessary for her to find time in her busy schedule to do so. The problem appeared to be the manner in which her husband paid the bills (i.e., paid only the minimum balance when it was possible to pay more). Mr. Fujitsu saw things differently. According to him, the problem was that his wife procrastinated in paying the bills so long that he had to do it. He might pay only the minimum amount, but at least he paid them! So, it appeared that the problem was more complicated than Mrs. Fujitsu had originally suggested. In this case, there were two problems: getting bills paid on time and paying an agreed upon amount.

Some practical problems (e.g., unemployment, financial problems, or schedule problems) are easily defined. More existential problems (e.g., dissatisfaction with life or low self-esteem) are more difficult. If patients make general complaints about themselves or their lives, therapists can help by inquiring about the situations in which their dissatisfaction is more apparent.

> "I hate my life," complained Ms. Louise. "Nothing is going right. Work, my social life, my body, my family—it all stinks." When asked to specify which element in each of these domains was troubling her, Ms. Louise replied, "All of it, the whole package." Her therapist was skeptical that there were problems in all aspects of the patient's life. A different tactic was necessary to hone in on

Ms. Louise's problems. Taking one topic at a time (e.g., work, social life), the therapist inquired about what was going right for Ms. Louise in each domain. What parts of her job did she like or dislike? Was it the task, the environment, the people, or the pay? What was it about her body, her family, and her social life?

Defining complaints about other people requires a somewhat different strategy. The offenses that people commit against one another are generally defined by the meaning that each party attaches to the event rather than by what is observable.

Mr. Magee made an extra effort to get home early to prepare dinner for his family. He made his specialty, set the table, and called everyone to dinner. His wife was not hungry and declined to eat. Mr. Magee was hurt and angry. There was no discussion about the dinner, but a quiet coldness pervaded the household. To Mrs. Magee, her husband shouldn't have been resentful. She just was not hungry. She appreciated his effort, although she may not have mentioned it at the time. So why was he so angry and hurt? He knew that his wife did not eat when she was not hungry. The problem was in Mr. Magee's interpretation of his wife's behavior. It conveyed to him that she did not care about the marriage, that she did not appreciate his efforts, and that she did not care about him or love him. When the therapist asked Mr. Magee to explain this to his wife, she understood, clarified her feelings, and apologized for contributing to his hurt.

Generating Solutions

Once the difficult task of defining the problem has been accomplished, efforts can be initiated to resolve it. It is particularly useful to assess a patient's coping resources, previous coping strategies, and obstacles to effective coping (i.e., strengths and weaknesses) before attempting to generate new solutions. Brainstorming for potential new solutions should proceed without stopping to evaluate the merits of any one idea. In addition, because obstacles prevent the patient from making use of existing coping resources, the solutions generated to handle problems should include a plan for eliminating the patient's weaknesses while utilizing the patient's strengths. For example:

Mr. McNeeley's strengths included:
1. Creativity
2. Organizational skill
3. Assertiveness

4. Ability to get along with others
5. Knowledge about aspects of work

His weaknesses were:

1. Impatience
2. Irritability
3. Unwillingness to compromise
4. No time to deal with problems
5. Aggressiveness

Mr. McNeeley was angry about a new procedure implemented at his job site because it increased his work load and sacrificed quality for higher volume. He complained (weakness 5) to his superiors and demanded immediate action (weakness 1). He did not see any response to his complaints, so he returned to his boss's office, demanded to be seen (weakness 1), angrily (weaknesses 2 and 5) criticized management for their lack of foresight, and told them how to rectify their errors. Mr. McNeeley made little progress, but began to have stomach problems and tension headaches. He told his therapist that he thought he should quit his job (weakness 3).

The solutions that Mr. McNeeley attempted seemed to have no effect. His weaknesses appeared to have impeded his progress. Once he recognized this, he was able to use his creativity (strength 1) and organizational skill (strength 2) to generate a new plan that incorporated his strengths. He solicited the assistance of his colleagues (strength 4) to monitor their productivity and track occasions when they were unable to complete their work or had to compromise quality for speed (strength 5).

After documenting these findings, he made an appointment to talk with the management (strength 3) about his data and their implications. He and his therapist worked out a strategy that kept him from appearing angry and uncompromising.

Decision Making by Weighing the Advantages and Disadvantages

Life transitions, such as changing jobs, moving to a new neighborhood, and making new friends, can be very exciting. New opportunities often bring stress and uncertainty, however. Individuals may ask themselves, "Am I making the right decision? What if it doesn't work out? Am I just running away from my problems? What should I do?"

Patients with bipolar disorder often find themselves immobilized by indecisiveness. When poor concentration, low self-confidence, racing thoughts, and stimulus overload muddle their thinking, even the simplest decisions seem laborious. Fear of the consequences of each choice feeds rumination; in turn, past experiences, when change led to failure, feed this fear. Ideas, options, and fantasies flash through the mind of the manic or hypomanic patient. Disjointed details flood the patient's thoughts while the urge toward impulsive acts grows stronger. The depressed patient often makes decisions by default, when the failure to act becomes a decision or when others take over and make decisions. In either state, the outcome is not always in the best interest of the patient.

The clinician can facilitate decision making by teaching patients to slow down the process and organize their thoughts. Providing a structure for systematically evaluating choices can alleviate the mental wheel spinning and move patients toward active decision making. Committing these thoughts to paper allows the patient to make some constructive use of the mental energy spent ruminating about the options. It also buys the hypomanic patient some time to slow down and evaluate the choices objectively before impulsively acting.

The first step in this structured approach to decision making is to define each choice. For example, (1) I can change jobs, or (2) I can remain at the existing job. The second step is to list the advantages and disadvantages of each choice (see Figure 10.1). There will be some redundancy across lists, with the advantages of one choice paralleling the disadvantages of the other. The patient should explore all aspects of each choice, considering the pros and cons of each. When the four lists are complete, the patient can begin the third step, an evaluation of the choices.

As the third step in the decision-making process, the patient reads through the lists and places three stars (***) next to the items that he or she considers most important, two stars (**) next to items that are very important, and one star (*) next to those that are important. The patient can ignore the remaining items for the time being. Examining the starred items to determine the primary or strongest advantages and disadvantages of each choice (see Figure 10.1) simplifies the decision-making process by focusing the patient on the key issues. The patient can then compare the main advantages and disadvantages of the various choices relative to one another. When the evaluation is complete, the patient can proceed with the fourth step.

In this final step, the patient considers the possibility of maximizing the advantages of each choice (e.g., asking for a higher starting salary on the new job) while minimizing the disadvantages (e.g., negotiate for a limit on weekend work). This process often requires the

	Stay on This Job	Change Jobs
Advantages	It's close to home * Good secretary * I know everybody	*** Can make more money Larger office ** More independence in decision making Get away from boss
Disadvantages	Business has been poor *** Stuck with current boss *** No raise this year Bad neighborhood No room for creativity	The work schedule may require more weekend work *** May have to move the family The new boss could end up being a jerk

FIGURE 10.1. Advantages and disadvantages of job changes. ***most important item; **very important item; *important item.

patient to gather additional information on each option before making a decision.

These interventions for improving cognitive processing in bipolar disorder can be used even when patients are relatively asymptomatic. Those who developed bipolar disorder early in life often miss out on opportunities to learn basic problem-solving and decision-making skills. While their peers were learning how to solve psychosocial problems, they were fighting off depression or coping with mania. Even people who appear to be successful may lack systematic strategies for sorting through and resolving problems. Therefore, taking time in therapy to practice cognitive structuring methods can be very beneficial.

Key Points for the Therapist to Remember

♦ The clinician can facilitate decision-making by teaching patients to slow down the process and organize their thoughts. Providing a structure for systematically evaluating choices can alleviate the mental wheel spinning and move patients toward active decision making.

♦ When flooded with thoughts that include responsibilities, failures, regrets, incomplete tasks, and unaccomplished goals, all of which feel equally pressing, it can be difficult to choose a direction and make a plan. Selecting one task and ignoring the others is often uncomfortable if the person feels that he or she "should" accomplish them all or "should" stay on top of tasks at all times. Therapists sometimes have to give patients permission to do one thing at a time.

Points to Discuss with Patients

♦ Speed, clarity, logic, organization, perception, and decision making ability are compromised. These deficits can have a negative effect on a person's ability to cope with daily hassles and major life difficulties and in fact, can cause new psychosocial stressors.

♦ In depression, stimulation, both internal and external, can be overwhelming. In contrast to mild or moderate mania, where stimuli engage, distract, or inspire an individual, too much stimulation blocks cognitive processing in depression and interferes with taking action.

♦ The natural intelligence, creativity, and adventurousness of some people with bipolar disorder can sometimes lead to financial successes. Unfortunately, during mania a person's ability to distinguish between good ideas and grandiose delusions is compromised.

♦ As symptoms of mania worsen, thinking becomes more disorganized. There is a decreased ability to synthesize information into organized groups. That is, patients cannot pull ideas together to form a complete picture of a particular problem or task.

♦ As the cognitive symptoms of depression worsen, self-doubt tends to increase. People do not trust their decisions, fearing failure or disapproval if the "wrong" choice is made. Mental slowing and tunnel vision make it difficult to generate new solutions to problems. And as anxiety increases, it becomes easier to imagine the worst-case scenario for any solutions considered.

♦ Impaired judgment, grandiosity, and impulsivity can all affect the decisions made during hypomanic and manic episodes. As described previously, magnification of positives and minimization of negatives can interfere by providing an unbalanced view of the risks and benefits of any plan.

♦ A strategy for addressing cognitive processing problems is first to slow them enough to allow the patient to compensate for them. The second step is to focus attention on one problem at a time. And, finally, the third step is to impose some type of structure on cognitive processing to allow problems to be solved or decisions to be made.

CHAPTER 11

Stress Management

How Do Biological and Psychosocial Factors Interact?

Studies of the course of affective disorders (e.g., Leverich, Post, & Rosoff, 1990; Post, Roy-Byrne, & Uhde, 1988; Roy-Byrne et al., 1985) have consistently shown that episodes of mania and/or depression become increasingly frequent over the course of a person's life. Episodes that occur earlier in the course of the illness are more likely to be associated with the occurrence of stressful life events than later episodes.

Post (1992) suggests limbic kindling and behavioral sensitization as models to help understand the interaction of psychosocial and biological factors in the course of bipolar disorder. The notion of kindling (Goddard, McIntyre, & Leech, 1969) comes from observations that rats that received repeated electrical stimulations to the brain, each of which was not strong enough to cause seizures, eventually began having seizures. These seizures continued long after the electrical stimulation was stopped. Post proposes that these electrical stimulations may be analogous to life events or other psychosocial stressors; that is, an accumulation of stress eventually leads to depression or mania in a biologically vulnerable individual. Episodes of depression and/or mania may be like kindled seizures in that episodes which initially had an identifiable "trigger" (stressful life event) eventually occur spontaneously, when there is no longer a stimulus present.

Another possible explanation for the association between life events and episodes of depression or mania, particularly earlier in the course of the illness, is behavioral sensitization (Post, Rubinow, &

Ballenger, 1986). This is based on the observation that individuals who repeatedly take psychomotor stimulants (e.g., cocaine) seem, over time, to need smaller doses of stimulants to produce the same response as the person becomes sensitized to the drug. In patients with bipolar disorder, life events can be thought of as analogous to stimulants, with progressively fewer or less severe stressors needed to precipitate an episode of depression or mania as the illness progresses.

Because evidence from research with patients with affective disorders suggests that stressful life events can play a significant role in the course of illness, prevention of relapses and recurrences of depression and mania may, in part, be achieved by controlling stress. Therefore, this chapter focuses on managing stress commonly experienced by people with bipolar disorder.

Unfortunately with individuals who have suffered from bipolar disorder for some time, stress and illness do not have a simple cause-and-effect relationship. While distress, like that caused by loss of a loved one, can lead to depression, the depression itself can create other psychosocial problems for the individual.

Episodes of mania can occur without a particular precipitant, but the behavioral sequelae of mania can produce psychosocial stressors—for example, accrued debt due to financial extravagance and poor judgment, marital conflict due to hypersexuality and promiscuity, or legal problems resulting from illegal actions. When the mania clears, the individual sometimes finds that his or her life is in ruins. As the realization of the damage occurs, it is not unusual for the person to become increasingly distressed, frustrated, and hopeless. In this case, the residual psychosocial stressors produced during an episode of mania could help to instigate an episode of major depression. The distress or dysphoria can come from the self-deprecation and guilt for "creating" problems, the natural consequences of the events (e.g., losing one's home), and the inability to solve the problems effectively. The feelings of frustration, hopelessness, and being overwhelmed can block creative and effective problem resolution. When the problems remain unresolved, they sometimes worsen, growing in intensity (e.g., like interest on overcharged credit cards) or complexity (e.g., marital conflict developing over financial problems) until it seems impossible to identify any clear way to address the difficulties.

Recall again the cognitive-behavioral model of bipolar disorder presented in Chapter 2 (Figure 2.1, p. 24). When declines in functioning cause psychosocial problems, these problems worsen stress, interfere with sleep, and exacerbate symptoms of depression and mania. Breaking the cycle after problems have developed can include not only the problem-solving methods covered in Chapter 10 but some preventive techniques to keep stress levels low and managable so that it does not worsen the symptoms of depression and mania.

Stress does not always result from declines in psychosocial fucntioning due to symptoms. Sometimes the cycle begins with stress imposed on the patient, and subsequently the sleep deprivation and worry caused by it make the person more vulnerable to relapse. Therefore, stress management must include methods to prevent stress from occuring in the first place, methods for managing normal and inevitable life stresses and problems, as well as methods for handling acute episodes of stress.

Stress Prevention

Maintaining Balance

Beck et al. (1979) suggest that to fight off depression it is necessary both to experience a sense of accomplishment and to derive pleasure from day-to-day life. This concept is true for preventing stress from building as well. Life full of work, chores, and responsibilities will give a strong sense of accomplishment. But the stress that goes with those tasks can become overwhelming if not balanced with periods of rest, relaxation, and enjoyment. Likewise, a lifestyle without direction, for example, when unemployed or when there are no other responsibilities that structure time, can be equally stressful, as there are no experiences of mastery or achievement.

> Sylvester, for example, is on social security disability because his mental illness combined with some health problems make it difficult for him to work. While some of his family members and friends think he has the easy life, not having much to do each day is very distressing and unsatisfying. Sylvester would rather work than sit at home all day. He feels no real sense of purpose. He does not feel like he contributes to the community in any ways. He just thinks that he takes up space and is buying time until the end of his life.

This is a miserable existence for many people on disability. It is off balance in that little pleasure comes from inactivity and there is no sense of accomplishment. Most people need to feel a sense of purpose in the world and without it their lives lack meaning. This is fertile ground for emerging depression. Keeping balance means finding some activity that gives their life meaning and making specific efforts to experience pleasure. Activities that just pass the time, such as watching television or playing computer games, do not count as fun.

Those who are most vulnerable to living out of balance are the unemployed, workaholics, mothers who care for young children, and multitaskers—those who work, go to school, and care for their families. Activity scheduling is a traditional cognitive therapy intervention for restoring balance in day-to-day activities. It is a two-part exercise. In the first part, the patient tracks his or her activities for a week, rating each for the amount of pleasure experienced and the subjective sense of accomplishment experienced. Each is rated on a 0–7 scale with 0 indicating no pleasure and no sense of accomplishment and 7 indicating maximum pleasure and maximum accomplishment. All activities are documented and rated including the most mundane, such as bathing or eating. After keeping a week of ratings, the therapist reviews the schedule and ratings. If mastery and pleasure are balanced, there would be a variety of ratings from 0 to 7 across both categories for activities throughout the week. When people are depressed it is common to see the majority of items rated low for both categories. This can be due to the activity itself or the misperception of patients that minimizes positives and magnifies negatives.

The second part of the intervention is to schedule activities that have already proven to be high in mastery and pleasure or to add activities to the schedule that might help with restoring balance in both categories. If the person is not using time well and finds little sense of accomplishment, the activities from the GTA exercise, the "A" and "B" list exercise, the Goal-Setting Worksheet presented in Chapter 8, or any other behavioral intervention can be added to the list. If pleasure is lacking, fun activities can be added. If the patient is depressed, he or she may not fully experience joy or pleasure even with activities that had been enjoyable at another time in life. Therefore, the potential for pleasure should be discussed and realistic expectations set.

Activity scheduling is an exercise that need only be used during times at which the patient is out of balance with mastery and pleasure, with too little of one or both. It can also be used as an assessment tool to periodically check on the balances of work and pleasure.

Keeping It Simple

Margaret's idol is Martha Stewart. She watches her television shows, reads her magazines, and aspires to be as creative, organized, and perfect as she perceives Martha. Margaret has a reputation for providing wonderful meals, parties, gifts, and advice for others. She always tries to go the extra mile because she believes that is the right thing to do, even if it means going without sleep, getting frustrated, feeling like a failure when things go wrong, or not being fully appreciated. The energy boost that Margaret gets from hypomania makes it possible for her to do amazing things. She has learned to take full advantage of the highs, and because she is very organized and has a lot more energy than most people, she can force herself to be productive even when feeling low.

Margaret's family and friends have tried to help her with her projects in the past, but they would always get sent away. Margaret preferred to do things herself and they knew it so they left her alone when she was having a creative moment. Over time, Margaret's family had come to expect perfection from her and did not react with particular enthusiasm when it occurred. Of course things were beautiful, delicious, thoughtful, and creative. That was who Margaret was.

As Margaret's bipolar disorder progressed she found that more and more days were spent in depression. The hypomanias were short-lived and would sometimes come without any euphoria. Sometimes she just felt agitated and irritable. Doing things perfectly became more and more difficult for her, and the family's lack of enthusiasm grated on her nerves. Margaret knew that they didn't care if she put a small amount or large amount of effort into special occasions. They were just happy to be together. Margaret, however, thought that others would be disappointed in her if she did not do her very best. She became distraught when her energy was too low to put up holiday decorations, when she could not come up with a unique gift idea for each of her children, and when her husband had to pitch in to cook.

Life is hard for people with bipolar disorder who have high standards or who are perfectionists when they do not have the energy, motivation, or concentration to realize their ideals. They are often such high performers, however, that when they put out half effort it is still better than what most people can accomplish, but it is not satisfying. No one drives them as hard as they drive themselves. Having bipolar disorder frustrates the efforts of these people and makes them feel bad about themselves. Encouragement or support from others who are less demanding does not soothe the guilt and frustration of the patient.

Stress management for these people with bipolar disorder involves making a conscious decision not to go the extra mile every time, to settle for a good effort, and to keep it simple when they are not at their best. "Do less, but do it well" should replace their mantra of "be perfect." It is likely that therapists will receive some resistance to this notion in people who are used to having extremely high standards. They will view the idea of backing down as giving up, copping out, being average rather than being exceptional. The cognitive intervention to address this issue is to evaluate the advantages and disadvantages of always pushing themselves to a high standard versus relaxing their standards. Another strategy that is used with overachievers, those who go overboard in preparation for occasions or events, is to suggest that quality and not quantity be their goal.

Another approach is to identify and evaluate the negative automatic thoughts that emerge when they are feeling pressured to complete a task and when they are attempting to keep it simple. It is likely that these individuals' thinking errors will fall into the category of "absolutes" as they think in terms of success and failure as well as should and musts. When the analysis is complete, the person with bipolar disorder who pushes him- or herself to excellence will always have to make the decision whether or not it is worth the personal wear and tear, the risk of stimulating mania, and the time. Sometimes the event will be important enough to make the effort, like preparing for a child's wedding or planning a special holiday party, and sometimes it will not. Selecting where to put their energy may be a new concept for those who feel compelled to push themselves toward perfection.

Lifestyle Choices and Limit Setting

It is a popular notion that a way to manage stress is to know your limits. With bipolar disorder, limits can vary as the illness waxes and wanes. When depressed, most people have less energy and can do less. In euthymic states, energy, motivation, and organization are usually adequate and more can be done. In hypomanic states, there is more drive than usual and, therefore, more can be accomplished than usual. And with mania, it can seem that the sky is the limit. Therefore, what a person is capable of handling (i.e., his or her limit) is a moving target.

Stress can be triggered when a person's capacity and activity do not match. This occurs when energy, motivation, and concentration levels change, but expectations for oneself and responsibilities and activities are not adjusted accordingly. Instead of expecting less and reducing workload or burden, people are more likely to push themselves harder and feel exhausted and frustrated in the end. Stress can be managed more easily when activity is adjusted to meet the limits of available coping resources such as energy and motivation. Many people will say that they cannot do less, work slower, take on fewer tasks, or give up. They do not want to risk rejection, disappoint others, feel like a failure, or accept that they have an illness that alters their capacity to function.

Ideally, the intervention is to adjust activity to meet available coping resources. Concretely, this means that when people are depressed, they should not volunteer to organize the company picnic, cook the Thanksgiving dinner singlehandedly, or take on extra care-taking responsibilities until they are feeling significantly better. If heading toward mania, they should not burn the midnight oil to make a good presentation into a fantastic presentation, volunteer to chaperone kids at an amusement park, or take on tasks that others could easily do, until they are feeling more like their normal selves. This is what it means to set limits.

Sometimes setting limits means making larger decisions about what is best for them such as where to work, where to live, whether to have more children, or whether to invite family members to visit for the holidays. Jobs that disrupt sleep schedules or require a great deal of overtime hours may not be the best choice for someone who has bipolar disorder and is sensitive to sleep disruption. Jobs that require a person to perform optimally in front of others regardless of their mood states, such as classroom teaching and working in a retail store, may also be poor choices. It is easy for some to put on a happy face when feeling low or control irritability when feeling high, but for others the challenge would be too great.

Having children is a judgment call. Some people will not know that they have bipolar disorder until after they have had children, so their only choice is to adapt to the situation. Children can be wonderful, but they are also demanding and overstimulating. They can bring joy to life, but they can also cause sleep disruption and stress. Most important, parenting is a constant demand, particularly for mothers. It is difficult to take a time out from parenting to manage a depressive or manic episode. More kids can mean more joy, but also more work. People have to decide if they want to have children, when they can afford to be off medication to do so, and how many to add to the family. These are big decisions. The best-case scenario for stress management is for people to have no more children than they have the resources to manage. This includes not only finances but also energy, time, patience, and support from others.

Boundaries

Gloria feels as though she's carrying the weight of the world on her shoulders. She has been feeling less depressed lately but isn't back to her normal self. Her sister, Nancy, has recently been diagnosed with cancer and is beginning treatments soon. Nancy's teenage daughter has bipolar disorder too and is very stressed about her mother's illness. Gloria worries about them both just as she does her own children. Gloria's oldest son, Greg, got married last year, and he and his new wife are having trouble adjusting to life together. Greg calls on Gloria to ask for advice, but Gloria is never sure what to say. Her own two marriages didn't last long, and she doesn't feel like she's in any position to offer advice. Gloria's mom, Gladys, has been recently diagnosed with Alzheimer's disease. She lives in another state, near Gloria's brother, and Gloria is worried that Gladys will soon forget all about her. Gloria's best friend is having problems too. Her daughter was caught sneaking out of the house a few nights ago and after a fight with her mother is threatening to run away for good. Gloria prays for everyone, including herself, but it does not make her worry any less.

Despite her struggles with bipolar disorder, Gloria has always been a source of strength for her family and friends. They can come to her any time for comfort and understanding. She wipes their tears, loans them money, gives them a place to stay, and makes them feel cared for. When the stress gets to her she does a pretty good job of hiding it from everyone else. Gloria has more problems with depression than mania. In fact, she has not had another episode of mania since starting to take lithium more than 15 years ago. The depression can get severe. The only thing that has kept her from suicide is the thought of all these people needing her. Yet all these people needing her is what pushes her toward suicide. She realizes that her compassion is both her greatest strength and her greatest weakness, but she can't make herself stop caring about those she loves. She feels it is her responsibility to share the weight of their burdens so that they might feel a little relief and be better able to cope.

When a person takes on the stress of others it is often called compassion—unless it hurts that person, in which case it is called a boundary problem. It is not unusual for people who have bipolar disorder to have relatives who also suffer from mental health problems such as depression, anxiety, or substance abuse. People like Gloria try to take care of themselves while helping others along the way. Sometimes they ignore their own needs and tend only to the needs of others. For example, if resources are limited, a person might use his medication money to pay for the treatment of another family member. If this is a dependent child or disabled spouse, the decision may seem rational. But if the person in need is another adult who is as capable as the patient to acquire resources, then the assistance provided by the patient while neglecting his own health care needs may seem unreasonable or self-defeating.

There are many reasons why people put the needs of others above their own. Perhaps they view other people as having more value than themselves, fear rejection if they do not help, have strong maternal instincts, or believe that it is their duty or mission to help others. These beliefs can be subjected to evaluation to determine their validity or the therapist can guide patients to evaluate the advantages and disadvantages of maintaining this "helpful" position versus putting their own needs first. The analysis can help patients find a way to maximize their ability to be helpful to others while minimizing the risk to self.

Some people want to stop putting themselves out to help others because of the wear and tear it causes and because they see that even with their help, the other people are not getting any better, stronger, or independent. In this case, the patient may need permission from the therapist to pull back support as well as a rationale for doing so. The best rationale is that the process of going to the aid of others may only be fostering their dependence rather than encouraging their independence. In other words, they may actually be hurting the person rather than helping. Helpers never want to be hurtful and, therefore, they may be willing to allow others to suffer a bit and solve their own problems if they feel that it will be in everyone's best interest in the long run.

Acute Stress Management

In the previous section we talked about how to prevent stress from building, but for most people, acute stressors can occur despite efforts to prevent them. The following sections include methods for coping with psychosocial stressors once they have occurred.

Coping with Stress

People with bipolar disorder may have psychosocial problems in a number of different areas: family, work, health, finances, and so on. Stress from psychosocial difficulties can exacerbate symptoms such as impaired concentration, fatigue, and distractibility, which, in turn, can further interfere with effective coping. Therapists can help patients begin to cope with stressors by helping them to define and prioritize problems that need to be addressed in therapy. These become goals for therapy against which progress can be compared.

Patients have usually tried to resolve their problems on their own before presenting them to a therapist. Therefore, before developing a new treatment plan, it is helpful to determine what strategies patients have already used and how effective they have been in coping with stress. Therapists may ask questions such as:

- "How have you coped with problems in the past?"
- "How have you dealt with similar problems?"
- "Have you tried to apply those strategies to current problems?"
- "What kept those strategies from working for these new problems?"
- "What do you believe is the next strategy to try?"

Taking the time to inquire about past efforts to deal with stressors serves several purposes. First, it facilitates treatment planning; therapists can suggest interventions that patients have not yet tried or perhaps a modification of strategies that patients have attempted without success. Second, inquiring about patients' previous attempts at coping with problems makes it clear that the therapist respects the patient's intelligence and resourcefulness. Third, it establishes clinicians as consultants to patients in coping with stressors, providing expertise in areas in which patients need assistance. This emphasizes the view of the therapeutic relationship as a collaboration rather than a "fix-it shop" where patients passively bring in problems to be fixed and therapists do repairs and send bills.

Coping Resources

When developing a treatment plan to address patients' psychosocial stressors, the therapist generally thinks about ways to maximize patients' coping resources. The fact that patients are not coping well does not mean that they are devoid of internal and external resources. Internal resources include:

External coping resources include assistance from others, such as family, friends, therapists, coworkers, support staff on the job, and housekeepers. External resources can also include services that are purchased, such as a maid service, income tax services, clerical support services, babysitters, banks and other financial institutions, or real estate agents. Table 11.1 provides some examples of resources people might use in attempting to cope with stress.

Obstacles to Effective Coping

Although mobilizing patients' existing resources or acquiring new resources to cope with psychosocial stressors may sound simple, many

TABLE 11.1. Coping Resources

• Intelligence	• Resourcefulness
• Practicality	• Energy
• Analytical-mindedness	• Stamina
• Common sense	• Creativity
• Fortitude	• Patience
• Sensitivity	• Self-esteem
• Sense of humor	• Money
• Time	• Confidence
• Organizational ability	• Ability to ask for help
• Support system	• Perseverance

factors can interfere. To understand fully the context in which problems have developed and persist, patients' weaknesses and the obstacles to effective coping must be identified. In patients with bipolar disorder, the symptoms of the illness can produce problems. For example, the impaired judgment associated with mania may lead to ill-conceived financial ventures that leave the family in financial ruin. Sexual promiscuity can stress existing relationships. Similarly, the emotional distress and fearfulness associated with depression can create obstacles to effective coping by overriding patients' logic and keeping them from actively attending to their problems. Neglected problems can compound over time. Perhaps emotion is the most common obstacle to effective coping.

Several other internal and external factors can interfere with successful coping. Internal factors, such as fearfulness of the outcome, can keep patients from taking direct action to solve their problems. Not having sufficient information can impede problem solving, as can being unaware that there is a problem. External factors, such as other people over whom patients have little, if any, control, can produce, exacerbate, or maintain difficulties. When patients are faced with competing demands, impossible deadlines, and/or a mounting work load, they may not have time to resolve their problems. Instead, they struggle to keep their heads above water for another day. Some patients may have the time to work out their problems but may lack sufficient resources to do so. Money, for example, may be needed to solve financial problems and other problems of daily living. If patients are unemployed and have only limited sources of support, financial problems will linger.

The goal is for patients to recognize obstacles to effective coping, make use of existing coping resources, and attempt to reduce or eliminate the obstacles that preclude active coping.

Relaxation Training

Relaxation exercises can be used by patients to decrease mental stimulation and muscle tension at bedtime. For some individuals these exercises reduce physiological and mental arousal and, in turn, facilitate sleep. There are many different relaxation techniques. No one method works for all people. To help patients identify the most helpful relaxation exercise, provide a sampling of inductions during therapy sessions and allow them to select one or more methods to learn. For patients who have difficulty in "turning off" stressful thoughts, relaxation techniques that help to focus attention on the relaxation task and away from distracting thoughts are often most beneficial. For those patients with muscle tension, especially tension that produces muscle aches (back, shoulders, neck) or headaches, inductions that focus directly on release of tensed muscles may be best. Imagery exercises are useful for people who have the ability to create and sustain mental images.

Relaxation inductions can be done during exercise, while driving a car, or while sitting at a desk. To induce sleep, relaxation exercises can begin long before bedtime as the individual slows his or her mental and physical activity at the end of the day. In fact, the best relaxation inductions are those used throughout the day to reduce tension or overstimulation as it begins to build.

When prescribing a relaxation program, a clinician generally begins with those techniques the patient has found helpful in the past such as an evening walk or a warm bath. Some people with bipolar disorder relax by praying, meditating, or doing crafts, such as knitting. Reading helps some people slow down and fall asleep, but action-packed novels that are difficult to put down may not be ideal at bedtime. When tense or upset, it can be difficult to generate ideas to induce relaxation. A preplanned list kept at home can be helpful. Table 11.2 shows an example of a list of relaxation activities developed by a patient with bipolar disorder.

If new relaxation exercises are introduced, keep them simple (e.g., slow and controlled breathing). *Clinical Behavior Therapy* (Goldfried & Davison, 1994) includes several relaxation inductions that are easy for therapists to administer. Following is an example of a simple relaxation induction based on techniques presented in the book:

"Find a place to relax that will have as few distractions as possible. Turn down the lights. Turn off the television. Ask others to avoid interruptions. You can lie down or sit comfortably. Before you begin to relax, think of a number between 0 and 100 that describes how tense you feel. One hundred means the most tension you have ever felt and 0 means no tension at all. Write the number down somewhere so that when you have finished this exercise you can rate your tension level again to see if it has improved. Now take a deep breath in through your nose and let it out through your mouth very slowly (*pause*). You can close your eyes if you would like (*pause*). Try to let go of the tension in your body by allowing yourself to sink heavily into the bed or chair (*pause*). Loosen your fingers (*pause*). If you teeth are clenched, loosen your jaw and allow your lips to part slightly (*pause*). Let your arms and legs move into a more comfortable position (*pause*). Imagine yourself to be a rag doll or puppet lying limply on the bed or chair (*pause*). Feel the tension leaving your body. Your body feels more relaxed than before (*pause*). Now take another slow, deep breath in through your nose and out through your mouth (*pause*). You can let your eyes close if they are still open (*pause*)."

Some patients can relax when they close their eyes and imagine a relaxing scene. Others are more comfortable with their eyes open, as they find it harder to control rapidly moving thoughts with their eyes closed. In this instance, it may be more effective to use a technique in which the patient concentrates on a small object in the room while breathing slowly and deeply.

TABLE 11.2. Relaxation Activities

1. Take a walk.
2. Take a deep breath and slowly exhale. Repeat.
3. Got to my room and close the door.
4. Listen to music.
5. Lie down.
6. Take a warm bath.
7. Do an outside task (e.g., take out the garbage, take time to notice the stars.

Stress Control

People who have bipolar disorder have daily hassles with which to deal just as everyone else does. They must try to stay on top of problems to keep them from accumulating while they contend with their mental illness and their day-to-day responsibilities. Keeping stress under control may require periodic assessments of life circumstances and regular efforts at solving problems. In the sections that follow, we cover various ways to keep tabs on stress by resolving problems as they develop.

Times for Formal Problem Solving

Although people make decisions every day without going through each step in the problem-solving sequence, there are times when casual decision making does not adequately address the issues. The most common time to use formal problem solving is when there are obvious difficulties in everyday activities, for example, when there are unresolved problems at home, on the job, or in interpersonal relationships. Formal problem solving is most useful when (1) the problem persists despite the patient's efforts, or (2) the patient has been unable to identify a reasonable solution to the problem.

Cues To Action

Identifying and defining problems requires an awareness that problems exist. There are various internal and external cues to the need for problem solving. As part of their training in problem solving, it is useful to explore with patients the various types of cues and the ways in which these cues bring problems to their attention.

Physical Cues

Sometimes, the cues that problems need attention are physical discomforts, such as headaches, indigestion, muscle tension, fatigue, hives, and tightness in the chest. Even when individuals are not consciously aware that there is a problem, their bodies can speak for them.

Emotional Shifts

For patients with bipolar disorder, emotional shifts can serve as cues to initiate problem solving. At first, the focus should be on determining how to cope with the emotional shift itself. Defining the problem, in this case, means analyzing the situation and deciding whether the mood shift is an independent event or has resulted from a stressor. As noted in earlier chapters, the events, cognitions, and actions associated with the mood shift can provide clues about its source. The solutions generated to cope with the mood shift will depend on the identified source of the problem. If the cause of the mood shift is a belief or negative cognition regarding an event, the solution may be to use cognitive restructuring strategies. The patient can then evaluate and modify the emotion-laden thoughts about the event that are fueling the mood shift.

If the source of the emotional shift is a stressful event or problem itself, formal problem solving may be required. It is best if, before they begin the problem-solving process, patients try to reduce the intensity of the emotional shift by gaining emotional distance from the problem or by using other mood-stabilizing methods. The solutions that patients generate while they are extremely upset are often colored by the intensity of the emotion. Gaining emotional distance reduces the likelihood of impulsive responding and gives patients more control over troublesome situations.

Input from Others

Input from others can take the form of complaints and criticism. It is common for people to see complaints from others as unjustifiable and unworthy of concern. Although the complaints or criticisms from others may indeed be unsubstantiated, they are cues that something is wrong. Patients should be encouraged to hear criticism as a cue that a problem exists, whether it be in their own behavior, in the behavior of others, or in their relationships. Defining criticism as a cue may allow the patient to move beyond defensiveness to begin to evaluate the situation objectively. If the problem can be identified, it has a better chance to be solved.

Family members, friends, and significant others are often good observers. They may be able to identify problems before they become noticeable to the patient, particularly when the patient's judgment and insight are colored by mania or hypomania. Unfortunately, patients in this state do not always welcome the observations and comments of significant others. Many therapists discuss with their patients ways in which significant others may help patients identify areas in which active problem solving can be useful. It can be very useful to include the family in such a discussion if the patient is comfortable with the plan. During a conjoint meeting, the therapist can address (1) when the family should talk with the patient about problems, (2) how to present problems in a way that the patient can hear them, and (3) what to do when the patient is unable or unwilling to respond to the family's concerns. The therapist may also:

- Explain how the symptoms of the disorder interfere with the process of information.

- Find out how the family has dealt with similar communication problems in the past and how successful their attempts have been. Use the problem-solving model to generate solutions to any difficulties that may arise in the family's communications with the patient about anticipated or observed problems.

Scheduled Assessment

Patients need not wait until problems emerge before using formal problem solving. While it is most often used for putting out fires in the patient's life, problem solving can be *proactive* rather than *reactive*. Patients and their significant others can schedule time at regular intervals (e.g., every 3–6 months) to evaluate their progress and to address problems, either with the assistance of a therapist or on their own. At these scheduled progress checks, patients take stock in their lives, compare their goals with their progress, and identify any areas of dissatisfaction. Difficulties or impediments to progress can become targets for change.

After each self-evaluation or progress check, patients can decide when the next evaluation is to occur. It can be helpful to pair the exercise with a regularly occurring event, such as the next medication clinic visit. For example, Mr. Peters and his wife make time at the end of the month, when they are paying their bills, to check on their progress.

- *Symptom control.* To what degree is the patient maintaining his or her treatment gains? Is he or she taking the medication as prescribed? Are the symptoms of depression and/or mania under control?

- *Interpersonal sphere.* Are relationships progressing as expected and/or as desired? Are there any sources of tension in ongoing relationships? If so, what attempts have been made to resolve problems? Is there any need for professional intervention?

- *Occupational sphere.* Are there any problems on the job? Is the patient able to function on the job as expected? How is job attendance? Are there any problems in getting along with others on the job?

- *Social sphere.* Are social relationships progressing as desired? Is the patient maintaining an active social life consistent with his or her goals, needs, and desires? Is there sufficient social support? If not, what is keeping the patient from gaining support from others?

Predictable Times of Change and Stress

Major life events are associated with increased stress and can precipitate an exacerbation of symptoms in the patient with bipolar disorder. Stressful events, especially catastrophic events such as the death of a friend or family member, severe financial crises, major accidents, or illnesses in patients or their significant others, can tax a patient's internal coping resources. Positive life events can also be stressful. They require alterations in routine, including eating and sleeping patterns, and may affect symptom control. During these times, the patient may need to rely on more formal problem-solving strategies to cope with the changes associated with the event.

Life changes generally have an impact beyond the arena in which they are occurring. For example, job changes can affect life at home and vice versa. Periods of change, therefore, are also times in which more formal problem solving can be useful.

Expected role transitions can be similarly stressful and place the patient at increased risk for an exacerbation of symptoms. Role transitions can affect the patient directly (e.g., getting married) or indirectly by means of changes in other family members (e.g., the youngest child moving away from home). Developmental role transitions, like any other change or event, can be disruptive to the patient's mental health. One reason that life transitions produce stress is that they often change the amount and content of interactions and communication between patients and their significant others. In the next chapter, common interpersonal problems experienced by people with bipolar disorder are covered, including methods for preventing and resolving relationships stresses.

Key Points for the Therapist to Remember

♦ For many people who are unable to work because of disability, little pleasure comes from inactivity and there is no sense of accomplishment. Most people need to feel a sense of purpose in the world and without it their lives lack meaning. This is fertile ground for emerging depression.

♦ Life is hard for people with bipolar disorder who have high standards or who are perfectionists when they do not have the energy, motivation, or concentration to realize their ideals.

♦ The person with bipolar disorder who pushes him- or herself to excellence will always have to make the decision whether or not it is worth the personal wear and tear, the risk of stimulating mania, and the time. Selecting where to put their energy may be a new concept for those who feel compelled to push themselves toward perfection.

♦ Some people want to stop putting themselves out to help others because of the wear and tear it causes and because they see that even with their help, the other people are not getting any better, stronger, or independent. In this case, the patient may need permission from the therapist to pull back support as well as a rationale for doing so.

♦ Patients usually try to resolve their problems on their own before presenting them to a therapist. Therefore, before developing a new treatment plan, it is helpful to determine what strategies patients have already used and how effective they have been in coping with stress.

♦ People who have bipolar disorder have daily hassles to deal with just as everyone else does. They must try to stay on top of problems in order to keep them from accumulating while they contend with their mental illness and their day-to-day responsibilities. Keeping stress under control may require periodic assessments of life circumstances and regular efforts at solving problems.

Points to Discuss with Patients

♦ Prevention of relapses and recurrences of depression and mania may, in part, be achieved by controlling stress.

♦ Stress management includes methods to prevent stress from occurring in the first place, methods for managing normal and inevitable life stresses and problems, as well as methods for handling acute episodes of stress.

♦ Life full of work, chores, and responsibilities will give a strong sense of accomplishment. But the stress that goes with those tasks can become overwhelming if not balanced with periods of rest, relaxation, and enjoyment. Likewise, a lifestyle without direction, for example, when unemployed or when there are no other responsibilities that structure time, can be equally as stressful as there are no experiences of mastery or achievement.

♦ It is a popular notion that a way to manage stress is to know your limits. With bipolar disorder, limits can vary as the illness waxes and wanes.

♦ Stress can be triggered when a person's capacity and activity do not match. This occurs when energy, motivation, and concentration levels change, but expectations for oneself and responsibilities and activities are not adjusted accordingly.

CHAPTER 12

Addressing Problems in Interpersonal Communication

Oversensitivity

For people with bipolar disorder, oversensitivity to rejection or criticism occurs more often during depressive or mixed episodes than during manic episodes. Patients often state that their feelings are hurt easily, that they anticipate rejection or criticism before it occurs, and that they overreact when these events do occur. It is difficult for these individuals to distinguish between real rejection or criticism and their own cognitive distortions. Sometimes, patients are able to recognize intellectually that others' behavior was not intended to be rejecting or critical, but they are unable to inhibit or reduce their strong emotional reaction (e.g., sadness, guilt, embarrassment, or anger) to that behavior.

Interpersonal conflict may ensue if the "offender" responds to the oversensitivity of the patient with bipolar disorder by becoming defensive or counterattacking in response to the "unjustified accusations" of the patient. For example, the offender may say defensively, "You always accuse me of criticizing you. I didn't say a damn thing." Even if an argument does not develop, the patient may withdraw, further exacerbating his or her depressive feelings, and likely antagonizing the offender.

Several interventions may be helpful for the overly sensitive individual and his or her partner. The first is to teach the patient to evaluate the validity of the assumption that he or she has been rejected or criticized. Appropriate action can then be taken, depending on the outcome of this assessment (see Chapter 9). The easiest way to determine if feelings of rejection are warranted is to discuss them with the offender. To introduce the topic, patients can use the following fill-in-the-blank statement: "When you said/did on [specify time] _____, it made me feel _____."

Sometimes, it is best simply to ask: "When you said/did _____ on _____ [specify time] _____, did you mean _____ [assumption of rejection]?"

> Ms. Salinas and two coworkers had lunch together on Wednesday. Ms. Cain had not been asked to go with them; she had been invited on other occasions, though she rarely accepted these invitations. When she saw the three ladies laughing as they entered the office after lunch, Ms. Cain felt left out, rejected, and saddened. Her therapist had instructed her to discuss her feelings of rejection with the suspected "offender" as a first step in coping with the lingering hurt that often followed these events. Following this instruction, Ms. Cain said to Ms. Salinas, "When I saw you and the other two ladies return from lunch today, I really felt left out. Are you mad at me or something? Is that why you didn't invite me?" Ms. Salinas apologized for leaving Ms. Cain out and added that it was not the group's intention to exclude Ms. Cain, nor was she angry with her. The group had planned to eat at a restaurant that they knew Ms. Cain disliked, so she was not included. Ms. Cain reluctantly accepted the apology and explanation. After a period of mild sadness, she was able to put the event behind her.

In a second intervention for coping with interpersonal sensitivity, the therapist may teach the offender to recognize when the patient is feeling hurt and to respond by attempting to understand the situation from the patient's perspective. Rather than explaining or defending his or her position, the offender can express sympathy for the patient's hurt. For example, a partner may say, "I'm sorry that your feelings are hurt. That isn't what I intended." Another effective response is to focus on the patient's emotional state; for example, "I know that when you are having a bad day you get your feelings hurt easily. I'm sorry if I accidentally hurt your feelings." For offenders inclined to respond to the patient in anger or frustration, these responses take a considerable amount of coaching.

Pessimistic View of Self, Others, and the Future

When depressed and, perhaps to some extent, when euthymic, patients with bipolar disorder see the world through blue, cloudy, and myopic lenses. They feel hopeless about their prospects for a happy life, disheartened by what they see as a slim chance for improvement in their relationships (and/or partner), and unhappy with their current status yet too immobilized by pessimism to consider, let alone attempt, change. When a pessimist and an optimist meet to work out the problems of daily life, plan for the future, or attempt to have fun, their fundamentally different views of the world can create tension and conflict.

Research on the negative views of patients and their spouses suggests that the pessimism of the patient is not contagious (Prager & Basco, 1995). That is, dysfunctional or negative attitudes, low self-esteem, and feelings of hopelessness reported by depressed patients are not reported by their spouses any more often than they are reported by individuals who have never suffered from depression. It is helpful for both the patient and his or her significant other to learn to recognize when their differences in perspective are influencing their interaction. The patient can then evaluate the validity of his or her pessimistic views by using cognitive restructuring interventions (see Chapter 9). The partner can alter his or her responses to the patient by discontinuing the discussion before it worsens or, with considerable guidance, by attempting very carefully to help the patient examine his or her thinking for potential distortions.

> Brett and Patty Smythe were married for 10 years. Despite treatment, Mrs. Smythe was depressed for much of their married life. She was well educated, very attractive, creative, and talented. When her depression remitted, she had a lovely sense of humor. She viewed herself very differently from the way that others viewed her. She was exquisitely aware of her own imperfections, faults, and errors. She believed that the praise she received from her husband was patronizing and insincere. She easily overlooked the positive features of her relationships but had a highly sensitive radar that identified and recorded most negative events.
>
> Mr. Smythe, a man who prided himself on his analytical thinking, attempted to explain to his wife how her pessimistic views of herself, of him, and of their future together had no logical basis. He pointed out her strengths, his love for her, and their potential for happiness. However, in her pessimism she was not only unresponsive to his attempts to reason with her, but he also angered her because she thought he lacked a true appreciation of her feelings. Despite his failure to convince her that she was a wonderful, intelligent, creative person, he continued to use analytical reasoning in his battle against her negativity. As the process continued, tension, frustration, and distance between them increased.

It can be very frustrating for the spouses of depressed patients to cope with their seemingly illogically negative outlook. Attempts at "talking them out of" their negativity generally fail and may even worsen the conflict. The pessimistic spouse accuses the optimistic spouse of overlooking problems, while the optimistic spouse accuses the pessimistic spouse of finding problems where none exist. It takes tolerance, commitment, and love to stay married in these situations.

Paranoia

One of the more severe symptoms of mania and, occasionally, of depression is paranoia. In the early stages of paranoia, the patient may appear overly sensitive or suspicious of others. Furthermore, the onset of paranoia feeds the process by which patients presume that others have malevolent intentions. Not all patients with bipolar disorder experience paranoia as part of their symptom picture, however.

> Mr. Patterson knew that one of the symptoms of his mania was paranoia. He often imagined people at work talking about him behind his back and even colluding against him. While he knew that he could be overly sensitive to things at times, several things had happened at work that could be construed as attempts to exclude him. For example, he had not been invited to attend several important policy-forming meetings at his company, even though they directly affected his department. People often talked and laughed in groups that quickly quieted and dispersed when he approached them. Someone heard a rumor that several management positions were about to be eliminated, and Mr. Patterson had less seniority than did other managers in the plant. When his superiors approached him to discuss productivity problems in his department, he was openly defensive.
>
> At home, Mr. Patterson was tense. He told his wife about the conspiracy to get rid of him at work. She was well acquainted with his paranoia and tried to help him reason through the events of the day. He sensed that she did not believe him and convinced himself that she was against him as well. An argument quickly ensued. His wife encouraged him to get a good night's sleep and agreed to talk more about the problem in the morning.
>
> The paranoia subsided after Mr. Patterson had sufficient sleep, and he was able to talk with his employers to determine if his job was in jeopardy. Feedback that his position at work was secure allowed him to look at his reaction more objectively and recognize that his suspiciousness, coupled with real events, had contributed to his distress.
>
> The paranoia affected his interaction with people at work.

Perhaps others sensed his irritability and tension, and they may have avoided him to escape his sarcasm and short temper. Having experienced his paranoia several times before, his wife had lost her ability to be sympathetic, especially when there was reason to believe he was overreacting to coincidental circumstances. Mr. Patterson was correct in his assumption that his wife was unsympathetic. Until he was able to gain some distance from the problem, however, he was unable to examine his contribution to the uncomfortable interpersonal events.

Irritability

Like paranoia, irritability can be a symptom of either depression or mania. It can accompany paranoia, oversensitivity, or a pessimistic view of the world, but it can also exist independently of other symptoms. Irritability affects the way messages are sent to others and colors the interpretation of messages received from others. It can make a person quick to anger, can precipitate arguments, and can lead to intense anxiety or agitation. No matter how "reasonable" or "careful" a spouse may believe that he or she is being, interacting with an irritable partner can be like walking through a minefield; even stepping lightly, the spouse never knows when the next explosion will occur. While irritability can affect many individuals, regardless of their psychiatric history, it is particularly troublesome for those experiencing depression or mania.

Mrs. Westin had a history of severe depression with bouts of irritability. During these episodes, she was edgy and quick to anger. In fact, she sometimes became so intensely angry that she said and did things that she later regretted, even physically assaulting her husband. Her husband, a generally nonaggressive individual, occasionally "restrained" her in self-defense to minimize injury to himself. On one of these occasions, his "restraint" broke her arm.

The extent to which Mrs. Westin could inhibit her irritability and aggressive behavior was not always clear. On occasion, her husband responded to her irritability with reason. The more he used reason, however, the more irritable she became. It was as if his insistence on reason fueled the fire of her irrationality. Mrs. Westin knew that her irritability was a symptom of her illness and that this emotional state distorted her perception of reality. He responded to each of her angry statements by attempting to change her view. He could not; instead, he became more angry and frustrated, which, in turn, contributed to the downward spiral of conflict.

In this situation, rather than engage an irritable person in a discussion or argument about the validity of their statements, it is preferable to not respond. One useful strategy is to refuse to fight and then leave the scene for some period of time. This gives the irritable person time alone to cool off and regain some control. Another strategy that may be used in conjunction with the first is to express empathy for the person's hurt or angry feelings and to apologize for contributing to the person's troubles. For example, "I'm sorry that I hurt your feelings by my statement earlier. I can understand how it would make you angry to be left out, but I did not intend to hurt you." Giving an apology after being unjustly criticized is very difficult, but it can prevent an altercation with the irritable person. A third strategy is to draw the patient's attention to the irritability before it reaches a high level and to talk about whether it is a warning signal of the onset of a depressive or manic episode. Suggesting to the patient that he or she call the doctor to discuss the irritability can do more to address the "real problem" than arguing.

Pressured Speech

Mr. Alegro talked his wife's ear off when he was hypomanic. When she came home after a long day at work, she was preoccupied with tending to the children, cooking dinner, or trying to unwind. Mr. Alegro wanted to tell her about all the things that happened during work that day. At times, he felt a strong "need" to talk that he just could not inhibit, no matter how hard he tried. "I just need to talk to someone or I'll burst." Mr. Alegro's wife needed quiet time, not an incessant monologue of stories, jokes, plans, or observations. This conflict of needs caused her to withdraw from him, diminished her tolerance, and increased her own irritability. She did not notice the pattern of symptoms that began with his pressured speech and developed into mania. Instead, she tried to ignore him.

Although generally a symptom of hypomania or mania, pressured speech or increased talkativeness can occur outside an episode of illness. This talkativeness can be socially adaptive in that it facilitates entry into new social groups, reduces social anxiety, and is often enjoyable to or even envied by others. At home, it may be less valued, burdening other family members particularly at the end of the day when energy is low and people may have had their fill of conversation. A quid pro quo agreement provides a way for couples to cope with their competing needs and can be applied to other types of relationship conflicts. For example, Mr.

and Mrs. Bronson made an agreement that he would listen to her talk for at least 30 minutes if she would give him time after work to unwind and relax so that he could be more receptive to her.

Cognitive Impairment

Changes in a patient's cognitive functioning can make it difficult for him or her to process information, formulate thoughts, or make decisions. Such a cognitive impairment may be evident in decreased concentration, mental confusion, indecisiveness, sensory overload, distractibility, and flight of ideas. These symptoms may accompany depression, mania, or hypomania and may interfere with the patient's ability to operate on the job, at home, or in social situations.

> Mr. Macias found that, when his thoughts were "jumbled," he could not think clearly. He made poor decisions that he later regretted, interpreted the actions of others incorrectly, and forgot what he was doing or what he had to do. To others, he appeared to be a "scatterbrain." His wife and his boss became irritated with him on such occasions. Mr. Macias's attempts to cope with a variety of problems (e.g., marital problems, job problems, decisions about moving, preparation for vacation or holidays, plans to begin weight loss or exercise) seemed to exacerbate his mental confusion. He knew that cloudy thinking might indicate a symptom breakthrough and that he must carefully monitor his symptoms to avert an early relapse of depression or mania.

Patients can be taught to use the symptoms of cognitive impairment as cues that the onset of an episode of depression or mania may be imminent. They should watch for other symptoms and consult their clinician. In the meantime, it is best to encourage patients who are experiencing a cognitive impairment to avoid making any important life decisions and to reduce the number of problems that they are trying to cope with until their cognitive functioning improves.

It is difficult to know whether it is the mental confusion that interferes with normal coping abilities or the attempt to deal with too many issues simultaneously. In either case, reducing stimulation may help to prevent the development of psychosocial and interpersonal problems and may reduce the severity of the cognitive impairment.

Dimensions of Communication

Even without the complexities of bipolar disorder, communication with others can be very complicated and often fails. One reason is that each message is actually made up of several different levels of messages that are communicated simultaneously. These levels can be thought of as dimensions of communication. The verbal dimension consists of the words that are said. For example, "Oh, I see you cleaned the kitchen." Communication can become problematic when the words imply more than the message sender is saying directly: "Oh, I see you *finally* cleaned the kitchen." The addition of one simple word can turn a neutral comment or an acknowledgment of a positive event into an implied criticism of the times that the individual had not cleaned the kitchen.

The nonverbal dimension of communication includes the tone of voice in which the message is conveyed (e.g., angry, pleasant, and sarcastic), as well as the message sender's facial expression (e.g., smiling and frowning), body posture (e.g., arms crossed), volume of speech (e.g., loud and soft), rate of speech (e.g., fast, slow, and frequent pauses), and the timing of the message (e.g., during an argument or as soon as the message sender walks into the house). A husband who comes home from work and, with a sarcastic tone, a smirk on his face, and his hands on his hips, says to his depressed wife, "Oh . . . (*with surprise in his voice and followed by a long pause*), I see you finally cleaned the kitchen," sends one message. A mother who comes home from work and, with a pleasant tone, a smile, and a pat on her child's shoulder, says, "Oh, I see you cleaned the kitchen," sends a very different message—even though she uses nearly the same words.

The third dimension of communication, content, involves not just the choice of words but the general idea that is being conveyed in a message. The husband, for example, sends a message that he cannot believe she has done something good; that he perceives her generally as a failure; and that he is, therefore, surprised that she cleaned the kitchen. In her message to her child, however, the mother is acknowledging that her child has done something to be appreciated and that the mother is very pleased.

The relationship value of the message, the fourth dimension of communication, is generally conveyed through the message sender's choice of words and nonverbal behaviors. This dimension of the message indicates the way in which the sender views his or her relationship to the receiver. For example, when teachers give information to a class of students, they are communicating that they are in charge, know more than the students, and expect the students to behave with respect. Messages sent from employer to employee, physician to patient, and parent to child may have a similar relationship value. Although the relationship message communicates something about the status of the sender and receiver(s) as perceived by the sender, this perception may not reflect the true status differences. For example, the sarcastic husband's message suggests that he sees himself as superior to her, when they may actually be more equal than his tone suggests.

The fifth dimension of communication is the consistency between the intended message and the received message. The intended message is what the sender wants to communicate to another person. Although the verbal message that is sent may be accurate, the nonverbal information sent along with the words may alter the meaning in a way that makes the received message different from the intended message. The husband's intended message, for example, may have been to acknowledge his wife's accomplishments, perhaps because her psychiatrist said that it is important for him to notice and acknowledge her positive activities and to give her credit for taking small steps toward recovery. The message that she received, however, was that her husband is disgusted with her. In addition, she received the nonverbal message that he thinks she is merely doing what she should have done long ago. Therefore, the message did not make her feel that she is taking positive steps toward recovery but that she is merely digging herself out of the deep hole of previous failures.

Not only can a sender convey much more than just words, but also the receiver can alter messages by "reading in" more than the sender is conveying. Sometimes a listener hears a different nonverbal tone or relationship message in a speaker's voice than actually occurred or hears the negative part of a message while "not hearing" the positive part. For example, a wife may kiss her husband and ask to hold hands while they watch television together. In these nonverbal and verbal messages, the husband hears, "She wants to have sex. She doesn't care that I've had a bad day, I'm tired, and I need to sleep. She's going to get her feelings hurt or be mad if I say no. This is so unfair."

Communication problems can result from the absence of information from any of these dimensions. For example, when one spouse says "I love you" and the other says nothing, the first may perceive the absence of a response as rejection. Failing to reciprocate nonverbal messages (e.g., not returning a smile or not responding to another person's attempt to make eye contact) can also cause tension between people.

When the various dimensions of a message are inconsistent with one another, the receiver may become confused. He or she usually "believes" the component of the message that is the most powerful or that resonates best with his or her internal mood state. A parent who is upset with a teenager for staying out too late may yell angrily (nonverbal message), "Can't you see that we love you and don't want you to get hurt?" (verbal message). The teenager is likely to hear the non-verbal message of anger rather than the verbal message of love and concern. If a physician says to a patient in a compassionate tone, "Just call me if you have any problems" (verbal message) but delays returning the patient's call (nonverbal messages), the patient is likely to hear insincerity, lack of concern, or rejection.

Diagnosis of Communication Difficulties

Context

The first step in evaluating a patient's communication difficulties is to identify the context in which communication problems occur. With whom does the patient have difficulties communicating, under what circumstances, how often, how predictably, and to what degree does it upset the patient? Some individuals find it difficult to communicate effectively at home, at work, and on social occasions. It is not unusual, however, for a patient to be an eloquent or effective communicator with friends, coworkers, and strangers but to have considerable difficulty in talking to his or her spouse.

It is also common for people to be able to communicate well about some topics but not others. For example, a couple may have no difficulty in discussing the children, work, finances, or current events but may see their communication deteriorate or explode into an argument when the topic of love, affection, or sex is raised.

Skill Deficit vs. Performance Deficit

In diagnosing the communication difficulty of an individual or couple, it is important to determine whether the difficulty arises from a skill deficit or a performance deficit. A skill deficit implies a lack of the basic speaking, listening, and/or problem-solving skills necessary to communicate effectively. A person who has a skill deficit is likely to have trouble communicating with several individuals, especially in stressful situations, such as those involving problems in a relationship or at work. In this case, the intervention should include teaching the individual some basic communication skills.

Individuals who communicate effectively, at least under some circumstances and/or with some individuals, already possess basic communication skills. Environmental contingencies or stimuli prevent these individuals from making use of their existing communication skills—that is, they have a performance deficit. The most commonly observed example of such a performance deficit is an argument between two verbally skilled individuals, often a husband and wife, whose emotional state (often frustration or anger) causes them to "forget" to use their skill and leads them to resort to more primitive attack and defend behaviors, such as blaming, name calling, or sarcasm. It is not necessary to teach these individuals basic communication skills but, rather, to help them identify the factors that interfere with their ability to communicate effectively. In identifying these factors, it is helpful to ask the following questions:

- Are there predictable situations in which their communication is less effective?

- Is there something that one person says that predictably elicits a strong emotional reaction in the other?

- Are there certain topics of discussion that regress into arguments?

The goal is to develop new coping strategies for the situations identified as problematic in order to diminish or eliminate the obstacles to good communication.

Manifestations of Communication Problems

The most common manifestation of communication difficulties is conflict. It can range in intensity from disagreement, petty sarcasm, or "dirty looks" to serious verbal aggression. Occasionally, conflict escalates into character assassinations, humiliation of others, and threats of rejection or physical harm. At its extreme, conflict can include physical violence. The less severe forms of physical violence, such as throwing objects, breaking things, and pushing or shoving others, are common in family arguments. A less frequent but more serious problem is physical assault, such as slapping, hitting, biting, kicking, or using a weapon. The intervention for the management of verbally or physically aggressive conflict involves the diffusion of anger and training in problem-solving skills.

Conflict avoidance is also a manifestation of communication difficulty, in which individuals fail to communicate with each other about important and often problematic issues. These individuals are generally uncomfortable with confrontation or fearful of conflict. Teaching communication skills to conflict-avoidant individuals can be more difficult than working with those who have a more verbally aggressive style. The conflict-avoidant person must first be willing to initiate discussion and, therefore, risk conflict. The interventions for conflict avoidance are (1) to deal with the concerns that maintain the avoidance; (2) to teach assertiveness and communication skills so that patients know how to discuss problems and to cope with anger, both their own and that of others; and (3) to provide opportunities for repeated practice with these skills. Practice in discussing difficult topics can be framed as an experiment to test the patient's hypothesis that discussing problems can be hurtful.

Assessment of Communication Skill

A structured evaluation of the individual's or couple's communication problems before any attempt is made to address those problems serves two functions. First, it guides the therapist in the decision to include communication training in the treatment plan. Second, a baseline communication assessment provides an objective standard against which to compare post treatment change. Such a standard is useful for the clinician and the patient to monitor the progress of therapy and to determine if changes in the treatment plan are needed, as subtle changes in communication behavior over a long period of time may be difficult to detect.

The two most commonly used methods for evaluating communication problems are self-report measures and direct observation. The Marital Satisfaction Inventory (MSI; Snyder, 1979) is a 10-subscale self-report measure of satisfaction in various areas of marriage (e.g., recreation or sexual relations). Husbands and wives independently rate each of 280 statements as true or false for their relationship at present; then their scores are compared. Higher scores indicate greater dissatisfaction in this area of the marriage.

The MSI contains two communication satisfaction subscales. The Problem-Solving Communication (PSC) subscale measures the degree to which the respondents are satisfied with the way in which they solve problems through discussion. It includes statements such as "Minor disagreements with my spouse often end up in big arguments" and "My spouse seems committed to settling our differences." The Affective Communication (AFC) subscale measures the degree to which each individual is satisfied with his or her partner's expression of feelings, affection, and caring; empathy and understanding from the partner; and self-disclosure in the relationship. Some examples of items on this subscale are "There is a great deal of love and affection expressed in our marriage" and "Sometimes my spouse just can't understand the way I feel."

Evaluating communication problems from direct observation can be as simple as casually watching the way in which the parties interact in the therapist's office or as sophisticated as the microanalysis of verbal and nonverbal behaviors.

Many different observations can be made about the interactional style of patients, couples, or the clinician–patient dyad. The dimensions of communication discussed earlier in this chapter can be assessed by looking at the individual statements made by each person or by the overall flow of the discussion. Specifically, the nonverbal messages can provide a wealth of information about the speakers. For example, it is possible to make some judgment about the status of each person with respect to the other(s). To make this assessment the questions to consider include the following: Does one person appear to have more control over the interaction? Are the participants of equal status? Does one defer to the other?

The speakers' choices of words and nonverbal messages can also provide information about the emotional tone of the interaction. Simply, emotional tone can be categorized as positive, negative, or neutral, or it can be more qualitatively defined as angry, loving, collegial, tense, productive, conflictual, and so on. Verbal messages can provide some clues about the communication skill of the speakers. Do they express themselves well? Can they make themselves understood? Are their thoughts organized?

It is also possible to make observations about the degree to which there is consistency between the messages the speaker intended to send and the information the listener received. Inconsistencies would be evidenced in an escalation of anger, misinterpretations of messages, defensiveness by the sender, and confusion by either party.

These casual observations about the communication process can be made by observing others interacting, observing oneself in relation to others, listening to reports from the patient about interactional events, or assessing the participants' responses to a structured communication task. A variety of communication games or tasks can be assigned. The interaction can be observed by the clinician in the office, from another room through a two-way mirror or video monitor, or at a later date from a videotape of the interaction. If the clinician is observing the interaction of others, it is best that he or she be minimally involved in the interaction.

In research on interpersonal communication, semistructured games or tasks are occasionally used to acquire a sample of the interactional behavior of couples or families. These tasks provide enough structure for the interaction to make the situation comparable across many subjects. For individual patients, however, their responses to these standardized tasks may not provide an accurate representation of their day-to-day behavior.

A stimulus task for assessing everyday communication problems should approximate typical real-life scenarios. An interaction that takes place in the clinician's office is not likely to be as natural as those that take place at home. However, this assessment can provide some clues about what the patient is capable of under relatively neutral conditions (i.e., without interruptions, with constraints on use of inappropriate language or actions, and with focus on a specific topic). This type of assessment will help the clinician to determine whether the patient or the couple has a communication skill deficit or a performance deficit. If the patient or couple does well at this task but has difficulty at home, it is likely that they have a performance deficit. In this case, the clinician's job is to determine what factors interfere with their ability to communicate effectively.

If the patient or couple have difficulty with the communication task, appear disorganized, fail to state the problem clearly, or are unable to make progress toward resolution, it is likely that they have a skill deficit. In this case, the intervention required is training in basic communication and problem-solving skills.

While much can be learned from observing people interact, it is helpful to formalize or structure the evaluation of communication behavior. Many researchers have tried to quantify good and poor communication behaviors. The pioneers in this area (e.g., Gottman, 1979; Hops, Wills, Patterson, & Weiss, 1972) developed elaborate coding systems for categorizing each verbal statement and significant nonverbal behaviors made by couples, family members, or strangers participating in standardized communication tasks. Gottman's (1979) Couple Interaction Scoring System and Hops et al.'s (1972) Marital Interaction Coding System, two of the earliest coding schemes, continue to be used in interactional research today. The categories of behavior in these coding systems include positive statements such as praise or agreements, neutral statements such as definitions of the problems, and negative statements such as blame or insults. A tally of the total number of statements falling into each category and summed across groups of happy couples (presumably good communicators) and unhappy couples (presumably ineffective communicators) allows for the investigation of systematic differences between these groups. From this early research much has been learned about the behaviors that show effective communication skills. Communication training, a hallmark of the behavioral approach to marital and family therapy, stems in part from this early research.

Microanalytic coding schemes, while important in research, are not practical for the individual clinician, nor is a summary of a couple's individual behaviors easily interpretable. Several more portable assessment measures have been developed that can be used with individual couples. These include the Communication Skills Test (Floyd & Markman, 1984) and the Communication Rapid Assessment Scale (Joanning, Brewster, & Koval, 1984). These measures, while easier to use, also require special training in communication assessment. The Communication Style Q-set (Stephen & Harrison, 1986) is a card sorting task which assesses interactional "style."

The Clinician Rating of Adult Communication scale (CRAC; Basco, Birchler, Kalal, Talbott, & Slater, 1991) is a "user-friendly" clinician rating scale developed by clinicians for clinicians. This 20-item scale helps clinicians to structure their assessment of couples' interaction by focusing their attention on verbal and nonverbal behaviors important to good communication and problem solving. The original CRAC (Basco et al., 1991) includes six background information items for clinicians to document their clinical impressions of the couple. The abbreviated version of the CRAC presented in Figure 12.1 consists of only the 14 behavioral items that include involvement in the discussion, clarity of communication, listening skill, verbal aggression, problem solving, and attribution of blame. After watching a 10-minute sample of communication, clinicians rate couples' levels of skill in each of the 14 behaviors and sum the scores for each spouse (both spouses summed provide a total couple score). Each skill is rated as being better (1 point), similar to (2 points), or worse (3 points) than that of typical couples who present for treatment. The therapist can use this information to determine if communication training is necessary and, if so, what behaviors should be the focus of training. This structured assessment provides a standard against which posttreatment progress can be compared.

Errors in Communication

Communication Filters

Thoughts and feelings filter messages, influencing each of the five dimensions of communication and accounting for discrepancies between the message the sender intends and the message the listener actually receives. A communication filter can be a mood, a belief, an attitude, a physical state, or any other thing that influences the way a person speaks to others and interprets messages from others. When a person is angry, for example, the messages sent can sound harsh, sharp,

Couple _____ Rater _____ Date _____

From a standardized sample of marital communication (with therapist absent), rate husband and wife separately on each of the following dimensions. In rating these items, consider the average couple presenting for treatment. Rate the present couple as they might compare to that population.

For the purpose of this communication sample the topic of discussion is _____

---

1. Degree of Participation in the Discussion

   Husband Wife
   - ( ) ( ) contributed/participated more in the discussion than the average distressed spouse
   - ( ) ( ) contributed/participated as much in the discussion as the average distressed spouse
   - ( ) ( ) contributed/participated less in the discussion than the average distressed spouse

2. Communication Defensiveness: Overtly defending self against real or imagined attack as in making excuses, denying wrongdoing, or rationalizing

   Husband Wife
   - ( ) ( ) less defensive than the average distressed spouse
   - ( ) ( ) as defensive as the average distressed spouse
   - ( ) ( ) more defensive than the average distressed spouse

3. Communication Clarity: Rater is able to clearly comprehend content level of spouses' messages

   Husband Wife
   - ( ) ( ) conveyed message more directly and clearly than the average distressed spouse
   - ( ) ( ) conveyed message as directly and clearly as the average distressed spouse
   - ( ) ( ) conveyed message less directly and clearly than the average distressed spouse

4. Listening/Attending Skills: Maintained eye contact, acknowledged messages, demonstrated interest

   Husband Wife
   - ( ) ( ) listened/attended better than average distressed spouse
   - ( ) ( ) listened/attended as well as the average distressed spouse
   - ( ) ( ) listened/attended less than the average distressed spouse

cont.

---

*Top item = 1 point, middle item = 2 points, bottom item = 3 points. **Agreement on who is responsible = 1 point (each says that responsibility is shared or both agree that one spouse is to blame), total disagreement = 3 points (e.g., each blames the other), partial agreement = 2 points (e.g., husband says responsibility is shared, wife says it is her fault).

FIGURE 12.1. Clinician Rating of Adult Communication (CRAC).

5. Communicated Understanding: Demonstrated appreciation of and/or empathy for spouse's thoughts/feelings

Husband Wife
( )   ( )   communicated understanding better than the average distressed couple
( )   ( )   communicated understanding as well as the average distressed couple
( )   ( )   communicated understanding less than the average distressed couple

6. Quality of Nonverbal Behaviors*
Husband Wife
( )   ( )   generally positive (e.g., eye contact, smile, touch, positive voice)
( )   ( )   generally neutral (e.g., neither overtly positive nor negative)
( )   ( )   generally negative (e.g., harsh voice tone, arms crossed, little eye contact)

7. Display of Verbal Aggression: Blaming, sarcasm, name-calling, criticism, shouting

Husband Wife
( )   ( )   less verbal aggression than the average distressed spouse
( )   ( )   as much verbal aggression as the average distressed spouse
( )   ( )   more verbal aggression than the average distressed spouse

Does the couple report history of physical violence when arguing?
                  Yes ( )   No ( )

8. Overall Emotional Tone of Discussion*
( ) generally positive
( ) generally neutral
( ) generally negative

9. Amount of Agreement between Spouses
Husband Wife
( )   ( )   agreed with partner more than the average distressed spouse
( )   ( )   levels of agreement and disagreement similar to the average distressed spouse
( )   ( )   disagreed with partner more than the average distressed spouse
( )   ( )   lack of data

10. Effectiveness of Observed Level of Participation in Facilitating Problem Solving
Husband Wife
( )   ( )   more effective than most distressed spouses in facilitating problem solving
( )   ( )   as effective as most distressed spouses in facilitating problem solving
( )   ( )   less effective than the average distressed spouse in facilitating problem solving

FIGURE 12.1. cont.

11. Ability to Stay on Original Topic as Specified by the Task*
    ( )   generally stayed with topic throughout the discussion
    ( )   significant digression by one or both spouses, but eventual return to
          original topic
    ( )   failed to focus on original topic or multiple topic changes

12. Closure*
    ( )   reasonable solution(s) verbalized and agreed upon
    ( )   solution(s) verbalized with no specific agreement or plan of action
    ( )   no solutions verbalized

13. If Solutions Generated, Should Husband or Wife Change?**

    Husband Wife
     ( )   ( )   self
     ( )   ( )   both spouses are responsible for change
     ( )   ( )   spouse
     ( )   ( )   no data

14. Attribution of Blame**

    Husband Wife
     ( )   ( )   this spouse accepted primary responsibility for the problem
     ( )   ( )   responsibility was shared
     ( )   ( )   blame attributed primarily to spouse
     ( )   ( )   blame attributed to outside circumstances or individuals outside
                    of the dyad
     ( )   ( )   attribution of blame not established

FIGURE 12.1. *cont.*

negative, or sarcastic; anger becomes the filter through which that person sends messages. Similarly, oversensitivity to criticism or rejection can be a filter that distorts messages as the listener receives them; in this case, the sensitive person's filter can magnify a minor negative comment.

Communication filters can be transient, such as a "bad" mood or fatigue, and only temporarily alter communication. They can also be more permanent, such as a belief or an attitude (e.g., "People will take advantage of you if they can" or "Men are superior to women"). Filters can also be specific to communication with particular individuals. For example, a husband and wife who often argue may be on the defensive when speaking to one another. As a result, they can become hypersensitive to perceived attacks, fail to listen to one another, and initiate counterattacks. No one else may feel that these two individuals are defensive or argumentative, because the filters that are influencing their interaction with each other are not present with others outside the home. The intervention for reducing communication filters is to identify their existence and then to factor them in when communicating with others. Practically, this means that when people are "feeling bad" they compensate for it by monitoring their words and nonverbal behaviors when speaking to others. This can mean controlling an angry tone of voice or sarcasm. When listening to others, the "feeling bad" filter can affect how messages are interpreted or received. The listener has to tell him- or herself, "When I'm feeling bad, I'm a lot more sensitive. I get my feelings hurt more easily. Maybe I am reading more into what others are saying because I'm feeling bad."

This process takes time, effort, and the coaching of a therapist. Usually, people are unaware of their communication filters and need others to help them identify and label them correctly.

Incorrect Assumptions

Mrs. Clark complained that her husband was angry with her because she had worked late two nights ago. "It's just not fair. He expects me to work hard all day and still be there to cater to his every need. He has no right to be angry. After all, my earnings helped to buy his new golf clubs. Oh, he claims he's not angry, but I know that look. He's just saving it up to let me have it later. We argued about it all night." The therapist, being uncertain about the reason that Mr. Clark would be so angry, inquired about the interaction. "What did your husband say to you that indicated he was angry at you for working late?" "He didn't have to say a word," she replied. "I could just tell. And besides, he didn't even bother to kiss me when I came in from work." In fact, Mr. Clark had been talking on the telephone with a coworker about a problem on the job just before Mrs. Clark came home. Because he was upset about work, he was frowning and was not very interested in talking when Mrs. Clark came home. Mrs. Clark personalized his nonverbal behavior and assumed that he was angry with her.

Mind reading, a common communication error, stems from the incorrect assumption that, after knowing another person for some time, it is possible to know what that person thinks and how he or she feels—sometimes even before that person knows. If another person responds to situations in a consistent fashion, it may be possible to make good guesses about that person's thoughts and feelings, but there is always room for error in guessing. It is true, for example, that Mr. Clark has been angry with his wife in the past when she worked late, but he was not angry with her at all this time. Her anticipation of his anger prepared her to behave defensively when she returned home. This set the stage for the argument that followed. Clearly, mind reading or making assumptions can produce conflict.

Teaching people to ask questions instead of making assumptions is the key to reducing mind reading. In this example, Mrs. Clark needed to ask her husband, "Are you angry at me?" It is difficult to get people to ask questions. Their assumptions will be correct some of the time. This reinforces the notion that they know others well enough to not have to ask questions. Patients must be convinced that mind reading can create trouble. Practice in asking questions to evaluate the validity of their assumptions can begin the therapy.

Misattributions

Attributions are guesses or explanations about people and situations that help an individual to understand the cause of a given event. Misattributions are erroneous or inaccurate attributions (e.g., "You slammed the door just to irritate me"). A misattribution may not be verbalized, however, so there is no means of evaluating its validity. It feels right to the person holding the attribution and, therefore, in the mind of that person, it is right. As with mind reading, reacting as if the misattribution is correct can lead to misunderstandings, tension, and even arguments.

Some common types of misattributions are certain to cause bad feelings or conflict with others. Most commonly, misattribution of the negative or malicious intentions of others may occur when a person feels that others caused a troublesome situation. Some examples of misattributing intentions are "she wanted to make me late for my appointment" or "he did that just to be spiteful." The person who makes this type of assumption often does not discuss it openly with the source but, instead, may share these thoughts with others, keep them to him- or herself while silently fuming, or act them out in an angry countermove.

The source of the problem can also be misattributed. Blaming others for things they may not have done generally precipitates an attack-and-defend interaction that resembles a tennis match, where each person sends blame across the net and the receiver defends against it. The defense can take the form of a rational explanation or justification of a particular position, or it can take the form of a counterattack. For example, "You made me late for my appointment, and I looked like an idiot walking in after the meeting started" (blame). "I did not make you late; you were the one who couldn't find your keys" (explanation). "That's because you moved them" (blame). "I had to move them; they were in the middle of the dinner table" (justification). "Well, if you were a better housekeeper, there would be a clear space on the counter near the door where I could put my keys" (counterattack). "Well, if you weren't so cheap, we could hire a housekeeper . . ., etc." (counterattack).

The presumption of the deliberateness or purposefulness of the actions of others is another misattribution that can lead to conflict. An extreme example is paranoia. Patients with paranoia assume that others have malicious intentions to be hurtful. In everyday interaction, it is not unusual for these patients to assume that others purposefully acted to produce a negative outcome when, in fact, there may be no evidence to support this assumption. "You did that on purpose." "No, I didn't. It was an accident." "I don't believe you."

The intervention for correcting misattributions is the same as that for correcting negative automatic thoughts (see Chapter 9). First, misattributions are identified. Second, their validity is evaluated by gathering evidence for and against the attribution. An alternative approach is to generate other explanations for the event for which there may be some evidence. If the therapist is working with a couple for whom misattribution is a common communication problem, the misattribution can be discussed in a way that allows the accused person to explain his or her position without counterattacking the partner.

Failure to See the Reciprocity of Behavior

When examining how a problem has evolved, how an argument started, or why a problem continues despite attempts at discussion and resolution, it is easy to see how *others* are responsible. Most interpersonal problems, however, result from the actions of two or more individuals. This is especially true for communication problems. Each statement made by an individual is both a response and a stimulus for the next response, which, in turn, is a stimulus for the next response, and so on. This is called reciprocity.

Although most people would agree with the basic concept of reciprocity if it were brought to their attention, few people, even very skilled people, are aware of it when they are in the middle of an interaction that is going badly. If individuals could recognize their own contribution to poor communication, they could alter their responses so as to change the course of the interaction. For example, if the husband and wife described earlier knew that each defensive counterattack was escalating their anger and frustration, one or both could take another direction that might lead to a resolution of the conflict.

Helping Patients
to Improve Their Communication

Communication problems occur between at least two individuals, and it is easier for a therapist to help resolve such problems if both parties are present. This is not always possible or appropriate, however. In some cases, the second party is a boss, someone who lives a great distance away, or someone the patient is not likely to see again.

When it is possible and appropriate for a therapist to work with both parties in helping to resolve communication problems, the role of the therapist is similar to that of a referee. (It may be useful to come to the session equipped with a whistle and a striped shirt.) The therapist's job is to help the two participants follow the rules of the communication game and play fairly. If things get out of hand, the therapist blows the whistle, calls a time-out, and redirects the interaction by informing each player of the type of foul that he or she committed and the way to proceed differently.

Playing the Communication Game

Before the communication game starts, the therapist may find it helpful to assume the role of coach. The therapist teaches the players the basic rules, demonstrates each behavior, has them practice in and between sessions, watches them play, and provides feedback on ways that they can improve their skills.

Rules of the Communication Game

In normal daily interaction, it is not usually necessary to impose any structure on communication. Structure is useful when communication is ineffective or exacerbates relationship difficulties, however. When preparing to discuss potentially conflictual issues, it is useful to review the basic rules of the communication game as listed in the following:

• *Be calm.* It is counterproductive to attempt to discuss difficult issues when angry or stressed in any way. An angry person may let emotions dictate the choice of words and the solutions offered. Solutions that seem reasonable in the heat of anger may prove inappropriate when examined later. It is better to wait until the emotion subsides than to risk making bad decisions.

• *Be organized.* It is best to approach the discussion of troublesome issues after having taken the time to think through what the problem is and what must happen in order to resolve it. Furthermore, it is useful to have a plan for discussing the issue.

• *Be specific.* Global complaints (e.g., "I'm not happy," "You're irresponsible," and "I just can't take this anymore") cannot be easily resolved. It is necessary to specify the action, event, or process that is problematic: What does it look like? How would I know it was happening if I were watching you? What causes the discomfort?

• *Be clear.* Beating around the bush or speaking in vague terms leaves much room for misinterpretation of the message. It may appear that the intended message was received, but the message may not have been received accurately.

• *Be a good listener.* The best way to be heard is to be a respectful listener. Attentive listening without interrupting is important. The listener should not merely use the other person's talking time as an opportunity to prepare a response (or defense).

• *Be flexible.* The resolution of problems between individuals requires give and take. Although a plan to resolve the problems may have been developed before the actual discussion began, it is important to consider others' ideas before selecting a solution. Moreover, others are likely to have a different view of the problem, and all participants should approach the discussion as if the others' perspective is as valid as their own.

• *Be creative.* In generating a solution to a specific problem, it is useful to look beyond strategies used in the past, to be imaginative, and to try out new plans. If they do not work, another method can be used.

• *Keep it simple.* Those with communication difficulties should solve one problem at a time. When discussing a problem, they should describe it as simply as possible. If the conversation begins to digress into other areas, stop and redirect the conversation back to the original topic.

Communication Game Strategy

The first step in the communication game is to prepare for the discussion. Each person should prepare a clear definition of the problem and a list of who is affected by it and in what way each person is affected. Statements of the problem that do not criticize or blame others are most constructive. For example, an objective statement such as "The problem is that our bills aren't getting paid on time, and I'm worried that our utilities may be turned off" is more effective than a blaming statement such as "You are being totally irresponsible. Don't you care about anything but yourself? You said you'd pay the bills, and you haven't even bothered to touch them. You won't be happy until the electric company turns off our electricity."

As part of the preparation for discussion, it is also useful for each party to consider what actions may be necessary to solve the problem and to generate a list of potential solutions. Timing is important in successful communication, and the discussion should be scheduled at a time that is convenient for all parties. As a final preparatory step, each party should take time to be in a calm emotional state before beginning the discussion of troublesome issues.

The first goal in the problem-solving discussion is to define the problem. Each party may have a different definition of the problem and should have an opportunity to give his or her perspective. The clinician can help the participants to generate a mutually agreeable definition of the nature of the problem. It is essential that there be agreement on the definition of the problem before resolution is attempted.

The second goal of the discussion is to select a solution to the problem. The participants may begin this process by simply listing all possible solutions to the problem without stopping to evaluate the feasibility of each. After eliminating from the list those solutions that are unlikely to resolve the problem, the parties should evaluate the probability of success, the practicality, and the acceptability of the remaining suggestions. The best solutions are those that require action from all parties involved. For example, "I'll pay the bills on time, if you will remind me when it is time to pay them." The solution chosen must specify (1) who will take action, (2) what that action will be, and (3) when the action is to be accomplished.

It is helpful to specify a means for evaluating the success of the intervention. That is, how will the parties know if the solution was effective? It is also helpful to set a time to evaluate the success of the intervention. For example, "Let's try this out for the next 2 months to see if it works."

Overcoming Communication Failure

The most common source of disruption in communication is emotion. As discussed earlier, intense emotion such as sadness, frustration, or anger can influence the way in which information is conveyed and received. If any person's emotional level becomes uncomfortable or appears to interfere with the interaction, the discussion should stop until the intensity of the emotion has substantially decreased. It is essential that a plan be made to resume the discussion at a specified time. To stop the interaction, the individual can say, "I'm getting too upset to talk about this. Let's stop and talk about it again after dinner." Another way to stop the interaction is to talk about the communica-tion process itself. "This isn't going the way I hoped it would. We're getting angrier instead of working out the problem. Let's stop for now and try it again later."

It may be possible to save the discussion by following the commu-nication rules in a structured way. A "cheat sheet" or list of problem-solving steps can provide this kind of structure. If the discussion con-tinues to flounder, it may be helpful for the parties to write down the information that they want to communicate to each other. For exam-ple, it may be helpful for each to write down a definition of the prob-lem, as well as a list of potential solutions.

If it becomes clear that the parties cannot resolve an issue through discussion, it may be necessary to bring in a third party, such as the therapist. The mediator should not be someone who is deeply involved in the problem, a family member who is likely to "take sides" (e.g., the mother-in-law), or someone who may be negatively affected by the process of discussion (e.g., a child). It may be helpful if each party talked individually with the therapist to gain assistance in defin-ing the problem or in generating solutions.

Other Common Relationship Problems of Patients with Bipolar Disorder

In addition to communication problems, there are several symptoms of depression and mania that can interfere with their relationships with others. These include cognitive distortions such as tunnel vision or selectively monitoring negative events while ignoring positive and neu-tral events in relationships as well as having unrealistic expectations for the relationship. Decreased sex drive can limit intimacy and reduce pos-itive interactions that can offset the stress from negative events. In the sections that follow, these symptoms are discussed with some suggestions for addressing them with patients and their significant others.

Selective Monitoring of Negative Events

It is not unusual for people in unhappy relationships to be acutely aware of every error committed by their partner. Similarly, depressed persons seem to attend to negative events selectively, "missing" more positive events. Depressed individuals in troubled relationships may report with absolute certainty that "nothing good" has happened in their relationships lately. To determine if this is true, the clinician may instruct the couple to keep a log of every positive thing each partner does. This exercise broadens the negative focus of both partners to include the tracking of positive interactions. A more balanced report on events allows the clinician to determine whether there is a perceptual inaccuracy or an actual imbalance in the number of positive and negative events in the marriage that needs attention.

Decreased or Increased Sex Drive

Depending on the intensity of the change in the sexual interest of the patient and the interest and drive of the partner, fluctuations in libido can place stress on relationships. The stress caused by decreased interest, which is more common in depression, differs from that caused by increased interest, which is more common in mania. Decreased sexual interest is generally accompanied by a reduced energy level, a lack of motivation, and a blunted ability to enjoy activities in general. For the partner, the patient's decreased libido can take on other meanings abut the relationship, for example, that the patient no longer finds the partner attractive, is no longer in love with the partner, or must be having an affair with someone else.

In counseling couples whose sexual drive has diminished, it is useful to ask each partner what he or she believes this shift in interest means. Often, the intervention most helpful to the couple is to provide them with an alternative and less damning reason for the diminished sexual interest. This can be accomplished by educating both partners about the common symptoms of depression and the way in which these symptoms interfere with sexual intimacy.

Increased sexual drive is particularly problematic if the patient is in a monogamous relationship but impulsively becomes sexually involved with others. The patient may never disclose his or her sexual promiscuity to the partner. If the partner finds out, however, it is often very difficult for him or her to accept and forgive such behavior as merely a symptom of the illness. In these cases, the couple may require counseling to resolve this issue and develop a plan for preventing its future occurrence.

Unrealistic Expectations for the Relationship

When two people enter a relationship, they generally have specific expectations for each other and for the relationship. Most expectations are unspoken and may even be outside the individuals' conscious awareness. They originate in what the individuals observed, learned, and imagined as they became adults. Some people expect to duplicate what they observed at home; others expect to do just the opposite in an attempt to have a lifestyle different from the one that they experienced as children.

If two people marry before the onset of the first episode of depression or mania, they have no way of knowing how the disorder will affect their lives. Old expectations may no longer be achievable. The spouses of patients describe feeling compassionate and concerned for their partner, while simultaneously feeling angry and "tricked" because the marriage they now have is not the one that they anticipated in the beginning. Spouses of patients with bipolar disorder understand that their mates are ill and feel obligated to stand by them despite the hardships. Some never know that their spouses have an illness, however, because the problems were so great that the marriage ended before a diagnosis was made.

Denial of the severity or recurrent nature of the illness by the patient and the spouse may prevent them from adjusting their expectations for the behavior of the spouse and for the stability of the marriage.

> Mrs. Okuma thought that she could manage the children, her job, and her many other civic and family responsibilities despite recurrent depressions. She assumed responsibilities with the same vigor that she had shown before the onset of the disorder. She took on more than she could handle, felt guilty and angry with herself for not being able to complete all tasks to perfection, and became immobilized.
>
> In contrast, Mrs. Iinuma set limits on the amount of work that she accepted, making adjustments to fit her energy, interest, and concentration levels. Her husband, however, had not adjusted his expectations of her and communicated with negative nonverbal behavior that he was disappointed when she failed to complete household tasks, prepare meals, or put in a sufficient number of hours on the job. She felt torn between trying to please him and trying to take care of herself.

In either scenario, it may be useful for the clinician to meet with both partners to renegotiate a relationship contract in which each person spells out what he or she expects from the other and is willing to do to make the marriage work. As with any contract, it is important to define the terms clearly so that both partners know what is expected of them and what they can expect of their partner.

Key Points for the Therapist to Remember

♦ It is difficult for people with mood disorders to distinguish between real rejection or criticism and their own cognitive distortions. Sometimes, patients are able to recognize intellectually that others' behavior was not intended to be rejecting or critical, but they are unable to inhibit or reduce their strong emotional reaction to it.

♦ Communication filters can include bad moods such as anger, negative attitude such as pessimism, a physical state such as fatigue, or any other thing that influences the way that a person speaks to others and interprets messages from others. Filters account for discrepancies between the message that the sender intends and the message that the listener actually receives.

♦ If the patient or couple have difficulty with communication exercises, appear disorganized, fail to state the problem clearly, or are unable to make progress toward resolution, it is likely that they have a skill deficit.

♦ If individuals could recognize their own contribution to poor communication, they could alter their responses so as to change the course of the interaction.

Points to Discuss with Patients

♦ It can be very frustrating for the spouses of depressed patients to cope with their seemingly illogically negative outlook. Attempts at "talking them out of" their negativity generally fail and may even worsen the conflict. The pessimistic spouse accuses the optimistic spouse of overlooking problems, while the optimistic spouse accuses the pessimistic spouse of finding problems where none exist.

♦ Not only can a sender convey much more than just words, but also the receiver can alter messages by "reading in" more than the sender is conveying. Sometimes a listener hears a different nonverbal tone or relationship message in a speaker's voice than actually occurred or hears the negative part of a message while "not hearing" the positive part.

♦ Mind reading, a common communication error, stems from the incorrect assumption that, after knowing another person for some time, it is possible to know how that person thinks and feels. Teaching people to ask questions instead of making assumptions is the key to reducing mind reading.

♦ When examining how a problem has evolved, how an argument started, or why a problem continues despite attempts at discussion and resolution, it is easy to see how *others* are responsible. Most interpersonal problems, however, result from the actions of two or more individuals.

♦ It is not unusual for people in unhappy relationships to be acutely aware of every error committed by their partner and report with absolute certainty that "nothing good" has happened in their relationships lately. This may be an example of tunnel vision.

♦ In counseling couples whose sexual drive has diminished, it is useful to ask each partner what he or she believes this shift in interest means. Educating both partners about the common symptoms of depression and the way in which these symptoms interfere with sexual intimacy provides couples with an alternative and less damning reason for the diminished sexual interest.

CHAPTER 13

Putting Together
a Treatment Program

In Chapter 1 we divided patients with bipolar disorder into three groups: those newly diagnosed, those who have had quite a bit of experience with the illness but have not yet reached symptom remission, and those patients who are for the most part symptomatically stable. Table 1.1 summarized the interventions suggested for each of these groups, but we repeat that table here as Table 13.1, for clarity.

Sequencing the Intervention

With patients who have never had exposure to cognitive-behavioral treatments it is reasonable to systematically progress through each set of interventions beginning with those suggested for the newly diagnosed, moving on to interventions for those who are symptomatic, followed by maintenance interventions suitable for patients who have achieved remission.

A second strategy is to select interventions that match the specific presenting problems of a given patient. If time is limited, clinicians can select those interventions they have time to complete and defer the others to another visit or to a therapist that has more time to work with the patient.

A third possibility is to use the session-by-session guide from the first edition of this book (Basco & Rush, 1996), which is presented in the Appendix A. The original CBT for bipolar disorder treatment protocol was based on the assumption that the intervention would be

TABLE 13.1. Suggested Interventions by Patient Group

Newly diagnosed

   Education

   Instructions on lifestyle management

   Symptom Summary Worksheet

Experienced, but not yet stable

   Mood Graphs

   Symptom Summary Worksheet

   Controlling triggers

   Management of cognitive symptoms

   Management of behavioral symptoms

   Compliance training

Symptomatically stable

   Relapse prevention

   Maintenance of adherence

   Achievement of life goals

delivered in 20 sessions each lasting a full 50-minute hour. What became apparent after training many people to do the original intervention is that most clinicians who treat people for bipolar disorder do not have the luxury of time to do 20 therapy sessions either because insurance companies will not pay for 20 sessions of psychotherapy or because the clinician is a psychiatrist with a heavy caseload and only has time to conduct 20-minute medication visits.

Learning from Experience

Remember that the strength of CBT is in altering the course of bipolar disorder over time. That is, with earlier and more aggressive intervention, times of illness should be shorter and times of wellness longer. Subsyndromal depressive symptoms that that often continue between episodes can be minimized and, therefore, satisfaction with life improved. Each time a relapse of depression, mania, or mixed states occurs it is an opportunity to learn more about the factors that precipitate recurrences for a given patient. With that information, both the patient and clinician can be better prepared in their efforts to thwart the next potential relapse. For example, if a manic relapse occurs following an increase in anxiety level over several weeks, the patient and therapist can note this so that the next time anxiety reemerges it can be watched more carefully as a potential sign of relapse and precautionary measures can be taken to keep medication adherence in check, regulate sleep, and reduce stimulation. If an escalation continues despite these efforts, an alteration in medication regimen may be needed to help contain symptoms.

Sometimes the patient knows the signs of relapse, is aware of the precautions that need to be made, and chooses not to make them. Because the risk of recurrence is not always 100%, people bet that they can beat the odds by pushing the limits, not taking care of themselves, or defying their doctor or parents or therapist. This is particularly true for teenagers and young adults who have not had a lot of experience with the consequences of letting mania or depression fully evolve. These people may have to go through several episodes before they are willing to accept the fact that the illness is recurrent and that they must take control over it rather than letting the illness control them. Jamie is a good example.

Jamie is a 23-year-old recent college graduate who has had bipolar disorder for 5 years. He had two major depressive episodes that interfered with his ability to function at school and required him to take two semester-long leaves of absence. He managed to graduate with his bachelor's degree and was accepted to business school for the following fall semester, but before he could start grad school he had his first severe manic episode. His previous episode of mania had been fairly easy to contain and was short-lived. The recent episode landed him in an inpatient facility for a week.

When Jamie was discharged he immediately began CBT as part of his follow-up care. At his first session it was obvious that Jamie was not quite ready to accept the diagnosis of bipolar disorder or the limitations on his social life that were suggested by his psychiatrist. He downplayed its severity and claimed not to recall his behavior during mania. Jamie was young and full of life and he and his friends loved to party several times each week. They all enjoyed smoking marijuana and drinking. After discharge Jamie started going out with his friends against his parents' and his doctor's advice and within 2 weeks, he stopped taking his medication and had a relapse of mania. He was found wandering around a shopping mall after hours by security who called the police claiming that Jamie was drunk. This was at first perplexing to Jamie, his parents, and his psychiatrist. He had seemed to be doing better, although he had lied to everyone about his substance abuse. Jamie was rehospitalized to "adjust his medication" and released again a few days later. For the first few weeks after this second hospitalization Jamie tried to be more consistent with his medication and even avoided alcohol. He told his friends that he was taking antibiotics for an infection and would have to stay away from alcohol for a while. His friends were fine with this idea. However, Jamie kept alcohol in his apartment for his friends so as not to give the impression that he could no longer drink. It did not take long for Jamie to succumb to the temptation of drinking and smoking again and before too long he had another relapse and was hospitalized. This time he had run into a light pole on a street corner and was arrested by police for drunk driving. After a night in jail he was transferred to a local psychiatric unit. By that time, Jamie's parents had been in his apartment and had figured out his partying habits and their contribution to his illness. They were angry with Jamie, frustrated with his doctor for not controlling the illness, and ready to give up on the therapist who had not been able to make Jamie change his behavior.

Jamie knew what he needed to do to stay well, but he was not ready to do it. His desire to be normal included being able to drink when he wanted to and to not have to rely on medications to control his mood. It took 9 months of mania, rehospitalizations, missing his admission to graduate school, and several encounters with the law before he was ready to accept the fact that he had a problem and he controlled his own fate.

The moral of Jamie's story is that if the patient is not ready to accept the illness, the treatment, and the lifestyle restrictions, CBT will not help.

Selecting Interventions

Table 1.2 in Chapter 1 (pp. 13–14) summarized patients' problems, suggested interventions, and the location of relevant instructions in this book. If a given patient has several of these problems, teach the interventions for newly diagnosed patients first before teaching the ones for experienced patients. It is acceptable to teach the interventions out of the sequence presented in this book if it better meets the needs of a patient. The guiding principle in selecting and sequencing interventions is to do what is in the best interest of the patient, addressing more pressing needs first.

Therapeutic Challenges

We provide a few examples of how we have coped with some common therapeutic obstacles or complexities within the constraints of this manual. We cannot hope to provide answers to all the questions therapists would pose. We can, however, provide a model for overcoming problems that stays within the framework of the manual. We end this chapter and the book with a number of false assumptions or beliefs that therapists might have about using this manual. Our rational responses to each of these dysfunctional beliefs are also provided.

Managing Comorbidities

Approximately 60% of people diagnosed with bipolar disorder suffer from one or more comorbid psychiatric disorders (McElroy et al., 2001). The most common secondary psychiatric diagnoses are alcohol and substance abuse (Weissman & Johnson, 1991) with estimates from 17–64% of patients with bipolar I disorder (Brady, Casto, Lydiard, Malcolm, & Arana, 1991; Strakowski, Tohen, Stoll, Faedda, & Goodwin, 1992). Up to 42% have a comorbid anxiety disorder with panic disorder being the most prevalent (McElroy et al., 2001) and many meet criteria for posttraumatic stress disorder (Strakowski et al., 1992). The treatment of comorbidities is beyond the scope of this book; however, there are many excellent books available that describe cognitive-behavioral treatment approaches to substance abuse (e.g., Beck, Wright, Newman, & Liese, 1993), social phobia, (e.g., Heimberg & Becker, 2002), obsessive compulsive disorder (e.g., Clark, 2004), panic disorder and generalized anxiety disorder (e.g., Barlow, 2001), and posttraumatic stress disorder, (e.g., Follette, Ruzek, & Abueg, 1998).

As in the example of Jamie described previously, substance abuse can greatly interfere with the treatment of bipolar disorder. However, it is equally valid to say that the incomplete treatment of the mood disorder is what makes substance abuse a bigger problem. Clinicians must use their best judgment to decide how to proceed with treatment. Conventional wisdom is that a comprehensive approach may be best if it allows for the management of both primary and comorbid disorders.

Alcoholics Anonymous (AA) and Narcotics Anonymous (NA) philosophies and methods work well in conjunction with CBT and are often recommended for people who have substance abuse problems. CBT methods can reinforce the changes in attitude required by AA and NA and the support provided by group members can greatly enhance the effect of CBT when loneliness or social isolation is worsening symptoms of depression. For those who have social phobia, group experiences provide a laboratory for testing out new skills for being with people.

The skills for identifying and controlling triggers to relapse described in Chapter 7 can be applied to substance abuse. The methods for catching, controlling, and correcting distorted cognitions covered in Chapter 9 can easily be applied to several comorbid problems including anxiety, eating disorders, and posttraumatic stress disorder. The stress management skills advocated in Chapter 11 are applicable to most psychological and psychiatric problems because elevations in stress generally make people more anxious, lead them to want to use substances of abuse to escape the discomfort, stimulate overeating in bulimia, and can trigger a return of symptoms of posttraumatic stress disorder.

Another skill that cuts across disorders is the involvement of family members or increases in other sources of social support when family is unavailable or unwilling to participate in treatment. Social isolation only feeds distress. Therefore, the interpersonal skills covered in Chapter 12 can help to improve patients' relationships. When possible, involvement of significant others in the therapy process can be very useful. It provides family members with an opportunity to meet the therapist and to be informed about what happens during therapy sessions. This demystifies the process of treatment and encourages supportive others to be facilitators of care rather than oppose it.

Sometimes additional family therapy is required when the illness has led to the development of psychosocial problems or when there are communication difficulties or other relationship issues not related to the illness. Because the family can be an important source of support to the patient undergoing treatment for bipolar disorder, any breaches in those relationships should be mended. If not, the family becomes just another source of stress that places the patient at risk for relapse.

Crisis Intervention

In the course of therapy, it is not unusual to be sidetracked by a major crisis in a patient's life, such as an unwanted pregnancy, a lawsuit, threatened divorce, a car accident, or behavior problem of the patient's child. The therapist has to decide when and how to deviate from the treatment package and then how to return to the planned agenda. Some patients always seem to be experiencing crises, both minor and major. Can protocols be followed in these cases?

Crises cannot be ignored or disregarded. They must be discussed to some extent during the session. To fail to acknowledge their importance is to risk damaging the therapeutic alliance with the patient. Sometimes the patient needs assistance in resolving the crisis. Sometimes he or she has already developed a plan or has taken action toward resolving the crisis and merely wishes to report to the therapist what has transpired. Telling the story, however, can fill an entire session. The therapist should quickly assess whether or not the crisis has been resolved and how much time will be needed for further discussion. This can be accomplished at the beginning of the session when the agenda is being set. Sometimes patients will begin telling their story as soon as the door closes and the session begins.

Sometimes the crisis can be the content around which a CBT intervention is taught. For example, a patient might present with a problem having to do with getting his or her income tax forms completed on time. Goal setting, graded task assignment, or problem-solving interventions can be taught using taxes as the example. If the therapist is lucky, a problem presented by the patient will match the planned agenda for the session.

Patients as Passive Recipients of Care

Unfortunately, many institutional settings inadvertently socialize people with bipolar disorder to be passive recipients of care rather than active consumers of or participants in their care. When severely ill, people with bipolar disorder are sometimes unable to care for themselves. These are times when hospitalization is often needed. While many institutions are working toward changing these environments so as to foster passivity less and advocate for active patient participation in care, those adults currently in treatment for bipolar disorder may have already "learned" to behave passively in their treatment.

A passive view of the patient's role in treatment is in opposition to the collaborative view espoused by this treatment manual. Therefore, in many cases, the therapist will have to take time to socialize patients to this new collaborative role early in the course of treatment. Countering the institutional belief of patients as passive recipients of care can be accomplished by eliciting active participation in the patient. This means encouraging them to ask questions, asking their opinion, and providing ample opportunities for them to tell their personal stories.

Patients who are accustomed to a passive role will sometimes ask the therapist for advice or guidance. The helpful therapist will feel inclined to provide such guidance. A strategy that is helpful and that encourages patients to be active problem-solvers is to ask them how they have coped with similar problems in the past.

Developmental Delays Due to the Illness and Their Impact on Therapy

For many people with bipolar disorder, symptoms of the illness began in young adulthood or adolescence. During these years, people also learn to relate to others in an adult manner, and begin to develop their own ideas about who they are and what they believe. They begin to examine and challenge the beliefs of their parents, forming instead, their own views of the world.

This growth process can be interrupted by depression or mania in people with bipolar disorder. The impact this has on the individual is delayed or retarded social, psychological, and emotional growth. What therapists often see in these patients are poor interpersonal skills, limited coping skills, immature views of relationships, a failure to separate sufficiently from parents, or poor problem-solving skills.

The relevance of these developmental delays to the therapeutic process is in the choice of interventions. As therapists, we often assume that our patients have basic social skills such as how to get information, how to cope with stress, how to interact with others in various social situations, or how to make decisions about activities of daily living. With some patients who may have had bipolar disorder prior to adulthood, it may very well be necessary to help them to develop these basic skills. This can take extra time in therapy. Patients may not know that they are lacking in basic life skills until they attempt new tasks or engage in unfamiliar social activities.

To accomplish the goals of this treatment manual, therapists must assess and teach patients skills necessary to carry out each intervention. When basic skills training is needed to best execute an intervention, take time to teach. It will be time well spent and provide patients with basic skills they may be able to apply to several aspects of their lives.

"I Can't Do It"

Living through several episodes of depression and mania leaves most people with bipolar disorder feeling fearful and lacking in confidence. The fear is that the symptoms will return especially if they stress or push themselves. The setbacks, losses, and devastation that many people experience affects their self-esteem. When working with these individuals, clinicians must find a place between pushing too hard and underchallenging. Particularly with the behaviorally oriented interventions, where therapists are asking patients to act, there may be resistance from those patients who are either fearful of the consequences or lack confidence in their abilities. "I can't do it" is a negative cognition that can be addressed with the cognitive restructuring exercises presented in Chapter 6. With this cognition, it may be particularly helpful to frame the behavioral interventions as experiments to test the validity of the cognition "I can't do it." These experiments should be simple enough to be accomplished by a given patient. Time should be taken to explore the potential obstacles to success of the intervention (see Chapter 5 for guidelines) with adjustments or precautions made as needed. After the intervention has been executed, the cognitive, "I can't do it" should be reevaluated given these new experiences.

Teaching these people to monitor mild, subsyndromal symptoms is difficult because the fear of recurrence is so great that any admission of even mild symptoms means to them that they are getting sick. When technical labels are used to describe symptoms, these patients will deny their occurrence (e.g. I do not have insomnia and I'm just having a little trouble falling asleep). The therapist can work with their denial by using more palatable labels. For a few patients we relabeled the anchors on the mood graph using words that were easier to acknowledge (e.g. "down in the dumps" instead of mild depression). The fear underlying the denial can be addressed with the cognitive interventions described in Chapter 6.

False Assumptions of the Therapist

"CBT Is for Intelligent and Verbally Skilled Patients"

Because of the emphasis on cognition, many therapists assume that CBT is designed for patients who are verbally skilled or highly intelligent. Our experience to date has been with patients with varying levels of intelligence, education, and verbal skills. We have not seen a strong relationship between how well people can execute the CBT interventions and these characteristics. As with any form of therapy, the presentation of the interventions by the therapist must be tailored to the needs of each patient.

One of the verbal skills we have found to be important in this intervention, is the ability to label emotional experiences. Some people have limited emotional vocabularies (e.g., they either feel good or feel bad). Refining these evaluations takes time and practice. Therapists have to listen to patients' descriptions and help them to define the emotions they experience, thus building their emotional vocabulary.

"If My Explanations Are Clear, Patients Will Understand Them"

Clarity in receiving information is only partially dependent on clarity of sending information. The therapist may feel that he or she is conveying information clearly, when, in fact, the patient does not understand. Common mistakes include giving too much information at one time; talking too fast; speaking too softly for the patient to hear clearly; or using slang, jargon, or words that exceed the sophistication of the patient's vocabulary.

Patients are often too kind to tell their therapists that they talk too much, too fast, or are otherwise difficult to understand. However, their lack of understanding will show when expected to use or repeat the information conveyed by the therapist (e.g., when attempting to complete a homework assignment). Rather than being a problem with homework compliance, the real problem may be that the homework was not adequately explained. *Assuming* the patient understands without asking is the therapist's first mistake.

"Patients Will Recognize the Value of Homework"

For many people, the term "homework" has a negative connotation. It reminds them of grade school, punitive teachers, and interruptions in their play time. The value of homework may be appreciated logically, but emotionally the notion of homework may continue to be tied to old and negative memories. The therapist using this treatment manual must take time to resocialize patients to the concept of doing weekly homework. The ultimate goal of this therapeutic intervention is to teach skills that patients can use one their own in attempting to combat symptoms of bipolar disorder. Therefore, practice at home, between sessions, is essential to the learning process. Unfortunately, just because the therapist believes that homework is important and assigns tasks each week, patients will not necessarily accept the instruction and comply with their therapists' requests. Before giving the first homework assignment, the clinician should take time to ask patients how they feel about doing homework between sessions. If their response is negative, the clinician should ask them to say more about it. Listen for negative automatic thoughts about homework. Help the patient to compare homework given in therapy to homework given in school. Underscore the critical difference that there will be no evaluation or "grade" given to therapy homework. Therapy homework is more like practice exercises done regularly to acquire a skill, such as shooting baskets or going to the batting cages to improve athletic skill. The practice itself is not graded but does influence the ability to acquire or refine a skill.

The clinicians should use the compliance intervention each time they give a homework assignment. First, the clinician must make sure that the patient understands how to do the homework. Second, he or she should help the patient to anticipate things that might interfere with completing the homework assignment—"What could keep you from filling out your mood graph this week?" Third, the clinician should develop a plan for avoiding or overcoming the obstacles when they occur. Patients will quickly learn this intervention and will walk through the three step process will little assistance from the therapist.

A related dysfunctional belief of therapists is that if patients have the skill to do the homework, they will do it. As suggested previously, many things can keep people from completing their homework assignments. Reread Chapters 4 and 5 on treatment compliance for a summary.

"This Intervention Will Work with All Patients"

The development of this treatment manual was based on a prototypical patient with bipolar disorder. The individual interventions should be applicable to the majority of patients with bipolar disorder. It is likely that in working with each individual patient, the procedures in this manual will not be inclusive enough to cover all patient presentations at all times. Therefore, the therapist will need to use other CBT methods.

It is also possible that for some patients, this form of treatment will not be helpful at all. This may be particularly true when the patient presents with a substance abuse problem that is more severe than the bipolar disorder. In this case, treatment of the substance abuse problem may be needed before this manual can be effectively used with a patient.

"This Intervention Is Simple and Does Not Require a Lot of Training"

Our goal in writing this manual was to make the instructions easy to follow. We assumed that clinicians with varying clinical backgrounds will read the manual; therefore, we tried to be explicit with directions and limit the "psychobabble" in the text. We also wanted patients and their family members and friends to be able to read along and understand the interventions. Sometimes our descriptions of interventions sound so simple that it would seem that patients could follow the directions on their own. In fact, this may be possible in some cases. The intention of the manual was to provide a package of interventions that addressed each of our treatment goals. We knew that to be successfully administered, clinicians would have to "improvise" to personalize the procedures to the special needs of their patients. Therefore, considerable clinical skill is needed to adequately administer this intervention. Trainees should seek supervision from trained cognitive therapists when learning this intervention.

Key Points for the Therapist to Remember

♦ The strength of CBT is in altering the course of bipolar disorder over time. Each time a relapse of depression, mania, or mixed states occurs it is an opportunity to learn more about the factors that precipitate recurrences for a given patient.

♦ If the patient is not ready to accept the illness, the treatment, and the lifestyle restrictions, CBT will not help.

♦ Sometimes patients have experienced a crisis but have already developed a plan or taken action toward its resolution and merely wish to report to the therapist what has transpired. Telling the story, however, can fill an entire session. When setting the agenda, the therapist should quickly assess whether or not the crisis has been resolved and how much time will be needed for further discussion.

♦ Many institutional settings inadvertently socialize people with bipolar disorder to be passive recipients of care rather than to be active consumers of or participants in their care. A passive view of the patient's role in treatment is in opposition to the collaborative view espoused by this treatment manual.

♦ As therapists, we often assume that our patients have basic social skills such as how to get information, how to cope with stress, how to interact with others in various social situations, or how to make decisions about activities of daily living. Some patients who have had bipolar disorder since prior to adulthood may need help to develop these basic skills.

Points to Discuss with Patients

♦ Sometimes the patient knows the signs of relapse, is aware of the precautions that need to be made, and chooses not to make them.

These people may have to go through several episodes before they are willing to accept the fact that the illness is recurrent and that they must take control over it rather than letting the illness control them.

♦ Involvement of family members in the therapy process can be very useful. It provides family members with an opportunity to meet the therapist and to be informed about what happens during therapy sessions; it demystifies the process of treatment; and it encourages supportive others to be facilitators of care rather than to oppose it.

♦ Countering the institutional belief of patients as passive recipients of care can be accomplished by eliciting active participation in the patient.

♦ Living through several episodes of depression and mania leaves most people with bipolar disorder feeling fearful and lacking in confidence. The fear is that the symptoms will return especially if they stress or push themselves.

Protocol for 20 Cognitive-Behavioral Treatment Sessions

Session 1: Overview of Cognitive-Behavioral Therapy

Purpose of the Session

The purpose of this session is to provide patients and their family members with a rationale for cognitive-behavioral treatment of bipolar disorder and with an overview of the treatment process, including the goals of therapy. Providing information about the treatment procedures will help patients prepare for the coming months. In addition, the family members and friends, if present, will learn what will be provided and what is expected of patients. Perhaps more important, this and the remaining educational sessions provide opportunities for the clinician to establish an alliance with patients and their family members.

Goals of the Session

1. Provide an overview of the treatment process.
2. Discuss patients' rights.
    a. High-quality clinical care.
    b. Confidentiality.
3. Clearly specify patients' responsibilities in the treatment process.
4. Clearly specify the clinician's responsibilities in the treatment process.
    a. Providing high-quality care.
    b. Being available for emergencies when needed.
    c. Providing honest feedback to patients.
5. Discuss families' responsibilities.
    a. Symptom detection.
    b. Encouragement and support of patients.

Procedure

1. Socialize the patient to CBT.
2. Review the treatment plans. Discuss responsibilities of patients, clinicians, and family members.
3. Review the purpose of providing homework assignments and provide copies of the assigned reading material.

Homework

Basco (in press), Chapter 1: Taking Control of Your Illness.

Session 2: What Is Bipolar Disorder?

Purpose of the Session

In this session, the therapist will provide information regarding the definition and etiology of bipolar disorder. This process will help to clarify misconceptions patients or family members may have regarding the nature of bipolar illness.

Goals of the Session

1. Provide descriptive definitions and examples of depression, mania, and bipolar disorder.
2. Briefly review the biological aspects of affective disorders.
3. Discuss the relationship between psychosocial factors, such as stress, and recurrences of depression and mania.

Procedure

1. Elicit feedback on the reading assignment from the previous session. If the homework was not completed, use the compliance intervention (Chapter 5) and add the reading materials to the next homework assignment.
2. Discuss how the diagnosis of bipolar disorder is defined. Provide examples of symptoms. Ask patients and family members to describe their experiences with mania, with depression, and any other symptoms.
3. Assign reading material as homework.

Homework

Basco (in press), Chapter 2: Facts about Bipolar Disorder.

Session 3: Mood-Stabilizing Medications

Purpose of the Session

During this session, the therapist will discuss the use of antimanic and mood-stabilizing medications such as lithium and anticonvulsants. Patients and their significant others may have questions and concerns about the long-term use of mood-stabilizing drugs and their intended effects. This session aims at providing such information and clarifying any misconceptions about medication.

Goals of the Session

1. To review the pharmacology, toxicity, side effects, and positive effects of lithium or other mood-stabilizing medications that have been prescribed for the patient.
2. To review the interaction of illicit drugs and alcohol use with psychotropic medication use and with symptoms of bipolar illness.
3. To correct any misconception about the use of antimanic medications, including issues of addiction and dependence.
4. To identify medication issues and questions that patients should discuss with their physicians.

Procedure

1. Assess treatment compliance.
2. Homework review: Elicit feedback on the reading assignment (if completed). Allow time for questions regarding the material. If the homework was not completed, use the compliance intervention (Chapter 5) and add the Mood Graph to the next homework assignment.
3. Discuss commonly used antimanic medications such as lithium, valproic acid, or carbamazepine, including benefits, side effects, and interactions with other medications and drugs of abuse.
4. Assign reading material.

Homework

> Miklowitz (2002), Chapter 6: What Can Medication and Psychotherapy Do for Me?; Chapter 7: Coming to terms with Your Medication.

Session 4: Antidepressant Medications

Purpose of the Session

The purpose of this session is to provide general information regarding the use of antidepressant medications. Antidepressants are commonly prescribed in addition to mood-stabilizing medications to help shortcut possible recurrences of depression or to treat depressive symptoms. This session reviews the appropriate use of such medications.

Goals of the Session

1. Review the pharmacology of antidepressant medication including when its use is indicated, expected effects, toxicity, and side effects.
2. Correct any misconceptions about antidepressant medications.
3. Identify issues or concerns that patients should discuss with their physicians.

Procedure

1. Assess treatment compliance.
2. Elicit feedback on the reading assignment from the previous session (if completed). Allow time for questions regarding the material. If the homework was not completed, use the compliance intervention (see Chapter 5) and add the reading materials to the next homework assignment.
3. Discuss commonly prescribed antidepressant medications, including their benefits, side effects, and interactions with other medications and with the symptoms of bipolar disorder. Discuss potential mania-inducing effects of antidepressant medications.
4. Assign reading material.

Homework

> Wright and Basco (2002), Chapter 8: An Insider's Guide to Medications for Depression.

Session 5: Individual Symptoms of Bipolar Disorder

Purpose of the Session

The purpose of this session is to help patients and their family members to understand how their daily experiences with the symptoms of bipolar illness are common sequelae of the illness shared by thousands of others. In addition, therapists will begin to teach patients and their family members how to distinguish normal mood variations from symptoms.

Goals of the Session

1. Help patients and their family members to begin to identify how their day-to-day experiences may be related to symptoms of bipolar illness.
2. Help patients and their family members begin to differentiate normal mood states from symptoms of depression and mania.

Procedure

1. Elicit feedback on the reading assignment. If the homework was not completed, use the compliance intervention (Chapter 5) and add the reading materials to the next homework assignment.
2. Ask patients and their family members how bipolar illness has affected their lives and home environment.
3. Complete the Symptom Summary Worksheet.
4. Assign homework to the patient and any other session participants.

Homework

Provide the session participants with copies of the Symptom Summary Worksheet that was completed during the session. Ask them to add to the list over the next week and return the list for further discussion.

Session 6: Symptom Monitoring

Purpose of the Session

To prevent full episodes of depression or mania from recurring, it is essential to identify the early-warning signs. Early identification can lead to early intervention and may "head off" a full-blown episode of mania or depression. Early detection requires that the patient and those around him or her be aware of the signs and symptoms of the disorder. Helping the patient and others to identify and label their experiences of bipolar symptoms is the first step toward early intervention. The second step is to regularly monitor key symptoms, such as changes in mood, that indicate a shift into mania or depression. This session will review mood graphing as a method for monitoring symptom fluctuations.

Goals of the Session

1. Introduce the use of Mood Graphs.
2. Design a Mood Graph that best suits the symptom presentation of the patient.

Procedure

1. Review procedure for completing the Mood Graph. Complete the graph for yesterday and today. Modify the graph design as needed.
2. Assign homework.

Homework

Ask patients and family members that are present to keep graphs of the patients' moods for 1 week. This will help patients and their family members to begin to discriminate between normal and symptomatic mood states.

Basco (in press), Chapter 4: Developing an Early Warning System.

Session 7: Treatment Compliance

Purpose of the Session

In this session, the therapist will introduce the idea that it is common for patients on a long-term course of prophylactic medication to have difficulty in fully complying with the prescribed treatment. Various factors can interfere with the patient's ability to follow through. This inevitable part of medication treatment should be expected and planned for by patients and clinicians. Increasing patients' comfort with the discussion of adherence problems will allow patients and therapists to assess and resolve any current or anticipated problems with adherence to the prescribed treatment plan.

Goals of the Session

1. Introduce the CBT treatment compliance model.
2. Assess for current or potential obstacles to following the treatment plan.
3. Develop a plan of action for addressing these obstacles.

Procedure

1. Invite questions regarding the mood graphing assignment from last session. If the mood graph was not completed, proceed with the compliance intervention. Have patients try to retrospectively complete the mood graph for the previous week. Assign the graph again as the next homework assignment.
2. Introduce the CBT model of adherence.
3. Assess under what circumstances are patients most likely and least likely to following their treatment plans explicitly. What are the outcomes?
4. Ask patients to describe their current treatment plan. Assess patients' attitudes and beliefs about their diagnoses and treatment plans. Identify any misconceptions about either their diagnoses or treatments and address any misconceptions with information and/or cognitive restructuring techniques.
5. Assess current level of medication compliance. Ask patients how they are taking their medications. Compare prescribed plan to actual behavior. Assess for difficulties with the plans and negotiate changes with patients to accommodate their schedules and lifestyles. Seek approval from their designated psychiatrists, if needed.
6. Assess for and resolve any current or anticipated obstacles to treatment using the problem-solving model. If patients deny having any current or anticipated difficulties, review problems encountered in the past, choose one, and proceed with the intervention.
7. Provide patients with the homework materials for this week.

Homework

1. Implement plan to overcome obstacles to adherence.
2. Ask patients to keep a Mood Graph for the next week.

Basco (in press), Chapter 4: Developing an Early Warning System; Chapter 6: Getting the Most Out of Treatment.

Session 8: Biased Thinking

Purpose of the Section

The intention of this session is to lay the groundwork for the teaching of cognitive-behavioral techniques for coping with depressive and hypomanic symptoms.

Although pharmacotherapy may control the majority of symptoms of bipolar illness most of the time, it is not uncommon for patients to experience breakthroughs of symptoms while on medication. Equipping them with some cognitive-behavioral techniques provides additional coping strategies when medication alone is not enough.

Goals of the Session

1. Introduce the concepts of negatively and positively biased thinking.
2. Emphasize how biased thinking can influence the interpretation of events and subsequent actions.
3. Help patients to begin to associate mood shifts with events, thinking patterns, and behavior.

Procedure

1. Assess treatment compliance.
2. Review the compliance assignment from last session. Did patients encounter any of the obstacles to compliance that were anticipated and planned for at the last session? If yes, was the intervention helpful? If not helpful, what interfered? Use the compliance intervention and revise the plan to address these obstacles.
3. Review the Mood Graph for the past week. Discuss any variations from the normal range including the circumstances under which the mood shift occurred.
4. Biased thinking. Define "mood shifts" and "negative automatic thoughts." Review the association between events, mood shifts, and automatic thoughts. Provide examples of negative and positive mood shifts and concomitant shifts in cognitions (e.g., views or outlook). Ask patients to provide several examples of such occurrences and list them on the Summary of Positively and Negatively Biased Thoughts.
5. Provide patients with the reading materials for this week.

Homework

Wright and Basco (2001), Chapter 3: Changing Your Thinking; Chapter 4: Rules of Depression—Rules of Wellness.

Basco (in press), Chapter 8: How to Change Your Thinking.

Session 9: Cognitive Changes in Depression

Purpose of the Session

The purpose of the session is to begin to train patients to monitor their thinking for negatively biased thoughts and to identify thinking errors when they occur. Identification of negative automatic thoughts can cue patients to monitor their symptoms more closely or to use one of the cognitive interventions for negative automatic thoughts that will be covered in the next session.

Goals of the Session

1. Review the concept of negatively biased thoughts.
2. Teach patients to monitor thoughts and to identify negative automatic thoughts.
3. Teach patients to identify thinking errors.

Procedure

1. Assess treatment compliance.
2. Review the homework assigned in the last session.
3. Review the concept of negatively biased thinking. Try to elicit an example of a mood shift that might have occurred in the last week and any accompanying automatic thoughts.
4. Use an Automatic Thought Record as a guide for teaching patients to identify their negative automatic thoughts.
5. Define "thinking error." Provide patients with the list of common thinking errors. Refer back to the Automatic Thought Record or the Biased Thoughts Summary and note any examples of thinking errors
6. Provide patients with the homework materials for the next week.

Homework

1. Keep an Automatic Thought Record for the next week.
2. Assign the task of looking for thinking errors if there was not sufficient time to complete it during the session.

Basco (in press), Chapter 8: How to Change Your Thinking.

Session 10: Logical Analysis
of Negative Automatic Thoughts

Purpose of the Session

The purpose of this session is to teach patients two cognitive therapy techniques for combating negative automatic thoughts and reducing the intensity of associated mood shifts—generating evidence for/evidence against the thought and generating explanations for events.

Goals of the Session

1. Teach patients the "evidence for/evidence against" technique to evaluate the validity of negative automatic thoughts.
2. Teach patients to generate alternative explanations for events as a means of combating negative automatic thoughts.

Procedure

1. Assess treatment compliance.
2. Review patients' Automatic Thought Record homework. Evaluate how well patients understood the procedure, clarify any confusion, and reinforce the association between events, thoughts, and feelings. If patients did not complete their assignment, ask them to fill in a diary sheet for how they are feeling now for use in the skills training exercise of this session.
3. Evidence for/evidence against. Give a rationale for evaluating the validity of negative automatic thoughts. Provide patients with the Logical Analysis of Automatic Thoughts worksheet for use in this exercise. Walk them through the procedure using the automatic thoughts generated in the Automatic Thought Record homework assignment from the last session.
4. Alternative explanations. Provide a rationale for this intervention. Use the third column of the Thought Record for Evaluating Your

Thoughts to generate alternative explanations for the event in question. Ask patients to choose the explanation that seems most likely. Generate evidence for/evidence against the alternative explanation if necessary.

5. Have the patient rerate the intensity of the emotion associated with and belief in the original automatic thought. Help the patient to review the process from the initial negative automatic thought through the logical analysis and summary. Reinforce the logic of this exercise and its purpose.

6. Provide patients with homework materials for the week.

Homework

Provide an Automatic Thought Record and an Evaluating Your Thoughts Worksheet. Ask patients to try using the two cognitive interventions during the next week.

Basco (in press), Chapter 8: How to Change Your Thinking.

Session 11: Cognitive Changes in Mania

Purpose of the Session

The purpose of the session is to begin to train patients to monitor their thinking for "positively biased" or irritable thoughts that might signal the onset of mania and to intervene with methods that contain and organize cognitive symptoms. When patients find their thinking is marked with increased interest in taking on a greater number of activities, increased self-confidence, and grandiosity or is more scattered or disorganized, they can use these thoughts as cues to begin monitoring these changes, which may herald a manic or hypomanic episode more closely and to intervene appropriately.

The cognitive changes associated with the onset of hypomania and mania are often subtle early in the course of the episode. In teaching patients to monitor these thoughts, consider the evolution of mania as symptoms become clinically noteworthy.

Goals of the Session

1. Review the types of thoughts that may serve as indicators of the onset of mania.

2. Train patients to identify positive mood shifts and associated hypomanic and manic thoughts.
3. Practice the application of cognitive restructuring methods to cognitions that may be distorted by hypomania.
4. Teach methods for evaluating plans before taking action.

Procedure

1. Assess treatment compliance.
2. Homework review: Review the logical analysis of automatic thoughts homework from last session.
3. Review the positively biased thoughts that are associated with the onset of hypomania or mania. Ask patients for personal examples of their thoughts when hypomanic or manic.
4. Use the Automatic Thought Record as a guide for teaching patients to identify their positively biased thoughts.
5. Discuss how and when to monitor thoughts that may herald mania. Apply a cognitive restructuring technique to evaluate biased thoughts and modify accordingly. Discuss when to notify their psychiatrists of these cognitive changes.
6. Teach advantages/disadvantages technique and goal setting.
7. Assign homework.

Homework

Ask the patient to keep a Mood Graph for the next week. When the patient's mood falls outside normal limits, ask the patient to complete an Automatic Thought Record. Emphasize monitoring positive changes in mood for this homework assignment.

Basco (in press), Chapter 9: Mental Slow-Down.

Session 12: The Behavioral Aspects of Depression

Purpose of the Session

The purpose of this session is to teach patients two cognitive-behavioral skills for coping with common behavioral consequences of depression. These are GTA and increasing mastery and pleasure.

Goals of the Session

1. Review common behavioral problems associated with depression (e.g., feeling overloaded and overwhelmed and in a lethargy cycle).
2. Teach patients two CBT strategies for coping with these problems (e.g., GTA and increasing mastery and pleasure).

Procedure

1. Assess treatment compliance.
2. Review the Mood Graph and Automatic Thought Record for the past week and discuss any variations from the normal range, including the circumstances under which mood shifts occurred.
3. Review the concept of being overwhelmed and overloaded and provide a rationale for the GTA intervention. Ask patients about times when they may have felt overwhelmed or overloaded. Find out how patients have coped with this type of problem in the past.
4. Describe the procedure for GTA. Choose tasks that patients are having difficulty in completing and apply the GTA exercise.
5. Introduce the importance of experiencing a sense of mastery and pleasure and its role in depression. Assess level of pleasure in the patients' lives at present. If clinically indicated, construct homework assignments aimed at increasing pleasure during the next week.
6. Describe the lethargy cycle. Ask patients to describe their experiences with lethargy. Explain the use of increased mastery and pleasure and GTA to break the cycle. If patients are currently in a lethargy cycle, develop a plan for breaking the cycle and assign this as homework.

Homework

1. Attempt the first step in the GTA if a current problem was identified. Review patients' progress in the next session and continue to assign parts of the task as clinically indicated. Fade out your involvement in monitoring the patients' progress and prompting them to continue as clinically indicated.
2. Assign an intervention to increase mastery and pleasure or to break a lethargy cycle if clinically indicated. Follow up on these assignments. Continue to assign these interventions as long as clinically useful.
3. Assign a Mood Graph for use in the next session.

Wright and Basco (2001), Chapter 5: Managing Your Symptoms.

Basco (in press), Chapter 5: Taking Action.

Session 13: Behavioral Changes in Mania

Purpose of the Session

The purpose of this session on behavioral changes in mania is to train patients to use fluctuations in their activity level as cues of the onset of hypomania or mania and to teach a method for limiting or containing the increased, but disorganized activity.

Goals of the Session

1. Train patients to monitor their activity level.
2. Teach patients to set goals as a technique for setting limits on their activity before reaching problematic levels.
3. Discuss how to make use of feedback from others.

Procedure

1. Assess treatment compliance.
2. Review the homework from last session.
3. Provide a rationale for monitoring variations in activity level as a cue to the onset of mania or hypomania. Using patients' mood graphing homework from the last session, have them graph their activity level for the past week using the same scaling as specified for mood.
4. Provide a rationale for using goal setting as a means of setting limits on activity level when it begins to increase outside normal limits. Complete the Goal-Setting Worksheet.
5. Discuss past experiences where others may have provided feedback to patients on their behavior changes. Was the information welcomed or rejected? Discuss how patients might be able to benefit from the feedback of others.
6. Compare and contrast the patient's experiences of mastery and pleasure in normal, depressed, and manic states. Use the two cognitive restructuring exercises introduced in Chapter 6 if positive biased thoughts are present.
7. Assign homework.

Homework

Have patients monitor their activity level and mood over the next week using a Mood Graph.

Wright and Basco (2001). Chapter 3: Changing your Thinking; Chapter 4: Rules of Depression—Rules of Wellness.

Basco (in press), Chapter 8: How to Change Your Thinking.

Session 14: Psychosocial Problems

Purpose of the Session

This session changes the focus of the therapy from symptoms of bipolar illness to discussion of their psychosocial consequences. It sets the stage for the next training segment, which includes the assessment of, interventions for, and resolution of psychosocial difficulties, including interpersonal problems.

The plan for this session is to begin to examine some of the psychosocial difficulties the patient may be experiencing as a direct or indirect result of bipolar illness.

Goals of the Session

1. Open discussion of psychosocial problems faced by people with bipolar disorder, by providing examples of common psychosocial problems associated with bipolar disorder.
2. Facilitate discussion of problems that patients may have experienced in the past or are currently facing that may be directly or indirectly related to their mental illness.

Procedure

1. Assess treatment compliance.
2. Review patients' mood and activity graphs. Discuss the association between feelings and behavior.
3. Provide an explanation of how psychosocial or interpersonal problems can exacerbate or be exacerbated by symptoms of depression or mania.
4. Ask patients to describe any psychosocial difficulties that they have experienced that were related to the illness. Inform patients that in the next session you will be discussing these difficulties in more detail.
5. Assignment homework.

Homework

Assign mood and/or activity graph.

> Wright and Basco (2001), Chapter 10: Can't Live with You, Can't Live without You.

Session 15: Assessment of Psychosocial Functioning

Purpose of the Session

In this session, we take the first step toward addressing psychosocial problems by conducting a thorough evaluation of patients' psychosocial and interpersonal functioning, both strengths and weaknesses. If patients identify acute problems/crises in their current interpersonal relationships, the therapist may wish to encourage them to bring their significant others to therapy sessions to attempt to work out these difficulties.

Goals of the Session

1. Assess for psychosocial problems that may be troubling patients.
2. Assess patients' interpersonal strengths (e.g., resources and skills) and weaknesses.
3. Establish treatment goals to address psychosocial problems.

Procedure

1. Assess treatment compliance.
2. Review mood and activity graphs.
3. Assess the quality of patients' current interpersonal relationships including social network, amount of contact with others, quality of these interactions, degree of perceived support from others, and any current difficulties in primary relationships.
4. Assess for any current psychosocial stressors.
5. Help patients identify their strengths that facilitate psychosocial adjustment and weaknesses that may interfere with everyday functioning.
6. Assess any sources of support available to patients.

7. Utilizing the aforementioned information, assist patients in setting treatment goals to be addressed in the remaining sessions.
8. Assign homework.

Homework

Ask patients to continue working on the problems list and goals sheet.

Basco (in press), Chapter 9: Mental Slow-Down.

Session 16: Problem-Solving Skills Development

Purpose of the Session

Patients and their significant others may have difficulty organizing their discussion of troublesome issues in a way that leads to effective problem resolution. It is often useful to follow a structured stepwise approach to addressing problems. The purpose of this session is to teach a structured procedure for resolving psychosocial problems. The procedure can be used with individual patients or in conjoint therapy sessions with family members or significant others.

This basic problem-solving procedure should be modeled by the therapist in resolving problems in session as they arise, including problems with compliance, scheduling, or crisis resolution.

Goals of the Session

1. Teach a structured procedure for identifying and defining problems.
2. Teach a structured procedure for resolving problems.
3. Practice the procedure in session.

Procedure

1. Assess treatment compliance.
2. Select a psychosocial problem identified in the last session and apply the problem-solving procedure.
3. Assign homework.

Homework

Apply the problem resolution procedure with a moderately troublesome issue. Implement the solution and evaluate the outcome.

Basco (in press), Chapter 9: Mental Slow-Down.

Session 17–20: Resolution of Psychosocial Problems

Purpose of the Session

The purpose of the problem-solving sessions is to attempt to resolve the ongoing psychosocial difficulties identified in the assessment phase which continue to be a source of stress for the patient.

At least one session should be allocated for each of the treatment goals outlined in the assessment phase. Multiple sessions may be necessary to address a complicated problem. To facilitate the process, divide the main treatment goal into subgoals, and address each individually using the problem-solving procedure.

Over the remaining sessions, discuss how and when the problem-solving procedures can be incorporated into everyday life. Although problem-solving procedures can be applied with the assistance of a therapist, patients must learn to apply these skills in the course of their everyday lives. Help patients to identify times when problem-solving should be initiated.

Goals of the Session

Address one problem area defined in the previous sessions using the problem-solving procedure.

Procedure

1. Assess treatment compliance
2. Follow the procedure outlined in the Problem-Solving Skills Development session. Take sufficient time to address one problem area. If time allows, move on to attempt resolution of a second problem area.
3. Discuss how problem identification and problem-solving methods can be used at times when increased stress is likely. This may include major life events or developmental role transitions. Other cues that problem evaluation and resolution may be needed are when symptoms worsen, stress increases, or others recognize problems that

involve the patients. Regularly scheduled assessments of psychosocial functioning can help to head off problems before they occur.

4. Assign homework.

Homework

Attempt implementation of the solutions generated during the problem-solving discussion. Evaluate how well the solution addresses the problem and implement a new or revised plan if the proposed solution proved ineffective.

Wright and Basco (2001), Chapter 11: How to Grow Stronger When Relationships Change.

Basco (in press), Chapter 9: Mental Slow-Down; Chapter 10: Working the Program.

References

Aagaard, J., & Vestergaard, P. (1990). Predictors of outcome in prophylactic lithium treatment: A 2-year prospective study. *Journal of Affective Disorders, 18,* 259–266.

Altamura, A. C., & Mauri, M. (1985). Plasma concentration, information and therapy adherence during long-term treatment with antidepressants. *British Journal of Clinical Pharmacology, 20,* 714–716.

Altshuler, L. L., Post, R. M., Leverich, G. S., Mikalauskas, K., Rosoff, A., & Ackerman, L. (1995). Antidepressant induced mania and cycle acceleration: A controversy revisited. *American Journal of Psychiatry, 152,* 1130–1138.

Ambelus, A. (1979). Psychologically stressful events in the precipitation of manic episodes. *British Journal of Psychiatry, 135,* 15–21.

American Diabetes Association (2004). American Psychiatric Association, American Association of Clinical Endocrinologists, North American Association for the Study of Obesity: Consensus development conference on antipsychotic drugs and obesity and diabetes. *Diabetes Care, 27*(2), 596–601.

American Psychiatric Association (1994a). *Diagnostic and statistical manual of mental disorders* (4th ed.). Washington, DC: Author.

American Psychiatric Association. (1994b). Practice guideline for the treatment of patients with bipolar disorder. *American Journal of Psychiatry, 151,*1–36.

Angst, J. (1981). Clinical indications for a prophylactic treatment of depression. *Advances in Biological Psychiatry, 7,* 218–229.

Arancibia, A., Flores, P., & Pezoa, R. (1990). Steady-state lithium concentrations with conventional and controlled release formulations. *Lithium, 1*(4), 237–239.

Barbee J. G. & Jamhour N. J. (2002). Lamotrigine as an augmentation agent in treatment-resistant depression. *Journal of Clinical Psychiatry, 63,* 737–741.

Barlow, D. H. (2001). *Clinical handbook of psychological disorders* (3rd ed.) New York: Guilford Press.

Basco, M. R. (in press). *The bipolar workbook: Tools for controlling mood swings.* New York: Guilford Press.

Basco, M. R., Birchler, G. R., Kalal, B., Talbott, R., & Slater, M. A. (1991). The Clinician Rating of Adult Communication (CRAC): A clinician's guide to the assessment of interpersonal communication skill. *Journal of Clinical Psychology, 47,* 368–380.

Basco, M. R., Bostic, J. Q., Davies, D., Rush, A. J., Witte, B., Hendrickse, W., & Barnett, V. (2000). Is there a place for structured diagnostic interviewing in community mental health settings? *American Journal of Psychiatry, 157* (10), 1599–1605.

Basco, M. R., & Rush, A. J. (1995). Compliance with pharmacotherapy in mood disorders. *Psychiatric Annals, 25,* 78–82.

Basco, M. R., & Rush, A. J. (1996). *Cognitive-behavioral therapy for bipolar disorder* (1st ed.). New York: Guilford Press.

Bech, P., Bolwig, T. G., Kramp, P., & Rafaelsen, O. J. (1979). The Bech–Rafaelson mania scale and the Hamilton Depression Scale: Evaluation of homogeneity and inter-observer agreement. *Acta Psychiatrica Scandinavica, 59,* 420–430.

Beck, A. T., Rush, A. J., Shaw, B. F., & Emery, G. (1979). *Cognitive therapy of depression.* New York: Guilford Press.

Beck, A. T., Wright, F. D., Newman, C. F., & Liese, B. S. (1993). *Cognitive therapy of substance abuse.* New York: Guilford Press.

Becker, M. H. (1974). *The health belief model and personal behavior.* Thorofore, NJ: Slack.

Bowden, C. L., Brugger, A. M., Swann, A. C., Calabrese, J. R., Janicak, P. G., Petty, F., Dilsaver, S. C., Davis, J. M., Rush, A. J., Small, J. G., Garza-Trevino, E. S., Risch, S. C., Goodnick, P. J., & Morris, D. D. (1994). Efficacy of divalproex sodium vs. lithium and placebo in the treatment of mania. *Journal of the American Medical Association, 271,* 918–924.

Brady, K., Casto, S., Lydiard, R. B., Malcolm, R.,& Arana, G. (1991). Substance abuse in an inpatient psychiatric sample. *American Journal of Drug and Alcohol Abuse, 17*(4), 389–397.

Brown, C., Dunbar-Jacob, H., Palenchar, D. R., Kelleher, K. J., Bruehlman, R. D., Sereika, S., & Thase, M. E. (2001). Primary care patients' personal illness models for depression: A preliminary investigation. *Family Practice, 18*(3), 314–320.

Brown, G. W., & Harris, T. (1978). *Social origins of depression: A study of psychiatric disorder in women.* London: Tavistock.

Brown, S., Suppes, T., Adinoff, B., & Rajan, T. N. (2001). Durg use and bipolar disorder: Comorbidity or misdiagnosis? *Journal of Affective Disorders, 65,* 105–115

Burns, D. D. (1980). *Feeling good: The new mood therapy.* New York: HarperCollins.

Byram, S., Fischhoff, B., Embrey, M., de Bruin, W. B., & Thorne, S. (2001). Mental models of women with breast implants: Local complications. *Behavioral Medicine, 27,* 4–14.

Calabrese, J. R., Bowden, C. L., Sachs, G. S., Ascher, J. A., Monaghan, E., &

Rudd, G. D. for the Lamictal 602 Study Group. (1999). A double-blind placebo-controlled study of lamotrigine monotherapy in outpatients with bipolar I disorder. *Journal of Clinical Psychiatry, 60,* 79–88.

Caldwell, H. C., Westlake, W. J., Schriver, R. C., & Bumbier, E. E. (1981). Steady-state lithium blood level fluctuations in man following administration of a lithium carbonate conventional and controlled-release dosage form. *Journal of Clinical Pharmacology, 21,* 106–109.

Choo, P. W., Rand, C. S., Inui, T. S., Lee, M. L. T., Cain, E., Cordeiro-Breault, M., Canning, C., & Platt, R. (1999). Validation of patient reports, automated pharmacy records, and pill counts with electronic monitoring of adherence to antihypertensive therapy. *Medical Care, 37,* (9), 846–857.

Clark, D. A. (2004). *Cognitive-behavioral therapy for OCD.* New York: Guilford Press.

Cochran, S. D. (1984). Preventing medical noncompliance in the outpatient treatment of bipolar affective disorders. *Journal of Consulting and Clinical Psychology, 52,* 873–878.

Cohen, D. (1983). The effectiveness of videotape in patient education on depression. *Journal of Biocommunication, 10,* 19–23.

Cohen, M. A., Tripp-Reimer, R., Smith, C., Sorofman, B., & Lively, S. (1994). Explanatory models of diabetes: Patients practitioner variation. *Social Science and Medicine, 38*(1), 59–66.

Colom, F., Vieta, E., Martinez-Aran, A., Reinares, M., Benabarre, A, & Gasto, C. (2000). Clinical factors associated with treatment noncompliance in euthymic bipolar patients. *Journal of Clinical Psychiatry, 61,* 549–555.

Connelly, C. E., Davenport, Y. B., & Nurnberger, J. I. (1982). Adherence to treatment regimen in a lithium carbonate clinic. *Archives of General Psychiatry, 39,* 585–588.

Cooper, T. B., Simpson, G. M., Lee, J. H., & Bergner, P. E. (1978). Evaluation of a slow-release lithium carbonate formulation. *American Journal of Psychiatry, 135,* 917–922.

Craig, T. J., Fennig, S., Tanenberg-Karant, M., & Bromet, E. J. (2000). Rapid versus delayed readmission in first-admission psychosis: Quality indicators for managed care? *Annals of Clinical Psychiatry, 12,* 233–238.

Danion, J. M., Neureuther, C., Krieger-Finance, F., Imbs, J. L., & Singer, L. (1987). Compliance with long-term lithium treatment in major affective disorders. *Pharmacopsychiatry, 20,* 230–231.

De la Osa, N., Ezpeleta, L., Oomenech, J. M., Navarro, J. B., & Losilla, J. M. (1997). Convergent and discriminant validity of the structured diagnostic interview for children and adolescents (DICA-R). *Spanish of Psychology, 1,* 37–44.

Dell'Osso, L., Pini, S., Cassano, G. B., Mastrocinque C., Seckinger, R. A., Saettoni, M., Papasogli, A., Yale, S. A., & Amador, X. F. (2002). Insight into illness in patients with mania, mixed mania, bipolar depression and major depression with psychotic features. *Bipolar Disorders, 4,* 315–322.

Dell'Osso, L., Pini, S., Tundo, A., Sarno, N., Musetti, L., & Cassano, G. B. (2000). Clinical characteristics of mania, mixed mania, and bipolar depression with psychotic features. *Comprehensive Psychiatry, 41,* 242–247.

Dunning, D., & Parpal, M. (1989). Mental addition versus subtraction in counterfactual reasoning: on assessing the impact of personal actions and life events. *Journal of Personality and Social Psychology, 57,* 5–15.

Fava, G. A., Bartolucci, G., Rafanelli, C., & Mangelli, L. (2001). Cognitive-behavioral management of patients with bipolar disorder who relapsed while on lithium prophylaxis. *Journal of Clinical Psychiatry, 62,* 556–559.

First, M. B., Spitzer, R. L., Gibbon, M., & Williams, J. B. W. (1996). *Structured Clinical Interview for DSM-IV Axis I Disorders, Clinician Version* (SCID-CV) Washington, DC: American Psychiatric Press.

Floyd, F. J., & Markman, H. J. (1984). An economical observational measure of couples' communication skill. *Journal of Consulting and Clinical Psychology, 52,* 97–103.

Follette, V. M., Ruzek, J. I., & Abueg, F. R. (Eds.). (1998). *Cognitive-behavioral therapies for trauma.* New York: Guilford Press.

Frank, E., Prien, R. F., Kupfer, D. J., & Alberts, L. (1985). Implications of noncompliance on research in affective disorders. *Psychopharmacology Bulletin, 21,* 37–42.

Frye, M. A., Ketter, T. A., Kimbrell, T. A., Dunn, R. T., Speer, A. M., Osuch, E. A., Luckenbaugh, D. A. , Cora-Ocatelli, G., Leverich, G. S., & Post, R. M. (2000). A placebo-controlled study of lamotrigine and gabapentin monotherapy in refractory mood disorders. *Journal of Clinical Psychopharmacology, 20*(6), 607–614.

Gelenberg, A. J., Carroll, J. A., Baudhuin, M. G., Jefferson, J. W., & Greist, J. H. (1989). The meaning of serum lithium levels in maintenance therapy of mood disorders: A review of the literature. *Journal of Clinical Psychiatry, 50*(Suppl.), 17–22.

Ghaemi, S. N., Boiman, E., & Goodwin, F. K. (2000). Insight and outcome in bipolar, unipolar, and anxiety disorders. *Comprehensive Psychiatry, 41,* 167–171.

Gitlin, M. J., Cochran, S. D., & Jamison, K. R. (1989). Maintenance lithium treatment: Side effects and compliance. *Journal of Clinical Psychiatry, 50,* 127–131.

Glassner, B., Haldipur, C. V., & Dessauersmith, J. (1979). Role loss and working-class manic depression. *Journal of Nervous and Mental Disease, 167,* 530–541.

Goddard, G. V., McIntyre, D. C., & Leech, C. K. (1969). A permanent change in brain function resulting from daily electrical stimulation. *Experimental Neurology, 25,* 295–330.

Goldfried, M. R., & Davison, G. C. (1994). *Clinical behavior therapy.* New York: Wiley.

Goodwin, F. K., & Jamison, K. R. (1990). *Manic–depressive illness.* New York: Oxford University Press.

Gottman, J. M. (1979). *Marital interaction: Experimental investigations.* New York: Academic Press.

Greenhouse, W. J., Meyer, B. & Johnson, S. L. (2000). Coping and medication adherence in bipolar disorder. *Journal of Affective Disorders, 59,* 237–241.

Heimberg, R. G., & Becker, R. E. (2002). *Cognitive-behavioral group therapy for social phobia.* New York: Guilford Press.

Himmelhoch, J. M., Thase, M. E., Mallinger, A. G., & Houck, P. (1991).

Tranylcypromine vs. imipramine in anergic bipolar depression. *American Journal of Psychiatry, 148,* 910–916.

Hirschfeld, R. M. A. (2002). The mood disorders questionnaire: A simple, patient-rated screening instrument for bipolar disorder. *Journal of Clinical Psychiatry, 4*(1), 9–11.

Hirschfeld, R. M. , A., Perlis, R. H., & Vornik, L. A. (2004). Pharmacologic treatment of bipolar disorder. *CNS Spectrums, 9*(3, Suppl.), 1–27.

Hirschfeld, R. M. A., Williams, J. B. W., Spitzer, R. L., Calabrese, J. R., Flynn, L., Keck, P. E., Lewis, L., McElroy, S. L., Post, R. M., Rapport, D. J., Russell, J. M., Sachs, G. S., & Zajecka, J. (2000). Development and validation of a screening instrument for bipolar spectrum disorder: The Mood Disorder Questionnaire. *American Journal of Psychiatry, 157,* 1873–1875.

Hollister, L. E. (1982). Plasma concentrations of tricyclic antidepressants in clinical practice. *Journal of Clinical Psychiatry, 43,* 66–69.

Hops, H., Wills, T. A., Patterson, G. R., & Weiss, R. L. (1972). *Marital Interaction Coding System.* Unpublished manuscript, University of Oregon, Eugene.

Jacob, M., Turner, L., Kupfer, D. J., Jarrett, D. B., Buzzinotti, E., & Bernstein, P. (1984). Attrition in maintenance therapy for recurrent depression. *Journal of Affective Disorders, 6,* 181–189.

Jamison, K. R., Gerner, R. H., & Goodwin, F. K. (1979). Patient and physician attitudes toward lithium. *Archives of General Psychiatry, 36,* 866–869.

Joanning, H., Brewster, J., & Koval, J. (1984). The communication rapid assessment scale: Development of a behavioral index of communication quality. *Journal of Marital and Family Therapy, 10,* 409–417.

Johnson, D. A. W. (1973). Treatment of depression in general practice. *British Medical Journal, 2,* 18–20.

Johnson, D. A. W. (1974). A study of the use of antidepressant medication in general practice. *British Journal of Psychiatry, 125,* 186–192.

Kahn, D. A., Sachs, G. S., Printz, D. J., Carpenter, D., Docherty, J. P., & Ross R. (2001). Expert consensus guidelines for the medication treatment of bipolar disorder: A new treatment tool. *Economics of Neuroscience, 3,* 49–57.

Kahneman, D., & Tversky, A. (1979). Prospect theory: An analysis of decision under risk. *Econometrica, 47,* 263–291.

Keck, P. E., McElroy, S. L., Strakowski, S. M., Stanton, S. P., Kizer, D. L., Balistreri, T. M., Bennett, J. A., Tugrul, K. C., & West, S. A. (1996). Factors associated with pharmacologic noncompliance in patients with mania. *Journal of Clinical Psychiatry, 57,* 292–297.

Kowatch, R. A. , Suppes, T., Carmody, T. J., Bucci, J. P., Hume, J. H., Kromelis, M., Emslie, G. J., Weinberg, W. A., & Rush, A. J. (2000). Effect size of lithium, divalproex sodium, and carbamazepine in children and adolescents with bipolar disorder. *Journal of the American Academy of Child and Adolescent Psychiatry, 39*(6), 713–720

Kranzler, H. R., Kadden, R. M., Burleson, J. A., Babor, T. F., Apter, A., & Rounsaville, B. J. (1995). Validity of psychiatric diagnosis in patients with substance use disorders: Is the interview more important than the interviewer? *Comprehensive Psychiatry, 36,* 278–288.

Kranzler, H. R., Tennen, H., Babor, T. F., Kadden, R. M., & Rounsaville, B. J.

(1997). Validity of the longitudinal, expert, all data procedure for psychiatric diagnosis in patients with psychoactive substance use disorders. *Drug and Alcohol Dependence, 45*(1–2), 93–104.

Kübler-Ross, E. (1970). The care of the dying: Whose job is it? *Psychiatry in Medicine, 1,* 103–107.

Kübler-Ross, E. (1974). The languages of the dying patients. *Humanitas, 10,* 5–8.

Kulhara, P., Basu, D., Mattoo, S. K., Sharan, P. & Chopra, R. (1999). Lithium prophylaxis of recurrent bipolar affective disorder: Long-term outcome and its psychosocial correlates. *Journal of Affective Disorders, 54,* 87–96.

Kwon, A., Bungay, K. M., Pei, Y., Rogers, W. H., Wilson, I. R., Zhou, Q., & Adler, D. A. (2003). Antidpressant use: Concordance between self-report and claims records. *Medical Care, 41* (3), 368–374.

Lam, D. H., Bright, J., Jones, S., Hayward, P., Schuck, N., Chisholm, D., & Sham, P. (2000). Cognitive therapy for bipolar illness—A pilot study of relapse prevention. *Cognitive Therapy and Research, 24,* 503–520.

Lam, D. H., Watkins, E. R., Hayward, P., Bright, J., Wright, K., Kerr, N., Parr-Davis, G., & Sham, P. (2003). A randomized controlled study of cognitive therapy for relapse prevention for bipolar affective disorder: Outcome of the first year. *Archives of General Psychiatry, 60,* 145–152.

Leverich, G. S., Post, R. M., & Rosoff, A. S. (1990). Factors associated with relapse during maintenance treatment of affective disorders. *International Clinical Psychopharmacology, 5,* 135–156.

Lyskowski, J., & Nasrallah, H. A. (1981). Slowed release lithium: A review and a comparative study. *Journal of Clinical Psychopharmacology, 1,* 406–408.

Magura, S., Laudet, A. B., Mahmood, D., Rosenblum, A., & Knight, E. (2002). Adherence to mediation regimens and participation in dual-focus self-help groups. *Psychiatric Services, 53,* 310–316.

McElroy, S. L., Altshuler, L. L., Suppes, T., Keck, P. E. Jr., Frye, M. A., Denicoff, K. D., Nolen, W. A., Kupka, R. W., Leverich, G. S., Rochussen, J. R., Rush, A. J., & Post, R. M. (2001). Axis I psychiatric comorbidity and its relationship to historical illness variables in 288 patients with bipolar disorder. *American Journal of Psychiatry, 158,* 420–426.

McElroy, S. L., Keck, P. E., & Pope, H. G. (1987). Sodium valproate: Its use in primary psychiatric disorders. *Journal of Clinical Psychopharmacology, 7*(1), 16–24.

McElroy, S. L., Keck, P. E., Pope, H. G., & Hudson, J. O. (1988). Valproate in the treatment of rapid cycling bipolar disorder. *Journal of Clinical Psychopharmacology, 9*(5), 382–384.

Meichenbaum, D., & Turk, D. (1988). *Facilitating treatment adherence: A practitioner's guidebook.* New York: Plenum Press.

Miklowitz, D. J. (2002). *The bipolar disorder survival guide: What you and your family need to know.* New York: Guilford Press.

Morgan, M. G., Fischhoff, B., Bostrom, A., & Atman, C. J. (2002). *Risk communication: A mental models approach.* Cambridge, UK: Cambridge University Press.

Murphy, F. C., Rubinsztein, J. S., Michael, A., Rogers, R. D., Robbins, T. W.,

Paykel, E. S., & Sahakian, B. J. (2001). Decision-making cognition in mania and depression. *Psychological Medicine, 31*, 679–693.

Nilson, A. & Axelsson, R. (1989). Factors associated with discontinuation of long-term lithium treatment. *Acta Psychiatrica Scandinavica, 80*, 221–230.

Park, L. C., & Lipman, R. S. (1964). A comparison of patient dosage deviation reports with pill counts. *Psychopharmacologia, 6*, 299–302.

Peet, M., & Harvey, N. S. (1991). Lithium maintenance: 1. A standard education program for patients. *British Journal of Psychiatry, 158*, 197–200.

Peralta, V. & Cuesta, M. J. (1998). Lack of insight in mood disorders. *Journal of Affective Disorders, 49*, 55–58.

Perry, A., Tarrier, N., Moriss, R., McCarthy, E., & Limb, K. (1999). Randomised controlled trial of efficacy of teaching patients with bipolar disorder to identify early symptoms of relapse and obtain treatment. *British Medical Journal, 16*, 149–153.

Peveler, R., George, C., Kinmonth, A., Campbell, M., & Thompson, C. (1999). Effects of antidepressant drug counseling and information leaflets on adherence to drug treatment in primary care: Randomized controlled trial. *British Medical Journal, 319*(7210), 612–615.

Physicians' Desk Reference. (57th ed.). (2003). Montvale, NJ: Medical Economics.

Plous, S. (1993). *The psychology of judgment and decision making.* New York: McGraw-Hill.

Post, R. M. (1992). Transduction of psychosocial stress into the neurobiology of recurrent affective disorder. *American Journal of Psychiatry, 149*, 999–1010.

Post, R. M., Roy-Byrne, P. P., & Uhde, T. W. (1988). Graphic representation of the life course of illness in patients with affective disorders. *American Journal of Psychiatry, 145*, 844–848.

Post, R. M., Rubinow, D. R., & Ballenger, J. C. (1986). Conditioning and sensitization in the longitudinal course of affective illness. *British Journal of Psychiatry, 149*, 191–201.

Post, R. M., Uhde, T. W., Ballenger, J. C., Chatterji, D. C., Greene, R. F., & Bunney, W. E. (1983). Carbamazepine and its -10, 11- epoxide metabolite in plasma and CSF: Relationship to antidepressant response. *Archives of General Psychiatry, 40*(6), 673–676.

Prager, K. J., & Basco, M. R. (1995). *Negative thinking and marital communication of depressed patients and their spouses.* Unpublished manuscript, University of Texas at Dallas.

Preston, J., O'Neal, J. H., & Talaga, M. C. (1994). *Handbook of clinical psychopharmacology for therapists.* Oakland, CA: New Harbinger.

Reich, W. (2000). Diagnostic Interview for Children and Adolescents (DICA). *Journal of the American Academy of Child and Adolescent Psychiatry, 39*, 59–66.

Robins, L. N., Helzer, J. E., Ratcliff, K. S., & Seyfried, W. (1982). Validity of the Diagnostic Interview Schedule, Version II: DSM-III diagnoses. *Psychological Medicine, 12*, 855–870.

Rosenbaum, J. R., Fava, M., Nierenberg, A. A., & Sachs, G. S. (2001). Tgreatment-resistant mood disorders. In G. O. Gabbard, (Ed.), *Treatments of psychiatric disorders* (2nd ed.). pp. 1307–1386. Washington, DC: American Psychiatric Publishing.

Roy-Byrne, P., Post, R. M., Uhde, T. W., Porcu, T., & Davis, D. (1985). The longitudinal course of recurrent affective illness: Life chart data from research patients at the NIMH. *Acta Psychiatrica Scandinavica, 71*(Suppl. 317), 1–34.

Rubinsztein, J. S., Fletcher, P. C., Rogers, R. D., Ho, L. W., Aigbirhio, F. I., Paykel, E. S., Robbins, T. W., & Sahakian, B. J. (2001). Decision-making in mania: A PET study. *Brain, 124,* 2550–2563.

Rush, A. J., Giles, D. E., Schlesser, M. A. Fulton, C. L., Weissenburger, J., & Burns, C. (1986). The Inventory for Depressive Symptomatology (IDS): Preliminary findings. *Psychopharmacology Bulletin, 22,* 985–990.

Rush, A. J. Gullion, C. M., Basco, M. R., Jarrett, R. B. & Trivedi M. H. (1996). The Inventory for Depressive Symptomatology (IDS): Psychometric properties. *Psychological Medicine, 26,* 477–486.

Sachs, G. S., Printz, D. J., Kahn, D. A., Carpenter, D., & Docherty, J. P. (2000). The Expert Consensus Guideline Series: Medication treatment of bipolar disorder. *Postgraduate Medicine, 107* (Spec. Issue), 1–104.

Sackeim, H. A. , Rush, A. J., George, M. S., Marangell, L. B., Husain, M. M., Nahas, Z., Johnson, C. R., Seidman, S., Giller, C., Haines, S., Simpson, R. K., Jr., & Goodman, R. R. (2001). Vagus nerve stimulation (VNS) for treatment-resistant depression: Efficacy, side effects, and predictors of outcome. *Neuropsychopharmacology; 25,* (5), 713–728.

Schwarcz, G., & Silbergeld, S. (1983). Serum lithium spot checks to evaluate medication compliance. *Journal of Clinical Psychopharmacology, 3,* 356–358.

Scott, J., Garland, A., & Moorhead, S. (2001). A pilot study of cognitive therapy in bipolar disorders. *Psychological Medicine, 31,* 459–467.

Scott, J., & Pope, M. (2002a). Nonadherence with mood stabilizers: Prevalence and predictors. *Journal of Clinical Psychiatry, 63*(5), 384–390.

Scott, J. & Pope, M. (2002b). Self-reported adherence to treatment with mood stabilizers, plasma levels, and psychiatric hospitalizations. *American Journal of Psychiatry, 159,* 1927–1929.

Segal, D. L., Kabacoff, R. I., Hersen, M., Van Hasselt, B., & Ryan, C. F. (1995). Update on the reliability of diagnosis in older psychiatric outpatients using the Structured Clinical Interview for DSM-III-R. *Journal of Clinical Geropsychology, 1,* 313–321.

Seltzer, A., Roncari, I., & Garfinkel, P. (1980). Effect of patient education on medication compliance. *Canadian Journal of Psychiatry, 25,* 638–645.

Silverman, E., Woloshin, S., Schwartz, L. M., Byram, S. J., Welch, H. G., & Fischhoff, B. (2001). Women's views on breast cancer risk and screening mammography: A qualitative interview study. *Medical Decision Making, 21*(3), 231–240.

Simon, H. A. (1956). Rational choice and the structure of the environment. *Psychological Review, 63,* 129–138.

Simons, A. D., Levine, J. L., Lustman, P. J., & Murphy, G. E. (1984). Patient attrition in a comparative outcome study of depression: A follow-up report. *Journal of Affective Disorders, 6,* 163–173.

Skre, I., Onstad, S., Torgersen, S., & Kringlen, E. (1991). High interrater reliability for the Structured Clinical Interview for DSM-III-R Axis I (SCID-I). *Acta Psychiatrica Scandinavica, 84,* 167–173.

Slovic, P. (1987). Perception of risk. *Science, 236,* 280–285.

Snyder, D. K. (1979). *Marital Satisfaction Inventory (MSI).* Los Angeles: Western Psychological Services.

Steiner, J., Tebes, J. K., Sledge, W. H., & Walker, M. L. (1995). A comparison of the Structured Clinical Interview for DSM-III-R and clinical diagnoses. *Journal of Nervous and Mental Disease, 183,* 365–369.

Stephen, T. D., & Harrison, T. M. (1986). Assessment communication style: A new measure. *American Journal of Family Therapy, 14,* 213–233.

Sternhell, P. S., & Corr, M. J. (2002). Psychiatric morbidity and adherence to antiretroviral medication in patients with HIV/AIDS. *Australian and New Zealand Journal of Psychiatry, 36,* 528–533.

Stone, E. R., & Yates, J. F. (1991). *Communications about low-probability risks: Effects of alternative displays.* Unpublished manuscript. University of Michigan, Ann Arbor.

Strakowski, S. M., Tohen, N. Stoll, A. L., Faedda, G. L., Goodwin, D. C. (1992). Comorbidity in mania at first hospitalization. *American Journal of Psychiatry, 149*(4), 554–556.

Suppes, T., Leverich, G. S., Keck, P. E., Nolen, W. A., Denicoff, K. D., Altshuler, L. L., McElroy, S. L., Rush, A. J., Kupka, R., Frye, M. A., Bickel, M., & Post, R. M. (2001). The Stanley Foundation Bipolar Treatment Outcome Network. II: Demographics and illness characteristics of the first 261 patients. *Journal of Affective Disorders, 67,* 45-59.

Suppes, T., Phillips, K. A., & Judd, C. R. (1994). Clozapine treatment of nonpsychotic rapid cycling bipolar disorder: A report of three cases. *Biological Psychiatry, 35*(5), 338–340.

Suppes, T, Rush, A. J. , Dennehy, E. B. , Crismon, M. L., Kashner, T. M., Toprac, M. G., Carmody, T. J., Brown, E. S., Biggs, M. M., Shores-Wilson, K., Witte, B. P., Trivedi, M. H., Miller, A. L., Altshuler, K. Z., Shon, S. P. (2003). Texas Medication Algorithm Project, phase 3 (TMAP-3): Clinical results for patients with a history of mania. *Journal of Clinical Psychiatry, 64*(4), 370–382.

Suppes, T., Rush, A. J., Jr., Kraemer, H. C., & Webb, A. (1998) Treatment algorithm use to optimize management of symptomatic patients with a history of mania. *Journal of Clinical Psychiatry; 59*(2), 89–96.

Suppes, T., Webb, A., Paul, B., Carmody, T., Kraemer, H., & Rush, A. J. (1999). Clinical outcome in a randomized 1-year trial of clozapine versus treatment as usual for patients with treatment-resistant illness and a history of mania. *American Journal of Psychiatry, 156*(8), 1164–1169.

Suppes, T., Swann, A. C., Dennehy, E. B., Habermacher, E. D., Mason, M., Crismon, M. L., Toprac, M. G., Rush, A. J., Shon, S. P., & Altshuler, K. Z. (2001). Texas Medication Algorithm Project: development and feasibility testing of a treatment algorithm for patients with bipolar disorder. *Journal of Clinical Psychiatry; 62*(6), 439–447.

Svarstad, B. L., Shireman, T. I., & Sweeney, J. K. (2001). Using drug claims data to assess the relationship of medication adherence with hospitalization and costs. *Psychiatric Services, 52*(6), 805–811.

Swanson, C. L., Freudenreich, O., McEvoy, J. P., Nelson, L., Kamaraju, L., & Wilson, W. H. (1995). Insight in schizophrenia and mania. *Journal of Nervous and Mental Disease, 183,* 752–755.

Tsai, S. M., Chen, C., Kuo, C., Lee, J., Lee, H., Strakowski, S. M. (2001). 15-year outcome of treated bipolar disorder. *Journal of Affective Disorders, 63,* 215–20.

Tversky, A. (1972). Elimination by aspects: A theory of choice. *Psychological Review, 79,* 281–299.

Tversky, A., & Kahneman, D. (1974). Judgment under uncertainty: Heuristics and biases. *Science, 185,* 1124–1130.

Tversky, A., & Kahneman, D. (1981). The framing of decisions and the psychology of choice. *Science, 211,* 453–458.

Tversky, A., & Kahneman, D. (1982). Judgments of and by representativeness. In D. Kahneman, P. Slovic, & A. Tversky (Eds.), *Judgment under uncertainty: Heuristics and biases.* Cambridge, UK: Cambridge University Press, 84–100.

Van Gent, E. M., & Zwart, F. M. (1991). Psychoeducation of partners of bipolar manic patients. *Journal of Affective Disorders, 21,* 15–18.

Vestergaard, P., & Amdisen, A. (1983). Patient attitudes toward lithium. *Acta Psychiatrica Scandinavica, 67,* 8–12.

Wallis, J., Miller, R., & McFadyen, M. L. (1989). A comparative study of standard and slow-release oral lithium carbonate products. *South African Medical Journal, 76,* 618–620.

Wehr, T. A., Sack, D. A., & Rosenthal, N. E. (1987). Sleep reduction as a final common pathway in the genesis of mania. *American Journal of Psychiatry, 144,* 201–204.

Wehr, T. A., & Wirz-Justice, A. (1982). Circadian rhythm mechanisms in affective illness and in antidepressant drug action. *Pharmacopsychiatry, 15,* 31–39.

Weiss, R. D., Greenfield, S. F., Najavits, L. M., Soto, J. A., Wyner, D., Tohen, M., Griffin, M. L. (1998). Medication compliance among patients with bipolar disorder and substance abuse. *Journal of Clinical Psychiatry, 59,* 172–174.

Weissman, M. M., & Johnson, J. (1991). Drug use and abuse in five US communitieis. *NY State Journal of Medicine, 91*(Suppl. 11), 19S–23S.

Welner, Z., Reich, W., Herjanic, B., Jung, K. G., & Amado, H. (1987). Reliability, validity, and parent–child agreement studies of the diagnostic interview for children and adolescents (DICA). *Journal of the American Academy of Child and Adolescent Psychiatry, 5,* 649–653.

Wright, J. H., & Basco, M. R. (2002). *Getting your life back: The complete guide to recovery from depression.* New York: Touchstone Books. Wright & Basco was published in hardback in 2001 by the Free Press. In 2002 it was printed in paperback by Touchstone.

Young, R. C., Biggs, J. T., Ziegler, V. A., & Meyer, D. A. (1978). A rating scale for mania: Reliability, validity and sensitivity. *British Journal of Psychiatry, 133,* 429–435.

Youssel, F. A. (1983). Compliance with therapeutic regimens: A follow-up study for patients with affective disorders. *Journal of Advanced Nursing, 8,* 513–517.

Zarate, C. A. (2000). Antipsychotic drug side effect issues in bipolar manic patients. *Journal of Clinical Psychiatry, 61*(Suppl. 8), 52–61.

Zaretsky, A. E., Segal, Z. V., & Gemar, M. (1999). Cognitive therapy for bipolar depression: A pilot study. *Canadian Journal of Psychiatry, 44,* 491–494.

Zis, A. P., & Goodwin, F. K. (1979). Major affective disorders as a recurrent illness: A critical review. *Archives of General Psychiatry, 36,* 835–839.

Zis, A. P., Grof, P., Webster, M., & Goodwin, F. K. (1980). Prediction of relapse in recurrent affective disorder. *Psychopharmacology Bulletin, 16,* 47–49.

Index